A Science for the Soul

A Science for the Soul

Occultism and the Genesis of
the German Modern

Corinna Treitel

The Johns Hopkins University Press
Baltimore and London

The Johns Hopkins University Press
2715 North Charles Street
Baltimore, Maryland 21218-4363
www.press.jhu.edu

Library of Congress Cataloging-in-Publication Data
Treitel, Corinna.
    A science for the soul : occultism and the genesis of the German modern
/ Corinna Treitel.
    p.   cm.
Includes bibliographical references (p.   ) and index.
    ISBN 0-8018-7812-8
    1. Occultism—Germany—History. I. Title.
BF1434.G5T74 2004
133′.0943—dc21
2003010642

A catalog record for this book is available from the British Library.

Contents

List of Illustrations — *vii*
Acknowledgments — *xi*

PART I: The Occult in Context

1 The Lure of the Psyche — 3
2 A Psychological Point of View — 29
3 The Occult Public — 56

PART II: The Occult in Action

4 Varieties of Theosophical Experience — 83
5 The Creative Unconscious — 108
6 Occult Sciences and Their Applied Doubles — 132

PART III: Policing the Occult

7 The Crimes of Anna Rothe — 165
8 Between Church and State — 192
9 The Spectrum of Nazi Responses — 210

Conclusion: A Voice from the Beyond? — 243

Appendixes — *249*
   A. Clubs — *251*
   B. Presses — *264*
   C. Other Institutions — *267*
   D. Periodicals — *270*

Notes   275
Selected Bibliography   327
Names Index   349
Subject Index   356

Illustrations

Figures

1	Zöllner's knot experiment	6
2	A street astrologer	58
3	Albert von Keller, *Auferweckung der Tochter Jairi*	112
4	A psychical research experiment	113
5	Albert von Keller, *Hexenverbrennung*	115
6	The dream dancer Madeleine Guipet	117
7	The Berlin trance-painter Wilhelmine Aßmann	123
8	Wassily Kandinsky, *Picture with a Circle*	127
9	Heinrich Nüßlein, *Phantastische Landschaft*	129
10	Bô Yin Râ, *Jesus*	130
11	A parapsychological experiment	137
12	Making parapsychology objective	138
13	The telepath Marie Günther-Geffers	147
14	Mrs. Wildhagen gripping a dowsing rod	151

Tables

2.1	A Timeline of Important Dates Related to the Early German Occult Movement	32
3.1	Occult Clubs, 1869–1937	59
3.2	Male Professionalism in Three Early Occult Clubs, 1884–1888	62
3.3	Occult Businesses, 1870–1937	69
6.1	Criminal Mediumism in Germany, 1911–1930	145

Acknowledgments

Many institutions and people helped make this book possible.

Financial support from the Minda de Gunzburg Center for European Studies (1994–99), Harvard University (Sheldon Traveling Fellowship, 1996–97), the Woodrow Wilson Foundation (Charlotte W. Newcombe Doctoral Dissertation Fellowship, 1998–99), and the American Historical Association (Bernadotte E. Schmitt Grant, 1999) freed me to research and write. Two faculty awards (Wellesley College, 2003) supported the end stages of book production. In addition to financial support, the Center for European Studies provided office space and a stimulating intellectual environment within which I worked out major portions of the book from 1994 to 1999.

Also invaluable was the assistance of librarians and archivists who helped me locate and interpret material in the United States and Germany. Particularly worthy of mention are Baerbel Mund of the Niedersächsische Staats- und Universitätsbibliothek in Göttingen, Michael Häusler of the Diakonisches Werk der Evangelischen Kirche in Berlin, Aaron Kornblum at the United States Holocaust Memorial Museum in Washington, D.C., and Laura Farwell of Harvard University's Widener Library. Also deserving of recognition are the various staff members who helped me on a daily basis at the Bayerische Staatsbibliothek, Stadtbibliothek, Stadtarchiv, and Staatsarchiv, all in Munich; the Bundesarchiv, the Geheimes Staatsarchiv Preussischer Kulturbesitz, and the Evangelisches Zentralarchiv, all in Berlin; and the Stanford University Library Archives.

I am also grateful to the presses, archives, and libraries that granted me permission to reproduce the illustrations included in this book. L. Staackmann Verlag, the Institut für Grenzgebiete der Psychologie und Psychohygiene, and Oldenbourg Wissenschaftsverlag gave permission to reproduce, respectively, figures 1, 4, 6, and 14. In addition, Heinrich Nüßlein's *Phantastische Landschaft* (fig. 9) appears courtesy of the Fine Arts Library, Harvard College Library;

Albert von Keller's *Auferweckung der Tochter Jairi* (fig. 3) appears courtesy of the Bayerische Staatsgemäldesammlungen in Munich; and Wassily Kandinsky's *Picture with a Circle* (fig. 8) appears courtesy of the Artists Rights Society (ARS), New York/ADAGP, Paris. I would also like to thank Franz Steiner Verlag for allowing me to reprint previously published material; "The Culture of Knowledge in the Metropolis of Science" in *Wissenschaft und Öffentlichkeit in Berlin 1870–1930* (Stuttgart: Franz Steiner Verlag, 2000) became chapter 7.

Many colleagues and friends gave of themselves generously. David Blackbourn furnished excellent advice and unstinting support as I worked on this project, first as a doctoral student and then as a young faculty member. Charles Maier and Allan Brandt also provided valuable input, first as thesis readers and then as professional mentors. Suzanne Marchand and Conevery Bolton Valencius deserve special mention; their belief in me and this project sustained me through long years of work, and their detailed critiques of my manuscript made it immeasurably better. Conversations and correspondence with Eberhard Bauer, Cornelius Borck, Andy Daum, Nicolas de Warren, David Ehrenpreis, Geoff Eley, Daniel Gasman, Peter Gay, Constantin Goschler, Anne Harrington, Ben Hett, Jennifer Jenkins, Ulrich Linse, Margaret Menninger, George Mosse, Richard Noll, Uwe Puschner, Lisbet Rausing, Diethard Sawicki, and Klaus Staubermann sharpened my ideas and broadened my analysis. Two sets of perceptive comments from an anonymous reviewer and down-to-earth feedback from my editor, Jackie Wehmueller, helped me restructure and strengthen my manuscript; the editorial help of many staff members and associates of the Johns Hopkins University Press then assisted me in polishing my manuscript into its final form. Three more people, finally, merit special note: Krister Knapp, who was always ready to discuss my ideas with great intelligence and enthusiasm or—when I needed a break—to crack a good joke and then uncork a bottle of wine; and Tom James and Joe Triebwasser, two friends who cheered this project on through the years and even helped give my book its title.

Finally, special mention must go to my parents Renata and Sven, who first awoke in me a love of the intellectual life when I was a child, and my siblings, Geoffrey, Michael, and Nadine, who probably never quite figured out what I was doing or why it took so long but helped me when they could and always gave me a healthy sense of perspective about myself and my work.

Thank you.

Part I / The Occult in Context

The Lure of the Psyche

Experiments with the Fourth Dimension

The first major controversy of the modern German occult movement erupted in 1878 when Karl Friedrich Zöllner published an account of his sensational sittings with the spiritualist medium "Dr." Henry Slade.[1] Slade, an American by birth, had become popular in the mid-1870s with British spiritualists for his ability to mediate "spirits" who wrote messages on slates for séance participants. Unfortunately for Slade, his séances also drew the attention of hostile investigators, and their case against him culminated in a trial for fraud in the fall of 1876. After a London court found the medium guilty and sentenced him to three months' prison with hard labor, Slade avoided punishment by fleeing England.[2] Still on the run a year later, he arrived in Germany in the fall of 1877.

Slade's fugitive status did not in the least deter Zöllner from inviting the medium to his home in Leipzig for a series of sittings in November and December 1877. A well-respected professor of astrophysics at the University of Leipzig, Zöllner also invited several colleagues to these sittings, among them some of the most illustrious German scientists of the time. They included the physicists William Edward Weber and Gustav Theodor Fechner, the mathematician Wilhelm Scheibner, and the psychologist Wilhelm Wundt. Slade treated these professors to phenomena of astonishing variety and character, and Zöllner thought the séances so scientifically significant that he rushed to publish detailed reports on them, beginning in 1878.

The following are the highlights of the story that unfolded between Slade's arrival in Leipzig in 1877 and the publication of Zöllner's reports from 1878 to 1880:

1877

Friday, November 16. Slade attends a weekly tea organized by Zöllner for his friends, who include Fechner and Weber. In a spontaneous experiment, Slade demonstrates that he can deflect a compass needle without a magnet. Later that evening, Zöllner, Fechner, and another professor observe a series of phenomena that unfold in Slade's presence. The phenomena do not occur through any detectable mechanical intervention by Slade. Knocks sound from the coffee table. Writing appears on a sealed slate. A knife flies through the air. A bed pushed up against the wall abruptly moves two feet.

Saturday, November 17. Zöllner, Weber, and Scheibner hold another sitting with Slade. More mysterious phenomena occur. The professors jump in surprise when a screen splits in half. The following message, presumably from Slade's "spirits," appears on a previously blank slate: "It was not our intention to hurt your feelings. Please excuse this event."[3]

Sunday, November 18. Zöllner invites Wundt and two other men to a sitting with Slade. Again, a knife flies through the air and messages appear on another sealed slate. After approximately half an hour, Wundt and his companions leave abruptly.

Early December. Slade travels to Berlin for a few days. He meets there with Samuel Bellachini, the court magician, who signs an affidavit on December 6 stating that after closely observing Slade's séances, he has been unable to detect any evidence of fraud.[4] Thus validated, Slade returns to Leipzig and resumes the sittings with Zöllner and his colleagues.

Tuesday, December 11. Zöllner, Weber, Scheibner, and Slade sit at a table. Slade's hands and feet, Zöllner reports, are clearly visible. A hand bell placed under the table begins to ring, then flies ten feet through the air. A small table begins to dance so forcefully that it knocks over a chair. A bookcase weighted down with books crashes to the ground. An accordion begins to play. A small, red-brown hand appears on the table for a few seconds.

Friday, December 14. Zöllner, curious about the mysterious hand, conducts an experiment to investigate further. Zöllner, Weber, and Slade sit at a table under which a bowl with white flour has been placed. Zöllner challenges Slade to ask his "spirits" to press their hands in the flour before touching the séance participants. Zöllner suddenly feels a large hand grasping his knee under the table, then the bowl of flour slides four feet along the floor. Zöllner finds the flour print of a big, four-fingered hand on his pant leg. The flour in the bowl shows the imprint of the same hand. Zöllner and his colleagues carefully examine Slade's hands and feet for traces of flour, but find none.

Monday, December 17. Zöllner uses a saccharometer and two prisms to test Slade's ability to change the polarity of a simple chemical solution. Instead of accomplishing this feat, Slade manages to use the experimental setup to read a book "clairvoyantly." Such results prompt Zöllner to hypothesize that intelligent beings from the fourth dimension are responsible for Slade's phenomena. He performs two experiments to test this hypothesis. In the first experiment, Zöllner places a sealed slate, previously coated on the inside with soot, on his lap. He then challenges Slade to ask his "spirits" to leave their prints in the soot. After waiting five minutes or so, Zöllner opens the slate and discovers the prints of two feet, one left and one right.[5] In the second experiment, Zöllner presents Slade with a cord, the ends of which have been knotted together and then sealed with wax. He challenges Slade to ask his "spirits" to tie a knot in this continuous circle of cord. A few minutes later, not one, but four knots appear in the cord (see fig. 1).[6]

1878

April. Zöllner publishes an article entitled "On Space of Four Dimensions" in the *Quarterly Journal of Science,* a British publication edited by the chemist William Crookes, who shares Zöllner's interest in spiritualist phenomena. Zöllner postulates that Slade tied knots in the sealed cord by recourse to the fourth dimension of space and suggests that this experiment constitutes empirical proof of the reality of the fourth dimension.[7] Zöllner offers to send the knotted cord to anyone who doubts his report "so as to convince them that not a subjective phantasma is here in question but an objective and lasting effect produced in the material world, which no human intelligence with the conceptions of space so far current is able to explain."[8]

Spring. Zöllner publishes the first two volumes of his *Wissenschaftliche Abhandlungen.* The volumes consist of more than two thousand pages, the

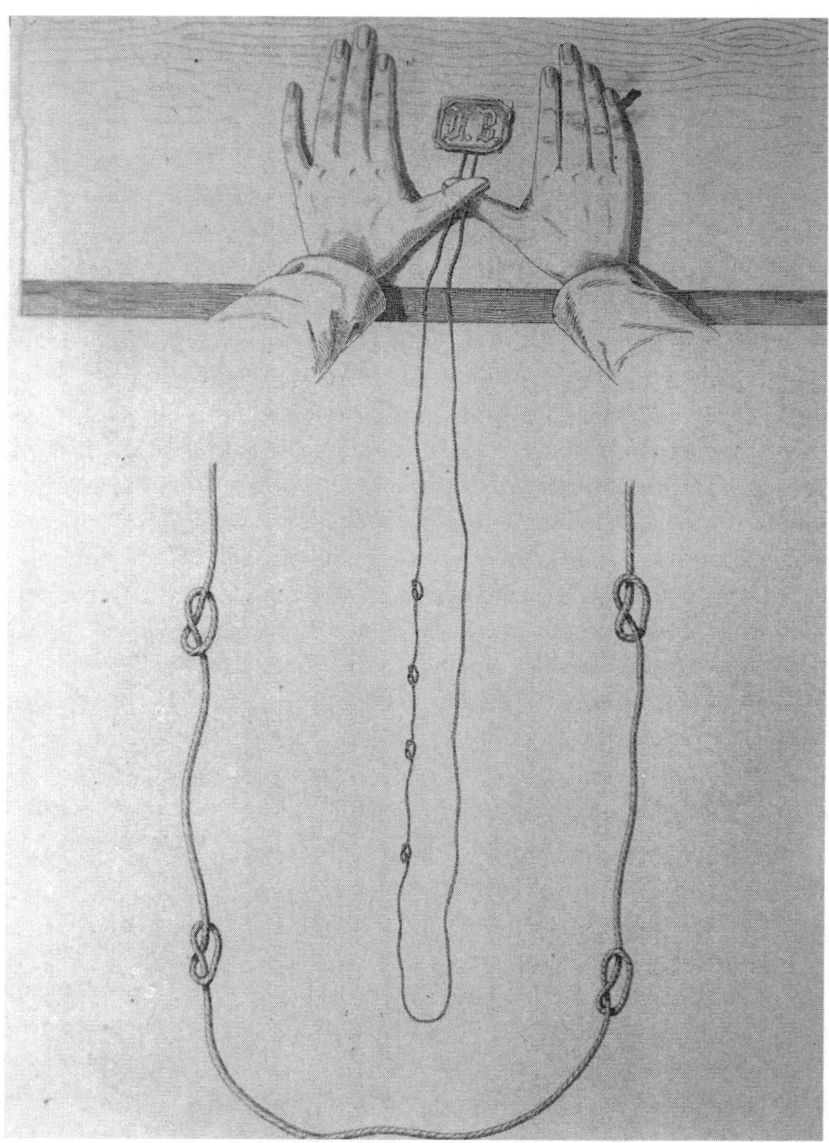

Figure 1. Zöllner's knot experiment (1877). After presenting the medium Henry Slade with a cord whose ends have been sealed together, Karl Friedrich Zöllner challenges the medium to have his "spirits" tie a knot in the cord. A few minutes later, four knots appear, prompting Zöllner to claim that the experiment has "proved" the reality of the fourth dimension of space. Friedrich Zöllner, *Wissenschaftliche Abhandlungen 2* (Leipzig: L. Staackmann, 1878–79).

bulk of which relate to the sittings with Slade. They also contain discussions of Kant's philosophy and the fourth dimension, criticisms of the German universities and the liberal press, and diatribes on the dangers posed by Jews to German culture.

1879

Zöllner publishes the third volume of his *Wissenschaftliche Abhandlungen.* Dedicated to Crookes, it consists of more than six hundred pages discussing the experiments with Slade and their implications for the founding of a new scientific field that Zöllner dubs "transcendental physics."

1880

C. C. Massey, the lawyer who defended Slade in London in 1876 and who still believes in Slade's honesty, assembles and translates into English Zöllner's various writings on the Leipzig experiments.[9] The book, appearing under the title *Transcendental Physics,* rapidly becomes a success with the international spiritualist community.

The Controversy over "Transcendental Physics"

The Zöllner episode quickly snowballed into an international controversy that lasted nearly a decade and continued to elicit commentary well into the twentieth century.[10] In Germany, the episode proved to be a key chapter in the early history of the modern German occult movement, which had its roots in the brief table-turning craze of the 1850s and resurged with popular interest in spiritualist séances. By the mid- 1870s the organizational center of German spiritualism lay in Leipzig, which was home to several spiritualist clubs, the spiritualist press of Oswald Mutze, the spiritualist journal *Psychische Studien,* and Dr. G. K. Wittig, the tireless organizer on behalf of German spiritualism.[11] From these beginnings, German occultism grew rapidly and by 1900 encompassed a wide variety of beliefs and practices—Theosophy, astrology, divination, psychical research, graphology, dowsing, and spirit healing, to name just a few. By the 1940s, when the Nazi regime shut the movement down, hundreds of occult clubs, businesses, institutes, and presses and thousands of devoted providers and consumers of occult goods and services had spread across Germany.

How are we to understand the rapid growth of this movement from the 1870s to the 1940s? And how are we to assess its significance for the cultural history of Germany in the turbulent years between national unification in 1871 and national defeat in 1945? The Zöllner episode presents an ideal entry point to such questions. Not only was it the first major controversy in the incipient German occult movement, it was also the means by which the new occultism of the late nineteenth century first came to the attention of a broad German public.

On the face of it, none of the men involved in the Leipzig sittings seemed likely candidates for experiments with a spiritualist medium, particularly one with Slade's tarnished reputation. This improbability began with the main investigator, Zöllner himself. Zöllner had helped found the new field of astrophysics, even giving the field its name. Presenting the first observational evidence that stars underwent a cooling sequence, his book *Photometric Investigations* (1865) earned him a chair at the University of Leipzig in 1866.[12] Fechner, to take another example, had been appointed professor of physics at the University of Leipzig in 1834 and opened the field of psychophysics in 1860 with his book *Elements of Psychophysics,* which is still considered one of the founding documents of the modern discipline of scientific psychology.[13] Wundt had pioneered the new field of experimental psychology with his book *Physiological Psychology* (1874). Following a campaign orchestrated by Zöllner, Wundt had been offered and accepted a chair in philosophy at the University of Leipzig in 1875.[14]

Why did these men, secure in their reputations not only as scientists but as pioneers of new fields of scientific study, bother with the investigation of a spiritualist medium like Slade? One important clue lay with Zöllner and his invocation of the fourth dimension of space to explain the startling phenomena he had observed. Here, the sequence of events was crucial. Zöllner's interest in the fourth dimension came first; only afterward did his desire to experiment with spiritualist mediums like Slade emerge.

Zöllner had been interested since at least the early 1870s in the non-Euclidean geometries developed earlier in the nineteenth century by mathematicians like Gauss, Riemann, Lobatschewski, Bolyai, and Klein. One channel for this interest must have been the physicist-turned-physiologist Hermann von Helmholtz, who had popularized this topic through numerous lectures and essays in Germany and Britain from the mid-1860s onward. Helmholtz had discerned in the fourth dimension both a weapon with which to attack Kantian idealism and a foundation with which to underpin a rigorous scientific empiricism.[15] Whereas Kant had argued that human understanding used transcendental categories of thought that were ideal, Helmholtz accepted Kant's categories but denied their ideal character. He set out to "naturalize" them by showing that geometrical axioms, supposedly derivable from Kant's categories, were not ideal but instead developed as a result of one's experiences in a particular space. Creatures living in a hyperspace of four or more dimensions, Helmholtz argued, would develop a geometry specific to hyperspace. They would be familiar with figures inconceivable to human beings, whose particular geometry was conditioned by sensory experience in a three-dimensional world. What looked like a sphere to a human observer, for example, would look quite different to a hyperspace creature, in just the way that the same sphere would appear to be a mere circle to an observer limited to two dimensions. Helmholtz's point was that although human beings could conceive of the possibility of the fourth dimension, they could not conceive of what a four-dimensional object might look like because they had no experience of such objects in their three-dimensional sense world. The geometrical axioms, Helmholtz concluded, had to be the result of experience.[16]

Like many intellectuals who came into contact with Helmholtz's discussion of hyperspace, Zöllner experimented with using the new geometry in other branches of science. In 1872, for instance, he applied this new geometry to the study of comets.[17] By the mid-1870s, he was hypothesizing that Kant's "thing in itself" was somehow associated with four-dimensional objects. Zöllner hoped that his experiments with the medium Slade would provide empirical evidence for the revision of contemporary notions of space and serve to challenge the Kantian heritage as well. Zöllner's hopes, of course, directly contravened Kant, who had argued forcefully that although humans could achieve firm knowledge about objects in the sense world, they could never achieve such knowledge about transcendent "things in themselves." Zöllner's attempt to overturn or at least modify Kant's limits on human knowledge belonged to a long history of such attempts in the intellectual life of nineteenth-century Germany. Helmholtz's exploration of the fourth dimension was one more, scientific psychology another, and modern occultism yet another.[18] Zöllner entered the séance room, in short, to engage some of the central philosophical issues of his time.

If these were the abstract issues that had prompted Zöllner to solicit the sittings with Slade in the first place, they were by no means the only issues that eventually coalesced around his published account of them. One major issue that emerged almost immediately in the controversy that broke out in 1878 concerned the nature of scientific authority, an issue that the German liberal press made a focus of scathing critique. An anonymous author writing in the bourgeois journal *Im Neuen Reich* in 1878, for instance, lambasted Zöllner for having lent his authority as a scientist to the outrageous claims of the spiritualists. Encouraged by the astrophysicist's eminence, the masses had been convinced of Slade's extraordinary powers and even seemed to regard Zöllner as the medium's prophet. Mockingly, the anonymous author noted that although German readers of the journal might thank Zöllner for the delicious amusement he had given them in offering such ridiculous explanations of such incredible phenomena, they had to deplore the example he set the scientific community and the public. The author acknowledged the right of every German to engage, in private, in any stupidity he liked, but called for state action—through the schools, police, and health authorities—to protect the wider public from infection with the spiritualist superstition.[19] Other bourgeois journals echoed the scathing, debunking tone of this article. Among these was the liberal Berlin paper *Berliner Volkszeitung,* whose coverage of the Leipzig sittings so incensed Zöllner that he accused the paper of orchestrating a campaign against him, and the family journal *Die Gartenlaube,* whose negative reports on Slade prompted Zöllner to launch an anti-Semitic attack on the article's author.[20]

While bourgeois periodicals attacked Zöllner for having misused his scientific authority to the detriment of a gullible public, the German academic community experienced deep embarrassment over the defection of one of its leading members to the seemingly crass superstition of spiritualism. A lively debate on the Zöllner fiasco ensued, and some professors went so far as to point an accusing finger at Helmholtz, who had done so much to popularize the fourth dimension in the first place. The most vocal was Professor Eugen Dühring, a philosopher at the University of Berlin, who berated Helmholtz for causing a "scientific scandal" and promoting "mathematical mysticism." Although his attack on Helmholtz cost Dühring his position, anecdotal evidence that the Zöllner episode had encouraged the lay public to associate spiritualism with the fourth dimension did exist. One report noted that a worker at a meeting of a Leipzig socialist circle had announced with some excitement that a famous professor in Berlin (presumably a reference to Helmholtz) had just discovered heaven. Someone else suggested that instead of speaking of the "fourth dimension" one should now speak of the "spirit world."[21] Against the background of such reports, Helmholtz joined the fray by denouncing Zöllner's explanations as a misappropriation of his arguments.

Soon, majority opinion in academic circles settled on the idea that Zöllner had clearly gone crazy, and here, too, there was evidence to support the possibility. Many professors recalled that Zöllner had already caused a stir in the German academic community in 1872 when, in a book on comets, he ended with a polemic on the negative effects of scientific professionalization in Germany. Looking back from the vantage point of the late 1870s, Helmholtz (who was an advocate of professionalization) and other colleagues saw this episode as the first sign of a mental illness that had eventually led to Zöllner's turn to spiritualism.[22] Supporting this assessment was the widely known fact that several of Zöllner's siblings had died while mentally ill.[23] But there were also colleagues willing to testify that Zöllner had been perfectly sane during the months he conducted the sittings with Slade.[24] In any case, Zöllner's possible insanity and his turn to spiritualism were obviously so embarrassing that the obituary notice that appeared in the local *Leipziger Illustrirte Zeitung* at Zöllner's death in 1882 avoided all mention of either topic.[25]

Unfortunately for those who would have liked to see an end to the discussion over the Leipzig sittings, the excuse offered by Zöllner's supposed insanity did not shut down debate in German intellectual circles.[26] In fact, a flurry of study, analysis, and writing that continued well into the 1880s reveals that it was not simply scientific authority, Helmholtz's responsibility, or Zöllner's sanity that was at issue. What was at stake, much more broadly, turned out to be the human soul or, as it was being called with increasing frequency, the human psyche: its significance for German culture, its amenability to scientific investigation, and the question of who in Germany was qualified to decide such weighty matters. The most revealing documents of this controversy were an open letter written in 1879 by Wundt to Hermann Ulrici, a professor of philosophy at the University of Halle, and a book published in 1885 by the philosopher Eduard von Hartmann at the avant-garde press of Wilhelm Friedrich. Wundt's letter attacked those—like Ulrici—who dared to use Zöllner's reports as empirical proof for religious beliefs. While not shying away from condemning the facile reasoning of spiritualists like Ulrici, Hartmann's book made the case that séance phenomena deserved sustained scientific and philosophical investigation. If Wundt's letter strove to undermine the debate by undermining Zöllner's report, Hartmann's book instead sought to keep debate open on an important if problem-ridden topic. These were the two poles between which the discussion of occult phenomena would remain for the duration of the German occult movement.

Wundt took Ulrici to task for having accepted Zöllner's interpretation of the phenomena solely on the basis of Zöllner's authority as an eminent scientist.[27] As Europe's preeminent psychologist, Wundt was of course well equipped with his own considerable scientific authority to comment on the scientific aspects of the spiritualist phenomena; because he had attended one of the Leipzig sittings with Slade, moreover, he had first-hand knowledge of the particular experiments in question. Scientists, he insisted, could only come to a correct judgment of an experiment after developing an intuition appropriate to the field of investigation. Neither he nor Zöllner were expert enough to render a definitive judgment concerning the spiritualist phenomena in general, Wundt wrote, but based on what he himself had seen at the Leipzig sittings, there seemed reason to doubt the genuineness of Slade's phenomena in particular. Grammatical errors in the messages written on the slates had aroused Wundt's suspicions, since their mangled German appeared appropriate to an English-speaker like Slade. He also remained unconvinced that the table that had levitated during the séance had not done so by means of a human shove from underneath. In the end, although Wundt did not dismiss all spiritualist phenomena as fraudulent, he held out little hope for their authentication. As Wundt put it, he would keep his trust in the authority of science, rather than in the authority of the scientists who had wandered into fields far beyond the realm of their expertise.[28]

But it was not simply the issue of misplaced trust that bothered Wundt. Still more troublesome was Ulrici's attempt to erase the boundaries separating religious faith and scientific knowledge. Ulrici had argued that the Leipzig sittings provided material proof for the certainty of human life after death— that spiritualism underpinned religious faith with experimental evidence from the natural sciences. Wundt attacked this line of reasoning by mocking what the spiritualists had learned. If the spiritualist explanation was correct, he pointed out, the spirits had given the living a rather grim foreknowledge of what they could expect in the afterlife: a loss of their earthly ability to spell and an eternal rest constantly interrupted by earthly mediums summoning them for séances.[29]

Mockery aside, Wundt came to the heart of the matter in his closing paragraphs, where he lambasted spiritualism as "a sign of the . . . cultural barbarism of our time." The spiritualist claim that séance phenomena provided material proof for the reality of life after death, he argued, was nothing more than an updated form of animism, a primitive form of belief that philosophy had progressively displaced. Spiritualism, in other words, was a reversion to an earlier stage of human cultural development.[30] In an afterword added in 1885, Wundt noted with satisfaction that Germany's relapse into cultural atavism had been halted in the six years since the letter to Ulrici. The German intellectual community at large had proven uninterested in spiritualist phenomena, and a public education campaign composed of antispiritualist demonstrations seemed to have been a success.[31]

It turned out that Wundt had expressed his relief too soon. Although it was true that by 1885 Leipzig had an antispiritualist club named Abila—the name of a medium who had been exposed as a fraud—spiritualism in particular and occultism more generally were still spreading across Germany. Moreover, although few German academics had dared to express interest in séance phenomena after Zöllner, intellectuals outside of the German university system had no such scruples. This became clear in 1885, when the popular philosopher Eduard von Hartmann entered the debate on Zöllner and the Leipzig experiments with the publication of his book *Der Spiritismus* (Spiritualism).

Like Wundt and Zöllner before him, Hartmann had the intellectual credentials to guarantee an audience on the topic. He had first become famous as a young man for his 1867 work *The Philosophy of the Unconscious*, where he combined philosophical analysis with observations drawn from neurology and psychology. A disciple of Schopenhauer, he considered pessimism the only tenable basis for a philosophical ethics and condemned liberal Protestantism for promoting an illusory faith in social progress. This philosophy drew a popular following during his lifetime and had many adherents among the early leaders of the German occult movement in the 1880s and 1890s. In addition, Hartmann was well respected in certain sectors of the academic community for his opposition to materialism and his inclusion of the unconscious as a factor in human psychology.[32] He thus had an audience both inside and outside academic circles.

When Hartmann entered the German debate on spiritualism in 1885, he echoed much of what Wundt had said in 1879. Like Wundt, Hartmann was appalled at the unbelievably low quality of debate on séance phenomena. Most people subscribing to the German spiritualist newspapers, he complained, had no interest in the scientific investigation of the phenomena but seemed to be searching rather for confirmation of their belief in an afterlife, a belief that precluded their critical investigation of mediumism as a psychological phenomenon.[33]

But whereas Wundt was content to call spiritualism a form of cultural barbarism and leave it at that, Hartmann believed that something worthy of salvage remained, that spiritualists had stumbled onto a new category of human experience deserving serious scientific study. He put it thus: "The public has the absolute right to know about such things, and since it is not in the position to form its own opinion, it must be instructed by the verdict delivered by the official leaders of science." Spiritualism, Hartmann conceded, had become a public problem in Germany, but he cautioned against trying to outlaw the movement (as had been done in Russia). Instead, he urged the state to use its authority to encourage scientists to investigate the phenomena in question and to push doctors, judges, and ministers to become acquainted with spiritualist activities in their districts.[34]

On the specific question of Zöllner's experiments with Slade, Hartmann declared himself unable to pass judgment. He had never attended a sitting and was reluctant to accept Zöllner's hypothesis about the fourth dimension. Still, he noted, Zöllner's experiments and reports were among the most scientifically rigorous accounts of the phenomena now available. Unlike most of his contemporaries, Hartmann was also perceptive enough to recognize that Zöllner had not in fact come out in support of the spiritualist hypothesis. A true spiritualist would have concluded that it was the spirits of the dead that caused the séance phenomena. Zöllner had never claimed this, preferring to limit his claims to the doings of mysterious beings commanding the fourth dimension.[35]

Ultimately, what Hartmann found most significant about the spiritualist movement was that it had recovered an entire realm of human experience that had been suppressed during the Enlightenment. This was the realm of the unconscious, and Hartmann believed that it was too important for scientists and philosophers to leave to the spiritualists. Indeed, even historians should take an interest in mediumism, Hartmann suggested, for such study would deepen their understanding of the human predilection for superstition and belief in miracles. Despite the layers of patent nonsense and fraud, Hartmann insisted, what the séance phenomena revealed was that there was more at work in the human organism than the exact sciences had yet discovered. Needed now were hard facts.[36] Thus, although condemning the spiritualist craze sweeping Germany, Hartmann nevertheless saw scientific merit in further investigations, and he had the courage to say so publicly.

Zöllner published his reports in 1878, Wundt wrote his letter to Ulrici in 1879, Zöllner died in 1882, and Hartmann came out with his book in 1885. In this span of seven years, the controversy over the Leipzig sittings had not died down, neither in Germany nor abroad. Indeed, Zöllner's reports had become a key part of the arguments offered by the international spiritualist community for the reality of the spirit world and the ability of human mediums to act as intermediaries between the worlds of the living and the dead.[37]

It was in this international context that the final chapter in the Zöllner episode opened in 1886, when the Leipzig investigators became the focus of a special inquiry mounted by the Seybert Commission. This commission had been established on a grant of several thousands of dollars from the late Henry Seybert, a devoted American spiritualist. Led by its secretary George Fullerton, the commission experimented extensively with Slade in the United States and concluded that the medium's phenomena were fraudulent. Because the Zöllner experiments had become such a useful prop to the international spiritualist movement and such a focal point of controversy, Fullerton also traveled to Germany to interview the surviving participants in the Leipzig experiments. He concluded that there were sufficient problems with the investigators to cast doubt on Zöllner's testimony. He summarized his findings thus:

> [O]f the four eminent men whose names have made famous the investigation, there is reason to believe one, Zöllner, was of unsound mind at the time, and anxious for experimental verification of an already accepted hypothesis; another, Fechner, was partially blind, and believed because of Zöllner's observations; a third, Scheibner, was also afflicted with defective vision, and not entirely satisfied in his own mind as to the phenomena; and a fourth, Weber, was advanced in age, and did not even recognize the disabilities of his associates. No one of these men had ever had experiences of this sort before, nor was any one of them acquainted with the ordinary possibilities of deception. . . . [T]he lack of such knowledge was unfortunate.[38]

As this passage demonstrates, Fullerton made the credibility of the scientists, not the authenticity of the phenomena, the focus of his attack. And since it was supposedly the investigators' credibility, grounded in their authority as eminent scientists, that had given the Leipzig experiments their significance, the Seybert report challenged the credibility of the entire spiritualist movement.[39]

In Germany, the response to the Seybert Commission report was cautious, even in the burgeoning occult movement. Writing in the newly founded German occult journal *Sphinx* later that year, for instance, the editor Wilhelm Hübbe-Schleiden noted that such reports were useful for alerting investigators to the pitfalls involved in the study of occult phenomena. But he also commented that should it turn out to be true that the Leipzig investigators had been deceived, Zöllner and his colleagues still deserved praise for having had the guts to stand up to materialism—the widespread belief that the world consists solely of matter in motion.[40]

Hübbe-Schleiden had identified the twin stakes of the controversy for occultists. These were to establish the truth of the phenomena and at the same time to combat materialism, a culturally loaded term evocative of both a Godless universe and the socialist menace. For better and for worse, all sides of the Zöllner controversy aspired to determine the truth of the phenomena. But the truth proved highly elusive, advancing toward some investigators and retreating from others depending on the questions being asked and the methods being applied. The phenomena remained indeterminate, their interpretation contested. Against this background, Hübbe-Schleiden's closing comment about Zöllner's courageous stand against materialism was especially significant, for it indicated that not only phenomena but entire worldviews were at issue. Occultists saw themselves as part of a counterculture, locked in battle against a dominant materialist tendency of the age, and this self-understanding gave their movement its dynamism and appeal. They aspired to use occult phenomena to establish new truths about the human soul and the world it inhabited, to construct on this basis a new worldview that would make materialism obsolete. Indeed, this hunger for a postmaterialist *Weltanschauung* was fundamental to the appeal of the occult in Germany right through the 1940s.

Long after the Seybert Commission had delivered the supposedly definitive blow to Zöllner's reputation, this sense that an entire worldview was at stake in the Zöllner controversy was confirmed by the Russian painter Wassily Kandinsky, who lived many years in Germany and contributed so much to the elaboration of German expressionism. Kandinsky saw himself as a warrior against materialism, and in his 1911 manifesto *Concerning the Spiritual in Art* he noted with approval that he was not alone in this fight:

> [S]uch facts as the science of yesterday greeted with the usual word "swindle" are
> on the increase, or are merely becoming more generally known. Even the news-

papers, those habitually most obedient servants of success and of the plebs, who base their business on "giving the people what they want," find themselves in many cases obliged to limit or even to suppress altogether the ironic tone of their articles about the latest "miracles." Various educated men, pure materialists among them, devote their scientific investigation to those puzzling facts that can no longer be denied or kept quiet.[41]

Among these "educated men" progressive enough to investigate "those puzzling facts," Kandinsky counted Zöllner, whose book *Transcendental Physics* he owned and whose name he cited in the footnote to this passage.[42] Zöllner's work, in other words, wound its way into the heart of German expressionism, and thereby also into German modernism. The links between Zöllner and Kandinsky are by no means exceptional, and one of the major goals of this book is to trace more such connections between the German occult and the larger history of the quintessentially modern.

From Transcendental Physics to Psychological Modernism

At first glance, Zöllner's appearance in Kandinsky's 1911 manifesto makes no sense. Zöllner, after all, had been dead since 1882 and discredited since 1887. Moreover, even while alive, he had never shown any particular interest in the fine arts or indicated that he thought transcendental physics might have aesthetic significance. What are we to make of the curious fact, then, that Kandinsky enlisted this long-dead scientist in a radical and highly influential effort to rejuvenate modern art? The short answer is that Kandinsky saw Zöllner's controversial experiments with Slade as the sign that a new, more spiritual age was dawning. What Kandinsky took to be the start of this new epoch, modern historians have called "the birth of the modern age." Whatever we call it, we should follow Kandinsky's lead in linking the Leipzig sittings to the dawn of something new. They belong, along with German occultism more generally, to the history of German modernism.

In order to clarify this point, which is central to this book, it is necessary to explore the larger history of late nineteenth- and early-twentieth-century Germany in more detail. At the outset, it is crucial to realize that these were years of massive political, socioeconomic, and cultural change. On the political front, they encompassed the rise of the German Empire and its devastating fall in the Great War, the creation of national political institutions like the Reichstag, and escalating political tensions surrounding the growth of mass political movements agitating for everything from democratic reform to radical nationalism. On the socioeconomic front, these were the years in which Germany emerged as a major economic power rivaling even Britain. This, along with her imperial aspirations, helped tip an already-precarious international order toward war in 1914. Fueling Germany's industrial economy was a population that had increased by 60 percent between 1871 and 1914 (to 68 million), more and more of it migrating to the large urban centers in search of work. In towns like Leipzig, where Zöllner lived, a core population of 63,000 residents in 1850 had nearly doubled by 1871, then mushroomed to a staggering 679,000 in 1910.[43]

These political and socioeconomic changes had wide-reaching effects on the cultural front as many Germans realized that they were witnessing the dawn of something new, what Eugen Wolff, of the naturalist movement, dubbed *"die Moderne"* ("the modern") in 1887.[44] Contemporary observers as different in temperament and focus as Friedrich Nietzsche and Max Weber concurred that a core cultural characteristic of this new, modern age was the rationalization of whole new areas of human endeavor. German businesses introduced techniques of scientific management and brought in scientists to study and solve problems like worker fatigue.[45] The newly nationalized state undertook to guard the public's health by instituting compulsory immunization and systematizing the inspection of food and water supplies. New technologies like typewriters, telephones, and sewing machines made workers more efficient, while cheap bicycles and urban transport systems made them more mobile. Universities grew larger as more and more Germans enrolled for advanced studies, and so, too, did commercial establishments as small shops gave way increasingly to chains and department stores selling mass-produced, brand-name items.

Germans recognized that what Wolff had called "die Moderne" in 1887 demanded their response, and one of the most widespread was anxiety. Anxiety could manifest itself in neurasthenia and hysteria, whose sufferers complained of exhaustion or overstimulation and became unable to conduct themselves in the rational and purposeful manner that the old bourgeois order prescribed. Anxiety also surfaced in the rising flood of literature purporting to diagnose the multiple ills plaguing Germany. Depending on the author's viewpoint, these might include Godless socialism, immoral materialism, self-centered individualism, cultural degeneration (signaled by the climbing rates of suicide and prostitution), Jewish capitalism, or liberal Protestantism. Although some Germans—the so-called antimodernists—parlayed their anxieties about this new age into wholesale rejection, many more struggled with an apparently irresolvable ambivalence. On the one hand, they applauded Germany's new order, wealth, and world status; on the other, they deplored the deep unease and disorientation that all these changes had brought in their train. From these ambivalent Germans emerged the so-called "modernists," who embraced the immense potential of the modern age while also working to correct what they saw as its deepest flaws. Among the most gnawing of these was a sense that although reason's triumph had made Germans materially wealthy, it had also impoverished them spiritually. That most famous modernist Max Weber called this process the "disenchantment of the world," and his Janus-faced phrase, which simultaneously celebrated and bemoaned reason's triumph, neatly captured the ambivalence that so many Germans felt about the new world emerging around them.[46]

Although Zöllner cannot truly be called a modernist since he died before this movement or its reason for existence had emerged, his restless dissatisfaction and his embrace of the occult sciences in the 1870s and early 1880s was symptomatic of what was to come. Zöllner and the ten-year controversy he sparked belonged to a crucial cultural moment. What, then, does the Zöllner episode teach us about this cultural moment and the place of the occult within it?

In the first place, it suggests that to Germans struggling to come to terms with their new world, the occult sciences beckoned as a useful new realm of study. As a typical member of Germany's educated middle classes, the *Bildungsbürgertum*, Zöllner had been a long-time supporter of the National Liberals and in 1871 he applauded Germany's unification. But as the 1870s developed, his enthusiasm for "progress" was tempered by a growing unease over the changes that he saw unfolding in the new Germany.[47] His anti-Semitic outburst during the Slade controversy and his earlier diatribes about the corrosive effects of academic careerism were symptomatic of this unease. Such expressions were not peculiar to Zöllner: middle-class anti-Semitism had been on the rise in Germany since 1873, when an economic downturn that hit craft- and tradespeople particularly hard generated a wave of rhetoric that linked creeping capitalism and immoral materialism to the new public prominence of Germany's Jewish citizens.[48] Similarly, professionalization had become the object of widespread critique in the 1870s and 1880s, when an earlier ideal of the university as an institution dedicated to the search for "pure truth" began to dissolve in the face of growing disciplinary specialization, increasing student enrollments, and ever more insistent demands for "practical results."[49]

But of all the causes for dissatisfaction that galled Zöllner, scientific materialism took pride of place. And it was this dissatisfaction that propelled him, like so many Germans after him, into the occult sciences. Zöllner entered the séance room to reclaim the transcendent both for modern science, which he saw mired in excessive materialism, and for modern life, which he believed had lost its moral compass as a result of this same materialism. Zöllner hinted at the first part of this agenda in 1878 when he wrote that he had embarked on the sittings with Slade "to investigate the *real* existence of a four-dimensional space . . . by *experience,* that is, by observation of *facts.*"[50] Even so circumscribed a statement indicated the larger issues at stake, particularly when we pay attention to the words Zöllner emphasized in the original: *real* existence, *experience,* and *facts.* He believed that the Leipzig sittings pointed to the reality of a higher dimension of space and that this higher dimension corresponded to nothing less than the Kantian realm of "things in themselves." How else, Zöllner asked, was the knot experiment to be explained?

But Zöllner's revolt against the natural sciences had definite limits, and these were limits that the occult sciences continued to follow long after his death. His challenge, it is crucial to realize, was metaphysical, but not methodological. He aimed to topple the hegemony of scientific materialism while at the same time reclaiming the transcendent, all by the modern means of scientific experiment. The significance of this project did not escape perceptive contemporary observers like Friedrich Engels, who noted in the wake of the Zöllner controversy that, if nothing else, spiritualism had demonstrated the surest way from natural science to mysticism. This was not the discredited romantic science of *Naturphilosophie,* as was commonly believed, but a shallow empiricism that mistrusted both theorizing and thinking.[51] Whether we accept his critical evaluation of spiritualism or not, we should nonetheless follow Engels in recognizing that Zöllner's empirical recovery of the transcendent was utterly contemporary, a most-characteristic expression of an age enthusiastic about modern science and its experimental method, but increasingly nervous about its life-changing accomplishments.

If the Zöllner episode suggests that séances were appealing because they offered a thoroughly modern route to the transcendent, it also helps us grasp that the occult sciences turned out to sit squarely in the middle of what was rapidly becoming a war zone. This was the no man's land of late-nineteenth-century psychological thought, a territory in which philosophers, psychologists, physiologists, physicists, psychiatrists, doctors, clerics, educators, spiritualists, and ordinary lay people were all staking their claims.

Why this territory was the object of such intense jockeying becomes clear if we pause for a moment to explore the role of four leading characters in the Zöllner episode—Fechner, Helmholtz, Wundt, and Hartmann—as key figures in the development of nineteenth-century psychology. Fechner, trained as a physicist and inspired by the romantic ideals of Naturphilosophie, had entered the field in the 1850s looking for a way to study the mind-body connection empirically. His elaboration of the psychophysical laws along with Helmholtz's development of sensory psychology helped initiate the destabilization of German psychology in the 1860s. An older German tradition that had made the study of the soul a subfield of philosophy began to give way to a new emphasis on psychology as an experimental science focused on the empirical study of sensation and perception. In the 1860s and 1870s, Helmholtz's former student Wundt became a vocal advocate of this trend, which came to be known as the "new psychology."[52] While this shift in academic psychology unfolded, non-academic psychology was also undergoing a transformation. Philosophers like Hartmann, building on insights gleaned from Schopenhauer and observations drawn from neurology and physiology, elaborated the notion of an unconscious mental life. These two trends merged in the last three decades of the nineteenth century, when psychological investigators working both in and out of university circles began to cast about for ways to study the unconscious mind experimentally. Hypnosis presented one avenue of approach; spiritualism was another. The "spirit communications" produced by mediums like Slade, some investigators hypothesized, were in fact psychological phenomena percolating up from the medium's unconscious mind, and these phenomena, some speculated further, might also prove empirically that the human soul was immortal.[53]

Such novel approaches to the experimental study of the human psyche were nothing if not controversial, particularly with new psychologists like Wundt. Mediums like Slade were notorious tricksters and thus offered an unreliable experimental subject. The spiritualists' belief that séances put the living in contact with the dead was even worse since it smacked of ignorance and superstition. Once the idea that séance phenomena might be psychological had been broached, however, men like Fechner, Helmholtz, Wundt, and Hartmann could not remain neutral for long since each man had a significant stake in the future direction of German psychology. What kind of science was German psychology to become, and under whose control was it to fall? Would the study of the soul continue to be a multidisciplinary effort dedicated, as it had been since the early 1800s, to establishing the "criteria for objective knowledge, while at the same time leaving room for intellectual freedom and moral values"?[54] Or would it become an institutionally distinct science with its own concepts, methods, narrowly framed questions, and professionally trained practitioners? Would it remain an open domain for nonpsychologists interested in philosophical questions about the ultimate nature of reality and the individual's role in the world? Or would it become a materialist science centered on the biology of the brain and the physiology of cognition and perception?

How each of the players in the Zöllner episode answered these larger questions about the future of German psychology helped determine their stance toward Slade's phenomena. Zöllner, with his concern over the corrosive effects of scientific materialism on human freedom and moral values, Fechner, with his lifelong philosophical interest in the links between mind and body, and Hartmann, with his commitment to making the unconscious relevant to modern ethics, were willing to consider the possibility that séances might be doorways to the deeper reaches of the human psyche. In contrast, Helmholtz and Wundt feared that spiritualism might derail attempts to establish the new psychology on a firm conceptual and institutional basis and regarded séances as a scientific dead end.

This fundamental disagreement among psychology's leaders pointed to psychology's still indeterminate status and left its mark on all aspects of the Zöllner episode. Consider, for example, the peculiar nature of the Leipzig sittings. Zöllner conducted the sittings in his own home, using a mixture of domestic props (coffee tables, bowls of flour, writing slates) and scientific instruments and concepts (compasses, prisms, experiment, the fourth dimension). The sittings were a hybrid affair, belonging wholly to neither the laboratory nor the home, neither physics nor philosophy, neither elite science nor popular practice. Their hybrid character, moreover, prompted one effort after another to police the boundary they crossed. As late as 1893, for instance, Zöllner and his defenders were being accused of having wrongfully taken possession of the "private property" of mathematicians.[55] *Private property* was an apt phrase, for participants in the Zöllner episode did often behave as if property were at stake. To whom, after all, did the fourth dimension or the human psyche belong? Mathematicians may have wished to obtain exclusive ownership over the fourth dimension, new psychologists over the psyche, but neither of these—nor x-rays, when they were discovered in the 1890s, nor quantum theory, when it emerged in the 1920s—ever functioned as the "private property" of any one group, either "within" the natural sciences or "outside" them in the larger realm of German culture. Just as Zöllner had appropriated the fourth dimension from Helmholtz, who had appropriated it from the mathematicians, German occultists in later years would continue to appropriate discoveries, practices, and concepts that many German scientists would have liked to regard as their exclusive preserve. Nor was this transmission process ever one way. Just as Zöllner's reports passed the fourth dimension on to the realm of general culture, they also helped pull mediums, not to mention magicians like Bellachini, into the service of scientific research.[56]

In the end, perhaps the aspect of the Leipzig sittings that most incited controversy was that they pointed to a range of human experience that many would have preferred to ignore. Slade's table-moving, knot-tying, and spirit-writing feats may have looked to skeptics like simple parlor tricks, but what was even a skeptic to make of other mediums—and there were plenty—who specialized in less-physical phenomena like telepathy, trance speaking, and clairvoyant imaging? These phenomena had been shunted aside earlier in the century under the banner of superstition and mysticism. Now, Zöllner's experiments threatened to open the door on them again. Zöllner, of course, had not begun the sittings with Slade with any such intention. Rather, his goal in 1877 had been to expand the metaphysical boundaries of the natural sciences: to topple the hegemony of scientific materialism and to make room for the reintegration of the transcendent into the modern worldview. But by 1885, commentators like Hartmann had linked séance phenomena to the unconscious, and more and more people joined him in insisting that investigators finally attend to this forgotten realm of human psychology.

What the new psychologists deplored, observers like Kandinsky applauded. For the Russian painter, as for so many other people, the Leipzig sittings and all the occult experiments that followed demonstrated quite simply that the human psyche was a world unto itself. It was a mysterious world with hidden depths and occult powers, but it was also a natural world amenable to techniques of modern experimental investigation. It was a world that each person carried inside his or her psyche, but it was also a world that somehow linked the individual to the transcendent cosmos. Caught between their assessment of their age as spiritually bankrupt and their commitment to scientific empiricism, modern-minded men and women turned to occult beliefs and practices in the hopes of ameliorating the "soul sickness" that plagued them. Could the occult powers of the psyche, many Germans wondered, reinvigorate those whom reason's triumph had flattened? This question sat at the core of the project of psychological modernism, and if Zöllner's experiments had helped broach this project in the first place, the occult movement that flourished in Germany until the middle of the twentieth century was its working out.[57]

Approaches to the German Occult: Old and New

Just as the Zöllner episode points the way to a new interpretive agenda linking German occultism to German modernism, it also suggests a new methodological approach. This becomes clear when we realize, perhaps with surprise, that the appeal of the occult was essentially pragmatic—that Zöllner, Hartmann, and Kandinsky each turned to the occult seeking solutions to specific problems. For them, the "truth" of the phenomena, as William James was saying on the other side of the Atlantic, lay with what the phenomena allowed them to do.[58] The occult helped Zöllner challenge the bedrock assumptions of nineteenth-century physics, helped Hartmann press forward with his attempt to open up the human unconscious to experimental probing, and helped Kandinsky create the blueprint for the new, more "spiritual" art that he believed the modern age demanded. To call their turn to the occult pragmatic, moreover, is in no way to demean their motivations or involvement with the occult as purely instrumental. For these three men, as for the thousands of less-famous Germans who followed them, the truth of the phenomena lay with the practical consequences of their belief in the phenomena. And these practical consequences were of the most momentous sort, for they involved strivings that each had dedicated a lifetime to fulfilling.

What all of this indicates is the absolutely central importance of *practice* to the appeal and dynamic of the German occult movement. Manifestations of the soul *in action*—in knot experiments, clairvoyant visions, telepathic communications, dream dances, automatic writing, and materialized spirits—were what fascinated Germans and propelled them to develop the potential they believed lay buried in the occult reaches of the mind and universe. Correspondingly, *A Science for the Soul* takes the issue of how, where, and why Germans put the occult to use as its organizational theme.

This approach to the history of the German occult contrasts strongly with the prevalent view among historians that the German occult movement is significant mainly insofar as it helps to explain the ideological roots of National Socialism. According to this school of thought, irrationalist philosophies of the late nineteenth and early twentieth centuries, including occultism, helped to clear a path for Hitler's rise to power and grounded his barbarous campaign to create a racially pure and powerful Germany.[59] George Mosse gave one of the most influential statements of this view in 1961 when he wrote: "In Germany the recovery of the unconscious, in reaction against the dominant positivist ideologies, laid the groundwork for the German form of XXth-century totalitarianism. This reaction combined the deep stream of German romanticism with the mysteries of the occult as well as with the idealism of deeds. What sort of deeds these turned out to be is written in blood on the pages of history." In Mosse's hands, occultism joined romanticism, antipositivism, and the return of the unconscious—irrationalism writ large—as part of the poisonous milieu that prepared the way for Auschwitz.[60]

Following Mosse's lead, historians have returned repeatedly to the key role played by Ariosophy, an early-twentieth-century doctrine that mixed occult and *völkisch* (racist, anti-Semitic, and nationalist) elements. Named by the Austrian Jörg Lanz von Liebenfels, Ariosophy combined spurious Teutonic beliefs and customs proposed by the Austrian Guido von List with Theosophical and other occult precepts. Based on the belief that there was a universal life force manifested most perfectly in blond-haired, blue-eyed Aryans, the society's primary objective was to study the history of the "blond" and "dark" races. Via a succession of esoteric circles, Ariosophy spread through Germany in the early years of the twentieth century. In 1919, one of these circles hosted the meeting during which the Deutsche Arbeiterpartei (the German worker's party), the predecessor to the National Socialist Party, was founded.

Pointing to these institutional connections and the resemblance between the racialist philosophy of Ariosophy and Hitler's ideas about race, many scholars have devoted themselves to studying these links more closely. Their efforts have been aided, in part, by the testimonials of Ariosophists who proudly saw their movement as a forerunner of National Socialism.[61] Looking for the ideological roots of Hitler's anti-Semitism, and thus for the worldview in which the genocide of Europe's Jews became thinkable, postwar historians have used such sources with varying degrees of success to make the case that German occultism, by way of Ariosophy, bears a measure of responsibility for some of the greatest atrocities of the twentieth century.[62]

Recently, however, this line of interpretation has begun to divulge its limits. Nicholas Goodrick-Clarke's important and exhaustive 1985 study on Ariosophy and the occult roots of National Socialism exposed both the strengths and weaknesses of the case. Aiming to provide new answers to old questions, Goodrick-Clarke drew on an impressive range of novel primary sources to expose "the myths, symbols and fantasies [bearing] on the development of reactionary, authoritarian, and Nazi styles of thinking."[63] He established that the occult figured in Ariosophical thought primarily to legitimate previously conceived notions of race and nation, but discovered that these notions appealed to Hitler as much as Ariosophical occultism repelled him. All of this led Goodrick-Clarke to conclude, rather anticlimactically, that Hitler and most of his colleagues were not occultists and that their infamous crimes were only loosely connected with occult doctrines.

This trend toward decoupling occultism and Nazism has continued in recent years as historians have begun to explore the völkisch milieu of Central Europe at the turn of the century in more detail. Particularly revealing are two essays in the pathbreaking *Handbook of "Völkisch Movements,"* a recent volume that concentrates on the imperial period (1871-1918).[64] Challenging previous interpretations on many points of fact, Ekkehard Hieronimus revisits Lanz von Liebenfels as a völkisch ideologue and concludes that his influence on National Socialism was minimal. Helmut Zander explores racial theories emanating from the occult underground and concludes that although völkisch ideas on race were certainly present in the occult underground, their effects are difficult to gauge. He makes the important point that historians should exercise caution in generalizing about German occultism, especially since many occultists did not turn their ideas and practices to anti-Semitic ends.[65]

Where do five decades of historical investigation of the theme "occultism and Nazism" or "occultism and völkisch milieus" leave us? In the first place, it has clearly established that there are links, both ideological and social, between Hitler and Ariosophical circles. But, at the same time, it has exposed the limits of these connections. Unable to make direct causal claims, historians have been forced to resort to the device of "affinities" to make their case. This body of literature also leaves one wondering whether German occultism has engaged historians' attention because of its intellectual distastefulness, a quality it shares with National Socialism in spirit and deed.[66] One might also speculate that locating Nazism's roots in the "lunatic fringe" and the occult "flight from reason" makes it that much easier to evade the hard question of what connects the proud heights of German (or even European) culture to the ignoble depths of Nazi barbarism.[67] Most importantly, finally, this body of literature has turned up several tantalizing signs that there was much more to German occultism than proto-Nazism.

This book is a systematic and detailed study of what this "other history" entailed. It focuses on the practice of German occultism in order to gain a fresh perspective on German modernism, but in doing so it does not neglect the links between the German occult movement and the völkisch milieu of Imperial, Weimar, and Nazi Germany. Rather than following the previous pattern of subordinating the occult to the völkisch, however, this study views them as distinct, if also partially overlapping, areas of cultural practice. It taps the recent historiographic trend that treats Germany during these years as "a crisis-racked, modernizing society in which teetering over the abyss was the norm and the resolution of conflict was the exception."[68] From this vantage point, both the occult movement and the völkisch milieu come into sharp focus as but two of a multitude of reformist attempts that sprang up in Germany to meet the novel challenges of living in the topsy-turvy modern age.[69]

In using the occult to examine Germans' experience of the modern, both their fear of its pitfalls and their engagement with its possibilities, I draw on a wide variety of novel primary sources. This material includes periodicals, investigative reports, memoirs, monographs, personal papers *(Nachläße)*, and archival holdings. Worthy of special mention are the collected papers of Wilhelm Hübbe-Schleiden, an early leader of the German Theosophical movement, at the library of the University of Göttingen; the collection at the Stadtbibliothek (city library) in Munich, whose former director, Hans Ludwig Held, observed the occult movement as it developed and assembled its texts for his library; and the Janos Frecot collection at Stanford University, which contains many of the movement's ephemeral documents and helps put them in their larger context of cultural reformism. In order to gain the perspective of contemporaries who were outside of but aware of the German occult movement, I have turned to a similarly diverse array of materials. These include published accounts and critiques as well as archival sources drawn from city police files in Munich and Berlin, Gestapo files at the U.S. Holocaust Memorial Museum in Washington, D.C., and files assembled by church bodies concerned with occult activities among their constituencies. Finally, newspaper articles drawn from contemporary periodicals have furnished reports on the important episodes and cases that reached the general public. They have also provided invaluable information not elsewhere available about the audiences before whom occultists offered their wares.

In this book, I assemble my material in a tripartite structure. The first part presents the groups and individuals who participated in the modern German occult movement and examines the conduits through which they developed and spread their beliefs. Chapter 1 has used the Zöllner episode to introduce occult phenomena and explore why Germans found these phenomena so alluring. Chapter 2 reconstructs the early organizational history of the German occult movement in the second half of the nineteenth century. Chapter 3 then examines economic and social factors responsible for the rapid spread of the movement from the 1890s onward and focuses on occultism as a facet of the emergence of twentieth-century mass consumer culture.

Building on this foundation, the second part of the book turns to the question of how German occultism acquired meaning in specific realms of practice. Here, the focus is on three venues in which ideas, techniques, and personnel from this movement acted: Theosophy, where occult studies were directed to the attainment of the spiritual enlightenment of the self (chapter 4); the arts, where occult states of consciousness were used to fuel the creative processes of avant-garde painters, writers, and dancers (chapter 5); and the applied sciences, where psychologists, detectives, engineers, and doctors used occult techniques to solve characteristic problems of the modern age (chapter 6).

The book's final part considers the meanings the movement had for contemporaries by focusing on the question of how different social groups attempted to police the occult. Chapters 7 and 8 examine the response of the churches, the state, and the general public in the imperial and Weimar periods and uncovers the reasons why efforts to control the occult during these years were so unsuccessful. Chapter 9 then turns to an extended consideration of the tangled affinities and antipathies that existed between German occultists and the Nazi regime and charts the movement's final decimation by 1945.

Throughout, the main purpose of the book is to examine the German occult movement in its broadest cultural setting; that is, to explore German occultism as a key facet of German modernism and thus to gain new insight into how modern-minded Germans met the challenge of living meaningful lives in their "disenchanted" age.

CHAPTER TWO

A Psychological Point of View

"The observations of the spiritualists, weird and questionable as they seemed to me, were the first accounts I had seen of objective psychic phenomena. Names like Zöllner and Crookes impressed themselves on me, and I read virtually the whole of the literature available to me at the time."[1] Thus did Carl Gustav Jung recall his first encounter with the modern occult sciences in the late 1890s. Still a medical student at the University of Basel at the time, Jung had been deeply disappointed by how little his professors had had to say about the human psyche. Overjoyed to discover that this silence did not extend to occult circles, he read the available spiritualist reports voraciously and soon began to sit with mediums. From 1895 to 1899, he conducted experimental sittings with his cousin Helly Preiswerk and, encouraged by his mentor Eugen Bleuler, eventually made these sittings the focus of his 1902 Ph.D. thesis. Reflecting back on these years later in life, Jung realized just how important his initial encounter with the occult had been: "All in all, this was the one great experience which . . . made it possible for me to achieve a psychological point of view. I had discovered some objective facts about the human psyche."[2] Occult phenomena, in other words, had been instrumental in launching his career as a scientist of the mind.

Jung's statement that his discovery of Zöllner and the spiritualists opened the way to "a psychological point of view" was highly significant since it explicitly linked the German occult sciences with a key modernist current within fin-de-siècle European culture. This was the widespread enthusiasm for plumbing the depths of human psychological experience so as to bring consciousness to an understanding of itself. As table 2.1 indicates, this enthusiasm built on decades of attempts to reconcile the previously transcendent realm of the human psyche with the methods and claims of modern science, an effort in which the occult had long been instrumental. Largely ignored or underplayed in accounts of the era, the history of how the occult helped bring science and the psyche into dialogue and thus facilitated the blossoming of psychological modernism circa 1900 is the subject of this chapter.

The Nightlife of the Soul

The "psychological point of view" embraced by Jung had its modern roots in the 1850s, a decade of political and cultural retrenchment in German-speaking Europe. The revolutions that began in 1848 had raised liberal hopes that a unified and more participatory state might emerge from the remains of the Holy Roman Empire, but the counterrevolutionary wave of 1849 had quickly dashed this dream. With political change blocked, at least for the moment, Germans turned to a wide variety of apparently nonpolitical pursuits. In the 1850s, they experimented with table turning and rediscovered animal magnetism; in the 1860s, they welcomed the American-born movement of spiritualism; and by the 1870s and 1880s, they had begun to lay the institutional foundations of the modern German occult movement. Informing all these developments were new answers to old questions. What were the relations of matter and spirit, body and mind? Were mind and spirit knowable in the same way as body and matter? From the 1850s onward, the occult helped reframe the mind/body problem for the modern age.

This pattern was visible from the very start in the German history of table turning, which began in January 1853 when a woman in Bremen received a letter from her brother, a businessman in New York. He reported on his successful table-turning experiments and, enclosing detailed instructions, urged his sister to make her own trials. A few days later, in the salon of a Bremen businessman, one of the first table-turning trials in Europe took place. Eight friends and family members came to the event laughing in skepticism, but good-naturedly built a human chain around a heavy table as the letter directed. After thirty minutes or so, the participants were amazed to feel peculiar currents passing through their limbs. Soon, the table began to crack and then to move so violently that the group was able to maintain its circle only with difficulty. As word spread of this successful experiment, more and more families in Bremen staged their own table-turning trials.[3] A local writer sent a report on the Bremen table-turning phenomenon to the *Augsburger Allgemeine Zeitung,* and the *Berliner Blatt* and *Vossische Zeitung* quickly reprinted it. Soon, table-turning experiments were being staged in German cities as far-flung as Berlin, Breslau, Nuremberg, Vienna, Hildesheim, Hannover, and Braunschweig. Everywhere, as the spiritualist Jacques Groll reported several decades later, "[t]he reliable witnesses, experts of all sorts—doctors, teachers, and even men in practical professions . . . businessmen, tradesmen, [and] all manner of artisans—did the experiment; success convinced them, often against their own will . . . all doubts necessarily fell away before the facts."[4]

Table turning provoked heated debates, but not because "the facts" themselves were in question.[5] As anyone attending a trial could affirm, the tables undeniably danced. Moreover, those who had no first-hand experience could count on the testimony of "reliable witnesses" (as Groll put it) from the German middle classes, on whose veracity and immunity to trickery one could depend. On the question of why tables moved, however, consensus broke down. One group of interpreters followed the author of the original Augsburg newspaper article in maintaining that there was a natural explanation involving the mechanical force of participants' hands.[6] Another group attributed the phenomena to the presence of spirits who used the table's cracks and creaks as a means for communicating with the assembled participants. This form of table turning, known as spirit rapping, was still being staged as late as the 1890s, when the Roman Catholic preacher Adam Rambacher convinced his followers that he could speak with the devil through the dancing table.[7] Yet a third group attributed the phenomena to the will of participants, whose hands communicated their unconscious wishes to the table itself.

These three explanations of why tables turned—the first stressing material causes, the second and third immaterial ones—reflected in microcosm one of the great cultural debates raging in German-speaking Europe from the 1850s onward. This was the debate over what status immaterial entities such as God and the soul would have in the modern age. In the first half of the nineteenth century, these immaterial entities had been understood to belong

Table 2.1. A Timeline of Important Dates Related to the Early German Occult Movement

Date	German Publications	German Events	Publications & Events Outside Germany
1779			F. A. Mesmer, *Memoir on the Discovery of Animal Magnetism* (France)
1781	I. Kant, *Critique of Pure Reason*		
1816		Prussian state creates university chairs of animal magnetism at Berlin and Bonn	
1829	J. Kerner, *The Seeress of Prevorst*		
1843			J. Braid coins *hypnotism* (UK)
1845	K. von Reichenbach, *Researches on Magnetism and Related Topics*		
1851	A. Schopenhauer, *Essay on Spirit Seeing*		
1853		Table-turning craze begins in Bremen	
1855	L. Büchner, *Force and Matter*		
1860	G. T. Fechner, *Elements of Psychophysics*		
1868	*Spiritualism Library for Germany*, ed. G. K. Wittig, begins publication		
1869	E. von Hartmann, *Philosophy of the Unconscious*		
1874	*Psychische Studien* founded		W. James founds first experimental psychology laboratory at Harvard
1877–78		K. F. Zöllner investigates Slade in Leipzig	
1878			J. M. Charcot begins using hypnosis at the Salpêtrière (France)
1879		W. Wundt founds Germany's first institute for experimental psychology in Leipzig	

Table 2.1. Continued

Date	German Publications	German Events	Publications & Events Outside Germany
1882			Académie des Sciences accepts Charcot's paper linking hypnosis to hysteria (France); Society for Psychical Research (SPR) founded (UK)
1884	E. von Hartmann, *Spiritualism*	Theosophische Societät Germania founded in Elberfeld	
1885			W. James begins experiments with the medium Leonora Piper (U.S.)
1886	*Sphinx* founded	Psychologische Gesellschaft founded in Munich	Seybert Commission report lambasts spiritualism (U.S.); Nancy School of psychiatry emerges under H. Bernheim (France)
1889	C. du Prel, *Philosophy of Mysticism*	Gesellschaft für Experimentalpsychologie splits from Psychologische Gesellschaft; Gesellschaft für Experimentalpsychologie founded in Berlin; M. Dessoir coins *parapsychology*	First International Congress of Physiological Psychology (Paris)
1890	A. Aksakow, *Animism and Spiritism*		W. James, *Principles of Psychology*
1896	*(Neue) Metaphysische Rundschau* founded as continuation of *Sphinx*		
1899			S. Freud, *Interpretation of Dreams* (Austria); T. Flournoy, *From India to the Planet Mars* (Switzerland)
1902			C. G. Jung, *On the Psychology and Pathology of So-Called Occult Phenomena* (Switzerland)

to the transcendent sphere ruled over by theologians and philosophers; by the 1850s, however, many natural scientists had begun not only to challenge the authority of theologians and philosophers to say anything meaningful on such matters but also to question whether or not the transcendent sphere (and the immaterial entities that populated it) existed at all. The differing answers to the question of why tables turned, in other words, belonged to this much larger debate over what status the transcendent would have in an age of science. This issue also lay at the heart of the heated debates that broke out in the 1850s over scientific materialism, whose unresolved issues Zöllner would revisit so provocatively just two decades later.

Materialism in its most basic form was the view that the world consists solely of matter. Its proponents preached that humans were like other natural objects in being composed solely of this substance and that no entities, whether God, soul, or mind, could exist apart from the material body. One important turning point in the popularity of materialism in German-speaking Europe came in 1855 with the publication of Ludwig Büchner's *Force and Matter*. Purporting to bring the truth about nature to the educated layperson, Büchner peppered his text with variations on the slogan "[T]here is, in the end, no fighting against facts." The facts proved that matter and force were the interdependent and determining elements of nature. Neither could exist without the other; neither could be created or destroyed. Thought, mind, and soul were not inhabitants of a transcendent sphere but products of matter in motion. Nature contained no design, divine or other, for human progress; in fact, the day would eventually come "when the physical forces now existing will be exhausted, and all animated beings plunged into night and death." To those who hung their hopes on proving the existence of a transcendent world through elucidation of the "night-life of the soul"—that is, by studying such phenomena as animal magnetism, somnambulism, and clairvoyance—Büchner replied with the dismissive observation that such hopes were but "idle fancies."[8] Knowledge came only through the five senses. Clairvoyants, somnambulists, and others who claimed to know a supernatural or transcendent reality by nonsensual means contradicted this iron law of nature.

What was it against which Büchner and the scientific materialists were raging, particularly when they belittled devotees of the "night-life of the soul"? One of their main targets was the legacy of Friedrich Schelling and his romantic philosophy of science known as Naturphilosophie. Beginning in 1799, Schelling had elaborated a metaphoric vision of nature as a living organism endowed with a "world soul," and his followers, eager to investigate the world soul directly, had embraced the study of psychological and occult phenomena. They had been particularly intrigued by the mysterious healing force known as animal magnetism (discovered by the Viennese physician Franz Anton Mesmer in the 1770s), and their enthusiasm had helped ensure the widespread acceptance of animal magnetism in the German states in the first half of the nineteenth century. Numerous small groups, schools, journals, and congresses devoted to animal magnetism had flourished.[9] Books by men like the doctor Justinus Kerner, who in 1829 published an account of his magnetic experiments with Friederike Hauffe (better known as the Seeress of Prevorst) and the chemist Karl von Reichenbach, who in 1845 attempted to explain magnetic phenomena by postulating a universal "Od" force, akin to gravity, had helped popularize the movement. Literary figures such as E. T. A. Hoffmann and Clemens Brentano had become vocal enthusiasts of the mysterious force, and animal magnetism had even found its way into leading German intellectual circles, where distinguished proponents included the philosophers J. G. Fichte and Schelling, as well as the theologians Karl Windischmann and Joseph Ennemoser. Perhaps most stunning had been the creation in 1816 of two university chairs of animal magnetism, at Berlin and Bonn, following the recommendation of an investigating commission convened by King Frederick William III of Prussia in 1812.[10]

When Büchner and the scientific materialists penned their materialist tracts in the 1850s, in other words, they saw Naturphilosophie and animal magnetism as indissolubly linked. The speculations of Naturphilosophie, they believed, had been highly detrimental to scientific practice: it was time to renounce the "world soul" and eschew any involvement with occult forces like animal magnetism. Scientists, they insisted, must reject metaphysical speculation and turn instead to the discovery of concrete facts about the real world of sense experience.[11]

But at midcentury, not everyone who rejected Naturphilosophie was willing to leave the "night-life of the soul" behind. As early as the 1840s, figures like the British surgeon James Braid were trying to sanitize animal magnetism for scientific use. Braid had coined the term *hypnotism* to denote an updated form of mesmeric practice that dispensed with philosophical speculation. His reformulation would become immensely important to medical practice in the 1870s, especially in France and Britain. The philosopher Arthur Schopenhauer mounted a parallel effort in German-speaking Europe in 1851, when he published an essay passionately defending animal magnetism in his reputation-making book *Parerga and Paralipomena*. His extended "Essay on Spirit Seeing" attacked those who doubted "the facts of animal magnetism and clairvoyance" as ignorant. These "facts," he argued, had an immense philosophical significance: "Considered . . . [from] the philosophical point of view, animal magnetism is the most significant and pregnant of all the discoveries that have ever been made, although for the time being it propounds rather than solves riddles. It is really practical metaphysics. . . . [A] time will come when philosophy, animal magnetism, and natural science . . . will shed so bright a light on one another that truths will be discovered at which we could not otherwise hope to arrive."[12] His use of the phrase *practical metaphysics* was key, for it indicated his intention to stake out a middle ground between Naturphilosophie and scientific materialism.

Although Schopenhauer concurred with the materialists in rejecting the speculative systems of Naturphilosophie, he and the scientific materialists parted company over the question of the "night-life of the soul." Whereas the scientific materialists turned their backs on this category of human experience, tainted as it was by association with Naturphilosophie, Schopenhauer saw its relevance to the transcendent world of what he called the "will" and what scholars now recognize as a forerunner to our own notion of the "unconscious." In short, in linking animal magnetism to "practical metaphysics," Schopenhauer was suggesting that occult phenomena might open a doorway to the transcendent, that grand philosophical category that the scientific materialists were attempting to dismiss as useless metaphysical speculation.

Although still poorly understood by historians, Schopenhauer's impact on the intellectual and cultural life of German-speaking Europe in the second half of the nineteenth century was immense. In the 1850s, Schopenhauer's work provided a viable alternative to the materialist cause, and his philosophy became immensely popular among the educated middle classes uncomfortable with the metaphysics of materialism but dedicated to the empirical epistemology of modern science.[13] In 1869, the publication of Eduard von Hartmann's *The Philosophy of the Unconscious* brought Schopenhauer's philosophy to an even wider audience. Within a few decades, such modernist icons as Friedrich Nietzsche, Thomas Mann, Sigmund Freud, and Jung would all acknowledge their debt to Schopenhauer's vision of human personality as a product of the arational force of "will." And this vision would also inspire many of the first generation of modern German occultists in the 1870s and 1880s. As these examples suggest, Schopenhauer's midcentury refusal to be bullied into renouncing either "the night-life of the soul" or the occult phenomena that accompanied it was instrumental to the emergence the modernist movement fifty years later.

Before turning to an examination of how the occult contributed to modernism by century's end, however, it is necessary first to attend to one more midcentury development in the occult field. This was the beginning of German interest in the American-born movement of spiritualism. According to spiritualist lore, the movement traced its beginnings to 1848, when unexplainable raps, clicks, bumps, and cracks had occurred in the presence of two young sisters named Kate and Maggie Fox in upstate New York. These mysterious noises became the phenomena around which a vast international movement began to form. Mediums inspired by the Fox sisters appeared across the United States, Britain, and France over the next decade. Wherever they appeared, mysterious noises, writing, motion of objects, and physical emanations followed. Flocking to these mediums by the thousands, people came to believe that the mediums were agents through which the immaterial spirits of the deceased could communicate with the living.[14]

The Zöllner experiments of 1877–78 were an important chapter in the history of spiritualism in German-speaking Europe. But long before Zöllner sat down to conduct his famous sittings with Henry Slade, other members of the German Bildungsbürgertum had worked tirelessly to adapt this foreign occult movement to German soil. And their work in the 1860s and early 1870s was important, for it linked the midcentury debates over materialism and the "night-life of the soul" directly to the modern occult movement that emerged a few decades later. Indeed, the Zöllner experiments, and all that followed in their train, are incomprehensible without some understanding of what these early German spiritualists did, and why.

One early German spiritualist of note was Georg von Langsdorff, who first felt the attraction of spiritualism in the 1850s in the United States, where he had settled into a dental practice following his participation in the unsuccessful Badenese revolution of 1848.[15] A man of science as well as an avowed atheist and materialist, he had always scoffed at the idea of life after death. But one day he had found his irreligion called into question. While idly reflecting that atheists like himself had no compelling reason to refrain from committing murder for personal gain, he had heard a mysterious voice. "Where does that leave morality?" it had asked. Unable to find the source of the voice, and disturbed by the question, Langsdorff had returned home to his wife, who showed him a newspaper article reporting the recent discovery of the spirit world. Soon thereafter, in 1859, he began to attend séances and to experiment with somnambulists, magnetists, and mediums, convinced now of the reality of the afterlife. Reflecting on this stage of political exile and spiritual awakening in later years, Langsdorff saw 1848 as a pivotal year, politically because in 1848 Germans had risen for the first time to erect a true republic, and morally because 1848 was the year in which modern spiritualism had first appeared in the United States.[16]

As Langsdorff's own life following his conversion in 1859 demonstrated, spiritualism involved much more than just communication with the spirit world. Deeply disappointed by the results of the revolution of 1848, but hopeful that eventually a republic would evolve in Germany, Langsdorff devoted the rest of his long life to furthering the cause of human progress. In this, his activities following his return to Germany in 1861 as both a spiritualist and a dentist ran on parallel tracks. As an innovative dental practitioner of the second half of the nineteenth century, for instance, Langsdorff achieved notoriety among his colleagues, but lavish praise from his more progressive counterparts, for advocating the use of fluoride compounds to prevent tooth decay. Langsdorff also campaigned successfully for the establishment of one of Germany's first university departments of dental hygiene, established at the University of Freiburg. The skills he developed as a publicist for these improving projects he also used to popularize the new improving religion he had brought from the United States, publishing more than eight hundred essays and articles on the topic over the rest of his long life.[17]

While Langsdorff labored to marry spiritualism to progressive social change in Freiburg from the 1860s onward, another group dedicated to making spiritualism relevant to German culture began to flourish on the eastern edge of German-speaking Europe, in Breslau and Leipzig. This branch of the early German spiritualist movement had its roots in the late 1850s, when the professor Christian Gottfried Nees von Esenbeck, of Breslau, discovered the writings of the American spiritualist Andrew Jackson Davis. A radical democrat and social reformer, Nees von Esenbeck had studied with Goethe and then gone on to become a prominent botanist in Schelling's romantic mode.[18] He had published on animal magnetism extensively in the first half of the nineteenth century and, in the hope that Davis's works would help revitalize German *Naturphilosophie*, he recruited the young Catholic theologian Gregor

Konstantin Wittig to oversee the effort of translation. Despite strenuous opposition by the Roman Catholic Church, the death of Nees von Esenbeck in 1858, and financial difficulties, Wittig kept this project alive. In 1868, he began to bring out the series *Bibliothek des Spiritualismus für Deutschland* (Spiritualism library for Germany), a collection of translations of works by Davis and other leading figures of the international spiritualist community that brought spiritualism to a wide German audience. By 1873 he had founded a spiritualist club in Leipzig, and by 1874 he had teamed up with the Russian spiritualist Alexander Aksakow and the German publisher Oswald Mutze to bring out *Psychische Studien,* for many years Germany's most prominent occult journal.[19]

As spiritualism spread across Leipzig, two factions with two different interpretations of the phenomena under investigation emerged. Enthusiasts of Davis in the 1860s and 1870s, Wittig and his circle began to embrace a novel interpretation of the phenomena in the early 1880s. Whereas Davis adhered to the so-called spiritualist interpretation, which held that spirits caused occult phenomena, Wittig and his circle now began to investigate what they called the "animist" view, which postulated an as yet undetected psychological force as the causal agent.[20] This interpretive difference became the basis of an ideological and institutional rift by the mid-1880s. Wittig and his colleagues at *Psychische Studien* became the proponents of what now became known as "psychical research," which sought a psychological explanation for séance phenomena. Their opponents, led by the publisher Wilhelm Besser and an apothecary's assistant, "Dr." Bernhard Cyriax, continued to advocate the spiritualist interpretation and founded two journals, *Sprechsaal* and *[Neue] Spiritualistische Blätter,* along with a variety of clubs to spread their views.[21]

The rift in Leipzig was symptomatic of developments across Germany. In 1884, the philosopher Eduard von Hartmann published his pamphlet *Der Spiritismus* (Spiritualism), in which he threw his prestige behind Wittig and psychical research. That same year, the first major Theosophical group in Germany, the Theosophische Societät Germania (Theosophical society Germania), came into existence with the express goal of mediating between the claims of the spiritualists and psychical researchers. Two years later, a series of scandals rocked the German occult community, including the publication of the Seybert Commission report that discredited Zöllner's Leipzig experiments with Slade. As mediums working both in and out of Germany were exposed as frauds, many occult circles like the Theosophische Societät Germania disbanded. In their place sprang up new groups dedicated even more fiercely to placing the "night-life of the soul" on an unimpeachable scientific foundation. Clearly, the incipient occult movement had reached a turning point.

Wissenschaft and the Psyche

Nothing signaled this turn toward the scientific study of the "night-life of the soul" more clearly than the founding of the Psychologische Gesellschaft (Psychological society) of Munich in 1886. A major venue for German psychical research over the next three decades, the Psychologische Gesellschaft attracted men from all sectors of the Bildungsbürgertum. Early members included the philosopher Carl du Prel, the psychiatrist Albert von Schrenck-Notzing, the lawyer Wilhelm Hübbe-Schleiden, the engineer Ludwig Deinhard, the curator of Munich's Alte Pinakothek, Adolf Bayersdorfer, and the painters Wilhelm Trübner, Gabriel von Max, and Albert von Keller.[22] Against such German materialists as Karl Vogt, best remembered for the brutal pithiness of his observation that "thought stands in the same relation to the brain, as bile to the liver, or urine to the kidneys,"[23] the men of the society sought to make *Wissenschaft,* or science in its broadest sense, relevant to the study of human psychological experience.

What attracted these men to mediums in particular? The group's manifesto, published in 1887 in the occult journal *Sphinx,* offered a multitude of answers. Philosophers, the manifesto declared, need no longer struggle to hold their own against the encroaching doctrine of scientific materialism since mediums would give them empirical evidence for the independence of the human soul from the human organism. Historians of human civilization *(Kulturhistoriker),* previously forced to dismiss numerous accounts of events either as incomprehensible or unreliable, would finally be able to resolve long-standing riddles in their field. Artists dissatisfied with traditional models who assumed their poses in a waking state would discover the high expressive content of gestures and facial expressions produced by mediums in hypnotic or somnambular states. The Psychologische Gesellschaft, its members believed, would help establish once and for all basic truths about the human psyche, truths that would revolutionize philosophy, history, art, and culture at large. And they would do so in a wholly modern way—that is, through rigorous application of the scientific method.[24]

Scientific experiments featuring the medium Lina Matzinger quickly became central to the group's identity. Reported widely in occult journals like *Sphinx* and *Psychische Studien* as well as the mainstream *Gegenwart, Über Land und Meer,* and *Universum,* these experiments were the fruit of the group's central collaboration between du Prel and Schrenck-Notzing. A typical series of experiments conducted by the two men in 1887 ran as follows: Schrenck-Notzing would hypnotize Matzinger, silently read to himself a simple command written down by du Prel, and then project this command mentally to the medium. Induced in this way to commit acts normally prohibited by social convention, Matzinger struck a visiting Baron Ferdinand von Hornstein on the hand and ordered the Baroness du Prel to bring her a cup of coffee. Although the collaborators were delighted with these results, their delight had different sources. Du Prel gloried in the medium's transgressions because he saw them as a decisive step toward toppling the materialist worldview.[25] Schrenck-Notzing, on the other hand, took a more narrow view. For him, it was not worldviews but the definition of what counted as science that was at stake. Matzinger's feats were astonishing, he admitted, but the rigorous scientific conditions under which they had been induced suggested that what had previously been relegated to the realm of mysticism now needed finally to be brought within the boundaries of "official science."[26]

This difference of interpretation between the two collaborators became a yawning chasm that split the Psychologische Gesellschaft in two in 1889. At issue were two competing visions of psychology and the place of occult phenomena within it. The break-off Gesellschaft für Experimentalpsychologie (Society for experimental psychology), led by du Prel, pursued the vision of "transcendent psychology," while the rump Psychologische Gesellschaft followed Schrenck-Notzing in turning its attention to the elaboration of what became the new science of parapsychology. As even a cursory examination of the thoughts and activities of these two men in the 1880s and 1890s reveals, the overlap and dissonance between these two visions was immensely significant, both for the subsequent history of the German occult movement and for the emergence of "new" psychology at century's end.

By the time he teamed up with Schrenck-Notzing in the mid-1880s, du Prel had been investigating the shadow side of human consciousness for decades. In 1866, he and several friends in Munich had founded a club called *Die Hoffnungslosen* (Those without hope). Passionate devotees of Schopenhauer and his popularizer Eduard von Hartmann, du Prel and his companions criticized both traditional Christian belief and the new faith of scientific materialism.

Searching for an alternative, they pursued the psychological as well as anti-clerical and antimaterialist implications of Schopenhauer's philosophy.[27] Du Prel continued to develop these interests with an 1868 doctoral thesis on dreams, and in 1874 he burnished his scientific credentials with *Der Kampf ums Dasein am Himmel* (The struggle for existence in the heavens), a book that brought him popular renown as a defender and developer of Darwinian ideas.[28] Soon, du Prel's enthusiasm for Schopenhauer, Hartmann, and Darwin merged with his dismay over the rampant materialism that had set in following German unification (1866–71). More crime among the lower classes and increasing suicide and insanity among the educated ones, he believed, were signs of Germany's spiritual devolution and could be attributed to the cultural malaise whose seeds the scientific materialists had helped plant at midcentury.[29]

"Transcendent psychology" soon became the cornerstone of du Prel's program for German spiritual renewal. At the heart of this program lay du Prel's understanding of human consciousness as Janus-faced. One face inhabited the waking world of everyday sense experience while the other lived in the unconscious world of dream, trance, clairvoyant vision, and telepathic suggestion. Between the two lay a barrier of awareness that normally blocked one face from knowing the other, a barrier on which all previous attempts to open the transcendent to scientific probing had foundered. Precisely here lay the scientific significance of mediums, du Prel believed, for mediums had the peculiar ability to displace this barrier fully. What had long remained occluded—nothing less than Kant's transcendental subject—now lay revealed. If mediums thus provided a novel approach to old philosophical conundrums concerning the mind/body problem, they could also function as a tool with which to vanquish scientific materialism once and for all. The scientific materialists, of course, had dismissed the second face of consciousness as an illusion; dreams felt real to the dreamer, they conceded, but since scientific experiments could not be performed on dreams, dreams could not be used to prove the existence of an immaterial reality. This objection had been nullified, du Prel believed, during the experiments conducted on Lina Matzinger. Matzinger's susceptibility to telepathic manipulation by Schrenck-Notzing proved that the unconscious existed and, more importantly, that it was accessible to experimental intervention and control. Kant's transcendental subject, now reinterpreted as the human unconscious, was finally open to objective scientific investigation.[30]

Du Prel's transcendent psychology made the unconscious and its occult phenomena the site where scientific concerns met spiritual ones, where cold truths met living meanings. If transcendent psychology was a legitimate science because it investigated real phenomena according to the most up-to-date experimental techniques, it was also an ethically oriented science because it offered answers to the "world riddle" *(Weltprätsel)* concerning the origins, nature, and purpose of human existence. As he explained to a popular audience in 1892: "The occult sciences in their modern form will not lead to a new faith but rather promote a new form of knowledge. . . . They are called upon to supply an essential component for the worldview of the future. . . . Once complete, this worldview will reveal its great meaning as a synthesis of religion and science, metaphysics, and natural scientific research."[31] This new worldview, centered around transcendent psychology and its interpretation of occult phenomena, would not promote dogma and blind faith, as religion did, nor exert a chilling cultural influence, as academic science did;[32] rather, by combining the best elements of both, it would provide just what late-nineteenth-century modernity required: scientific grounding coupled with spiritual uplift. For du Prel, this was no dead promise but a living fact, and for proof he pointed to the numerous letters he received from people testifying to the comfort and inspiration they derived from his scientific vision of the transcendent.[33]

But grand philosophical issues and cultural activism were of little interest to Schrenck-Notzing, who was two decades younger than du Prel and coming of age in an entirely different cultural context. As an aspiring philosopher in the 1860s, du Prel had embraced Schopenhauer and the antimaterialist cause, then came to the Psychologische Gesellschaft in 1886 as an established public intellectual. In contrast, when Schrenck-Notzing joined the group in 1886, he was a young doctor who still had his reputation to make. And make it he did, by introducing to Germany recent French work on the therapeutic uses of hypnosis associated with the doctors J. M. Charcot, at the Salpêtrière Hospital in Paris, and Hippolyte Bernheim, in Nancy. Charcot had begun to use hypnosis on hysterical patients in 1878; a few years later, in 1882, the French Academy of Sciences accepted Charcot's paper linking hypnosis to hysteria, thereby giving hypnosis its first official scientific recognition on the Continent. At the same time, another group of French investigators under the direction of Bernheim had begun to experiment with hypnosis for the treatment of various organic diseases. As international interest in this French work grew, German psychiatrists ignored or resisted it, largely because they still associated hypnotism negatively with animal magnetism and Naturphilosophie.[34] As a major exception to this trend, psychical research circles remained open to the French work and thus attracted Germans eager to experiment with the novel therapeutic tool. This was as true for Schrenck-Notzing in Munich as it was for two other pioneers of therapeutic hypnotism in Berlin, the psychiatrist Albert Moll and the philosopher Max Dessoir, who joined forces in 1889 to found Berlin's first psychical research group, the Gesellschaft für Experimentalpsychologie.[35] Schrenck-Notzing's participation in the Psychologische Gesellschaft of Munich made sense only against this background, for it was one of the very few German venues in the 1880s where he could have gone to pursue his passion for hypnosis.[36]

If Schrenck-Notzing came to the Psychologische Gesellschaft to experiment with hypnosis, what he found in du Prel was a mentor able to introduce him to an entire realm of psychological phenomena with which neither German psychiatry nor psychology wanted to engage. In the preceding decades, this mainstream aversion to the "night-life of the soul" had had as its positive counterpart the elaboration of a more materialist psychology, known as "physiological psychology" or "psychophysics." Building on Fechner's classic 1860 text *Elements of Psychophysics,* this materialist approach had yielded a plethora of theoretical insights, experimental discoveries, and institutional innovations, including Wilhelm Wundt's founding of Germany's first institute for experimental psychology in 1879.[37] For Wundt and other prominent practitioners of this new science, physiological psychology applied only to the study of psychological phenomena with a material basis, including reaction time, attention span, and sensation. Thought and other higher-order mental phenomena, they insisted, should remain beyond the scope of experimental investigation. Clearly, the success of physiological psychology had come at the cost of sidelining phenomena not readily assimilable to the materialist model. In this context, what du Prel did for the young doctor Schrenck-Notzing was to pose dream, trance, and a multitude of occult and mystical phenomena as scientifically significant and worthy of experimental study.

As quickly became apparent, however, Schrenck-Notzing and du Prel had very different agendas for psychical research. For one thing, materialism did not exercise Schrenck-Notzing to the degree it did du Prel. Schrenck-Notzing realized, of course, that the admission of higher-order psychological phenomena to the realm of scientific investigation required the passing of materialism. But he had no interest in making these phenomena the basis for a new worldview. Instead, he added his voice to a rising international chorus of psychiatrists and psychologists who were insisting in the 1880s and 1890s that the scope of experimental psychology had to be broadened beyond physiological psychology. In yet another departure from his mentor's outlook, Schrenck-Notzing explicitly rejected du Prel's hypothesis that occult phenomena originated with transcendent personalities. Instead, he spoke of his own interpretation of occult phenomena more tentatively, insisting that too little was known for researchers to offer any definitive explanations. He recommended that others follow his lead in taking a "psychodynamical" approach and a "purely observational attitude."[38] Finally, whereas du Prel had always pitched transcendent psychology as the solution to Germany's spiritual crisis, Schrenck-Notzing maintained a more narrow focus on the therapeutic potential of psychical research for individual patients. And it was on this score that his professional peers praised him, especially for his clinical innovations in the treatment of sexual dysfunction and neurasthenia.[39] The sexologist Iwan Bloch, for instance, credited Schrenck-Notzing as "the founder of modern sexual science," and the psychologist Willy Hellpach recognized the crucial influence that Schrenck-Notzing's theory on the etiology of homosexuality had had on German scientific psychiatry.[40]

Despite the differences that eventually pushed them apart, the coming together of du Prel and Schrenck-Notzing under the umbrella of the Psychologische Gesellschaft of Munich from 1886 to 1889 was an important chapter in both the history of the mind/brain sciences and the emergence of the modern German occult movement. Indeed, although historians have been strangely reluctant to examine these two developments together, there is much evidence to suggest that no history of German psychology will be complete without such an examination.[41] One line of support for this view comes from the fact that physiological psychology was never as far away from the occult sciences as its proponents would have liked. Fechner had originated the psychophysical laws underpinning physiological psychology, it was true, but Fechner himself had never truly been a pure materialist, and his willingness to cautiously endorse Zöllner's sittings with Slade reflected this fact. Wundt, to take another prominent example, had procured his influential post at Leipzig in 1875 only with the help of Zöllner, whose interest in Wundt and physiological psychology was inseparable from his growing excitement about spiritualist mediums. Yet another line of support for the view that a complete history of late-nineteenth-century German psychology will need to include an examination of the occult sciences can be found by exploring the many points of contact between du Prel, Schrenck-Notzing, and the gathering international movement to found a "new" psychology that emerged among scientific investigators of the psyche in the last decade or so of the nineteenth century.

From the perspective of the occult sciences, this reorientation received a very visible marker when the philosopher Max Dessoir coined the term *parapsychology* in 1889. The occasion for Dessoir's innovation had been yet another acrid debate over materialism that broke out in March, when the editors of *Sphinx* republished an essay by Ludwig Brunn entitled "The Prophet." Brunn's essay had cataloged as irrational a variety of common beliefs, including faith in God and the eternal existence of the soul, and located their appeal in the pathological brain states of saints, mystics, and seers who mistook their hallucinations for proof of a spiritual reality outside of themselves.[42] The editors followed Brunn's essay with a strongly worded reply, presumably written by or with the knowledge of du Prel, who was one of the main forces behind *Sphinx* at the time. Appropriately titled "The Curse of the Times," the editorial dismissed Brunn as a crass materialist and accused him and all other materialists of being responsible for the "bestiality" of the era.[43] This exchange then prompted the philosopher Max Dessoir three months later to publish a carefully worded rejoinder to both sides. To the editors, Dessoir observed mildly that theoretical discussions rarely had much of an influence on the masses. He suggested to Brunn that it was too hasty to lump visions and other such phenomena under the heading of mental illness. Might it not be more fruitful, Dessoir asked, to consider these phenomena as part of an "as yet unrecognized border zone between normal and abnormal [or] pathological states" of mind? The advantage of such an approach, he pointed out, would be to allow investigators more open-mindedness in exploring strange psychological phenomena manifested by otherwise psychologically average individuals. As a more felicitous term, Dessoir proposed *parapsychology* to designate the science of phenomena that "go beyond the everyday [but nonetheless] come out of the normal course of the life of the psyche."[44]

Schrenck-Notzing soon emerged as a leading investigator of this psychological borderzone, and his parapsychological activities quickly became allied to the international emergence of the new—and less exclusively materialist—experimental psychology associated with names like Charcot and William James. When the first International Congress of Physiological Psychology met under the presidency of Charcot in August 1889, for instance, Schrenck-Notzing and his parapsychological interests played a prominent role. A watershed in the history of experimental psychology, the congress focused on five topics: "Muscular Sense . . . Heredity . . . Hypnotism . . . an international census of Hallucinations on lines proposed by the English Society for Psychical Research . . . [and] Abnormal Association of Sensations [such as] 'coloured hearing.' " The mysterious psychological phenomena then being investigated in psychical research circles around the globe—including automatic writing, hypnotic suggestion, and the influence of magnets—provoked particularly intense interest and debate, and a committee including Schrenck-Notzing and James, the American philosopher who had been conducting experiments with the Boston medium Mrs. Piper since 1886, was formed to begin work on a "statistical study of hallucinations."

The roster of four hundred or so at the congress read as a virtual who's who of the new experimental psychology. In addition to Schrenck-Notzing, Charcot, and James, the list included the psychiatrists Bernheim and Alfred Binet, the physiologist Charles Richet, and the philosopher Pierre Janet, all from France. Also present were the Swiss psychiatrist Auguste Forel; the Belgian physician Joseph Delbouef; the eugenicist Francis Galton, the psychical researcher Frederic W. H. Myers, the Cambridge philosopher Henry Sidgwick and his wife Eleanor Balfour, a mathematician and sister of the prime minister, all from Britain; the American psychologist Hugo von Münsterberg; the German philosopher Max Dessoir; and the prominent Italian anthropologist and criminologist Cesare Lombroso. On the final night of the congress, this stellar cast ended up on the viewing platform of the Eiffel Tower, where they celebrated their many achievements, not least of which was the establishment of a congress to be named the International Congress of Experimental Psychology, which met under that name in 1892.[45]

Experimental psychology quickly emerged as the umbrella term under which many of these same names, including Schrenck-Notzing's, appeared together over and over again in the following years. Reflecting back on the most exciting scientific developments of the decade during his presidential address to the British Association for the Advancement of Science in 1898, for instance, the chemist William Crookes noted the close links between psychical research and new trends in psychology with approval. Long involved in psychical research circles (he had been a key contact for Zöllner in the Leipzig experiments with Slade), Crookes defended his interests by noting that "to ignore the subject would be an act of cowardice. . . . To stop short in any research that bids fair to widen the gates of knowledge, to recoil from fear of difficulty or adverse criticism, is to bring reproach on science." Lauding the studies of James, Richet,

Binet, Freud and his collaborator Josef Breuer, Bernheim and his collaborator Auguste Ambroise Liébeault, Schrenck-Notzing, Forel, and others, Crookes urged all the association members to support the new "Experimental Psychology."[46] This overlap between psychical research and the new experimental psychology also manifested itself in the membership list of the British Society for Psychical Research, which had been founded in 1882. By century's end, the group's impressive roster of corresponding members included Dessoir, Myers, the Sidgwicks, Liébault, Bernheim, Janet, Richet, Lombroso, Schrenck-Notzing, Théodore Flournoy, G. Stanley Hall, James, Morton Prince, and Freud.[47]

This recycling of the same names through the 1890s under the umbrella of experimental psychology was no accident: most of the named figures shared a common goal of bringing scientific rigor to the study of the human unconscious. Particularly salient in this regard were the many points of contact between psychoanalysis, psychical research, and parapsychology. Freud, like most of the scientifically trained psychiatrists of his generation, had initially regarded psychology (still considered a branch of philosophy) with suspicion. It was therefore highly significant that his 1899 masterpiece *The Interpretation of Dreams* contained many references to du Prel's philosophical works and that a 1914 edition included a special footnote praising du Prel as a "brilliant mystic" who had recognized that "the gateway to metaphysics, so far as men are concerned, lies not in waking life but in the dream."[48] Significant for a similar reason was Freud's homage to the philosopher Theodor Lipps—a professor at the University of Munich and chair of Schrenck-Notzing's Psychologische Gesellschaft at the turn of the century—as "the best mind among the present-day philosophical writers."[49]

The cautious sympathy between Freud and German occult circles also flowed in the other direction. Freud's *Interpretation of Dreams,* for instance, received its most sympathetic professional response in Germany from psychical researchers.[50] Among most German scientists and doctors, in contrast, Freud's masterpiece aroused little comment. Here again, hypnosis and its negative association with Naturphilosophie were to blame, for those who ignored Freud did so because they knew he had once used hypnosis therapeutically; German psychiatrists and philosophers, on the other hand, favorably disposed to the scientific elucidation of occult phenomena, were also precisely those few Germans inclined to take a positive view of hypnosis and extend a warm welcome to Freud. Thus, when Freud's *Interpretation of Dreams* was first published in 1899, Moll was one of the few German doctors to recognize it as a major scientific milestone.[51] Similarly, Schrenck-Notzing noted Freud's ideas with approval in his 1902 study of the dream dancer Madeleine Guipet (see chapter 5).[52] And Dessoir, who had coined the term *parapsychology* shortly before, carried a favorable review of Freud's dream book in the 1901 volume of his avant-garde periodical *Die Lotse,* alongside pieces by such modernist icons as Lou Andreas-Salomé, Rainer Maria Rilke, Georg Simmel, and Ferdinand Tönnies.[53]

Nor was Freud's relation to the occult limited to mere sympathy. Although he and his handlers kept it a closely guarded secret during his lifetime, Freud did in fact experiment actively with occult phenomena. With his colleague Sandor Ferenczi, for instance, Freud visited a clairvoyant in Berlin in 1909. He also treated several patients who had previously consulted occult seers for their psychological ailments. And in 1913 Freud sponsored a séance in his own home, along with three other psychoanalysts. Although he found the results unsatisfactory, he could not bring himself to reject occult phenomena as wholly fraudulent, an ambivalence he never made public. Freud's fascination with the occult finally emerged to public view after he died, when a 1921 essay taking a favorable view of telepathy surfaced among his papers and was published in 1941.[54]

Jung, for a time Freud's heir-apparent, had fewer scruples about divulging his fascination with the occult. His involvement had begun with the séances that became the focus of his 1902 Ph.D. thesis and had persisted throughout his long life. In 1919, for instance, Jung spoke at the British Society for Psychical Research about spirit phenomena. Taking the psychological point of view, he observed: "I must regard this whole territory as an appendix of psychology . . . [spirits must be] either pathological fantasies or new but as yet unknown ideas." Jung also knew Schrenck-Notzing personally. In Zurich in 1925 he and his old mentor Eugen Bleuler had attended a series of séances staged by the venerable parapsychologist and his medium Rudi Schneider.[55]

There were even links between Schrenck-Notzing's occult circle and the new philosophical movement of phenomenology that emerged under the leadership of Edmund Husserl after 1900. These came via Theodor Lipps, who collaborated with Schrenck-Notzing at the Psychologische Gesellschaft, circa 1900, while simultaneously training several students who went on to become denizens of phenomenology just a few years later. These students included Alexander Pfänder and Max Scheler, both of whom moved to Göttingen in

1905 to pursue study with Husserl. Once Pfänder returned as a professor to the University of Munich, the links between phenomenology and parapsychology persisted. Perhaps the most visible manifestation of this connection was Gerda Walther, who belonged to the loose circle of "Munich Phenomenologists" gathered around Pfänder and who had long collaborated with Schrenck-Notzing in his parapscyhological researches.[56]

Transcendent Lifestyles

While Schrenck-Notzing and his parapsychological interests wound their way to the heart of the new sciences of the mind, du Prel's project of transcendent psychology underwent its own transformation and soon emerged as a core part of the popular occult movement. The project had begun as an attempt to articulate a new science that took proper account of the "night-life of the soul." Du Prel had hoped that transcendent psychology would cater to modern-minded Germans who embraced the culture of scientific progress but nonetheless bemoaned its silence on pressing spiritual questions. Wherein did human life originate? To what ends did it tend? Although the natural sciences as yet offered no answers to these questions, du Prel promised, the new science of transcendent psychology could. It would incorporate modern scientific insights and discoveries but subordinate them to human spiritual needs. Du Prel's dream of marrying scientific method to human ethical development became a core theme of the German occult movement from the 1890s onwards.[57]

The ambivalence embedded in this view of a world in which scientific progress and spiritual loss went hand in hand had a definite modernist inflection. As the literary historian Marshall Berman has noted:

> Modernists . . . are at once at home in this world and at odds with it. They celebrate and identify with the triumphs of modern science, art, technology, economics, politics: with all the activities that enable mankind to do what the Bible said only God could do: to "make all things new." At the same time, however, they deplore modernization's betrayal of its own human promise. Modernists demand deeper and more radical renewals: modern men and women must become the subjects as well as the objects of modernization; they must learn to change the world that is changing them, and to make it their own.[58]

This dialectic of feeling like modernity's pawn yet desiring to become modernity's master describes the basic dynamic pushing du Prel and his co-workers to embrace the occult sciences. They were enthusiasts of modern science, yet anxious about the implications of the scientific enterprise—a cornerstone of German modernity—for human values. Bemoaning a world from which God, divine purpose, and religious meaning had fled, they sought not to return to a Christian past but rather to move forward into a future respiritualized on a scientific basis.

Du Prel and his followers were by no means alone in their ambivalence about fin-de-siècle modernity. Indeed, to grasp the place of the popular occult movement within the larger field of Wilhelmine cultural and political innovation, it is crucial to realize that attempts to theorize and practice what historians have begun to call "alternative modernities" were widespread in fin-de-siècle Germany. Adherents of "cultural Protestantism" *(Kulturprotestantismus)*, for instance, sought to bridge Christian tradition to modern scientific culture and liberal politics under the leadership of such left-leaning intellectuals as the philosopher Ernst Troeltsch, the theologian Adolf Harnack, and the sociologist Max Weber.[59] "Antipolitics" constituted a second fin-de-siècle social-reform movement. Associated with the political reformers Adolf Damaschke and Gertrud Bäumer, the economist Werner Sombart, and others, antipolitics sought to address the "social question" by using scientific research and planning to manage socioeconomic problems rationally before they could fester and become politically divisive.[60] Yet another reform movement dedicated to offsetting the negative effects of fin-de-siècle modernity was the politically multivalent *Zivilisationskritik,* or " critique of civilization." Proponents included the industrialist Walter Rathenau and the philosopher Ludwig Klages, both of whom castigated the new industrial capitalism for promoting a form of technological growth that degraded both the environment and the individual. Before 1914, they proposed solutions spanning everything from rehumanizing technology to reharmonizing humans' relation to nature through diet, clothing, and medical reform *(Lebensreform).*[61]

If the popular occult movement belonged to this larger spectrum of German attempts to elaborate "alternative modernities," it also had one distinctive feature. This was its embrace of a primarily *psychological* solution to the problems of modernity, an orientation it shared with all other non-German occult movements of the era. As the historian of British occultism Alex Owen has noted, the vogue for occultism circa 1900 was "deeply implicated in the contemporary innovative elaboration of subjectivity."[62] Normally associated more exclusively with names like Freud, James, or Jung, this attempt nonetheless also informed the popular German occult movement. But it did so in a distinctive way. Whereas the new scientists of the mind had insisted on the possibility of coming to an objective understanding of human psychological experience, occultists began to cultivate the subjectivity of their own psychological experience as an end in itself. They continued du Prel's value-seeking and empirical orientation toward the world, but stripped his project of its scholarly pretensions to Wissenschaft. In the process, they transformed the occult movement into a virtual cult of self-development and individual experience. In direct contrast to du Prel, occultists in the fin-de-siècle mode quested less after scientific knowledge than after a most-private wisdom and cultivated not experiment but rather a self-focused empiricism in which "occult arts" took center stage. By 1900 or so, they had created a truly transcendent lifestyle.

This shift from du Prel's rather scholarly project of building a transcendent worldview to the more populist elaboration of a transcendent lifestyle was clearly visible in the contrast between two major popular occult journals: *Sphinx,* which appeared from 1886 to 1896, and its successor *[Neue] Metaphysische Rundschau* ([New] metaphysical review), which published from 1896 onward. Under the editorial leadership of du Prel and Hübbe-Schleiden, *Sphinx* carried short articles on telepathy, hypnotism, magnetism, astrology, and magic, supplemented by essays exploring the cultural implications of these phenomena by well-respected authors like the biologist Alfred Russel Wallace, the anthropologist Adolf Bastian, and the philosopher Eduard von Hartmann.[63] The rationale for this mixture of technical and cultural articles was embodied in the journal's subtitle, which stated that *Sphinx* was "a monthly journal for the historical and experimental foundation of a transcendent worldview on a monistic basis," thus emphasizing the goal of "monistically" integrating matter and spirit, body and mind, into a scientifically ("historically" and "experimentally") grounded worldview appropriate to the modern age.[64]

A decade later, when *Sphinx* ceased publication and was superseded by *Metaphysische Rundschau* under the editorship of Paul Zillmann, the orientation of the popular occult movement had clearly shifted. Whereas du Prel and Hübbe-Schleiden had always stressed the scientific and scholarly underpinnings of the transcendent worldview and had indeed avoided using the word *occult* in the subtitle, Zillmann took a more populist approach. He made no bones, for instance, about the explicitly occult focus of his journal, subtitling it as a "monthly journal for the study of practical metaphysics, psychology, oriental philosophy, and general occultism."[65] With no pretensions about catering to an exclusively educated audience, he carried a jumble of articles and reports whose tone spanned everything from the scholarly to the sensationalist. Breathless reports on mediumism, astrology, Rosicrucianism, Theosophy, rays, phrenology, and yoga sat side by side with more serious pieces by Theodor Lipps and Carl du Prel. There were also diverse contributions from international authors, including the Austrian Ariosophical theorist Guido von List, the Russian-born Theosophical leader H. P. Blavatsky, and the British astrologer Alan Leo.[66] Supplementing these were bulletins on Nietzsche's deteriorating mental condition, a notice on an upcoming Zionist congress, obituaries for contemporary alchemists, and reports on recent scientific discoveries as diverse as the sighting of lights on Mars and a Düsseldorf magnetist's successful treatment of a case of eczema.[67] Portraits bundled with the periodical from the fifth volume onward pictured a diverse pantheon of heroes and heroines. Blavatsky, du Prel, Hoffmann, Cagliostro, Nietzsche, Davis, Schopenhauer, John Ruskin, Swami Vivekananda Ramakrishna Paramahamsa, Mary Baker Eddy, Justinus Kerner, Goethe, Mesmer, Richard Wagner, Guido von List, Leo Tolstoi, Friedrich Schelling, August Strindberg, Charles Darwin, and Helen Keller all had their turn in the metaphysical spotlight.[68]

This highly eclectic mixture of articles, news, and visual material had as its rationale the journal's purpose to bring "metaphysical research"—that is, the occult sciences—to wide public attention. Echoing the original goals of *Sphinx*, Zillmann noted that metaphysical research would challenge the materialist inclinations of modern science, medicine, and philosophy while at the same time promote the construction of a new worldview uniting science and religion on an empirical foundation.[69] But this statement lacked the emotional fervor that had once informed the pronouncements of du Prel and his followers. As the wider cultural context changed and materialism no longer loomed as large as it had a decade earlier, Zillmann became free to do what du Prel and his co-workers had not: to turn the transcendent worldview into a practical reality by actively promoting a new lifestyle that would lead individuals to self-knowledge and self-realization via occult means. Personal experience open to all now became the clarion call of the popular occult movement. As a 1907 statement of purpose for *Neue Metaphysische Rundschau* proclaimed, "We conduct cultural activities in which everyone can and should take part!"[70]

Zillmann himself embodied the populist and experiential occultism that characterized the transcendent lifestyle. A "professional" magnetist, he founded the Wald Loge (Theosophical forest lodge) in 1896 with the express goal of transforming ordinary individuals into powerful occultists. In an 1898 series of articles entitled "Letters on Mysticism to a Friend," Zillmann detailed the philosophy and activities of the lodge. Emphasizing the subjective element in occult practice, he defined occultists as people who, through developing the fullest possible command of their physical and mental powers, approached the ideal of human perfection or divinity.

In order to clarify what this meant more concretely, Zillmann highlighted the unique features of the occult sciences: "The occult sciences are not just unknown science but above all teach how the individual can strengthen the power of his soul and thereby penetrate regions that would otherwise be closed to him. . . . The occult sciences teach us to use our whole being. . . . Therefore, they deploy a method that is foreign to the other sciences. . . . From the occult sciences you can expect nothing less than the empowerment [*Potenzierung*] of your soul." Marking the occult as "science" yet also demarcating it from "the other sciences," Zillmann stressed the subjective yet scientific character of occult practice. At the lodge, he explained, members would come to know that "the goal is the full development of your soul, that is your self, for you are your soul." Aspiring occultists would learn to keep their thoughts pure, eat in moderation, avoid alcohol, caffeine, and tobacco, and spend time out in nature and the fresh air. As they learned to care for their physical bodies, they would also learn to develop their spiritual selves. By such means, they would eventually gain access to the transcendent world closed off to those perceptually limited to their five senses. They would, in other words, become true occultists.[71]

Zillmann's esoteric brand of occult self-enlightenment was not the only course open to those seeking a transcendent lifestyle. E. Honold, a spiritualist living in fin-de-siècle Berlin, pursued a different route. Her path to spiritualism began with a vision in which she confronted a white form bearing a cross on his right shoulder. When a sudden death in the family occurred four days later, Honold realized that the vision had been a premonition. At this point, she recalled: "[M]y life [took] an entirely new direction, I was drawn by a perfectly magical power to spiritualism. I was extremely unhappy, totally derailed from my life's path. Death had with one blow destroyed all my hopes. Only one thought remained alive in me: if possible, to put myself in contact with the dead. As many other lay people in this situation do, I went here and there but found satisfaction nowhere."

Honold's quest for satisfaction propelled her into Berlin's world of the occult, where she began to attend séances and develop her latent powers as a medium. Once she succeeded in contacting the deceased, her mediumship rapidly spread into other areas. To her surprise, she proved so adept as a trance healer that she and her family ceased going to the doctor. She learned to make art, write poetry, and sing religious music while in a trance. With her sister, now also a devoted spiritualist, she began to do an hour or so of daily trance dance. Describing the experience, Honold wrote: "There was a force pushing as if from the inside out that initially alarmed us, since the dancing was often so peculiar, the movement sometimes so perfectly strange and unexpected that we thought there was no longer a floor under our feet, and in anxiety we screamed aloud!" Terrifying as these spirited bouts of dancing were initially, the family soon learned to take them in stride, reassured that none of these trance activities interfered with the normal functioning of the household. As Honold herself recalled, she had once spent three days speaking only in verse without ceasing to perform the necessary household tasks.[72] Here was a woman little concerned with du Prel's original philosophical project but much invested in integrating her occult unconscious into everyday existence. Whether in the form of Jung's "objective facts about the human psyche" or the paeans to subjectivity voiced by Zillmann and Honold, by the turn of the century the "psychological point of view" had clearly emerged, and it had done so with half a century of crucial input from the occult sciences.

CHAPTER THREE

The Occult Public

The term *occult* derives from the Latin verb *occulere,* meaning to hide, or conceal. It is somewhat ironic, therefore, that although Germans were certainly fascinated by forces concealed from human sight or reason, there was nothing particularly hidden about the German occult movement itself. As the Zöllner episode demonstrated, indeed, occult topics could be very much in the public eye. And this was so not just because occultists and their critics engaged in heated debates on the pages of Germany's national newspapers. The fact was that occultists, even those who practiced a most esoteric form of occultism, lived in a modern society whose well-developed public realm left its mark on their endeavors.[1] Participants traveled by train to their occult congresses, communicated by phone about their clairvoyant experiences, and sold horoscopes on busy city streets (see fig. 2). Many went to specialized bookstores to buy texts that could teach them about modern occultism; others borrowed such material from public libraries set up by occult circles. Occultists mounted public exhibitions, established specialized journals available to anyone who could pay, and printed inexpensive editions of occult texts. German occultism, in short, was very much a public enterprise.

Previous chapters have questioned why Germans found modern occultism so appealing. This chapter examines where and how occultism spread, first by exploring the character of the occult public—its size and geographical diffusion, as well as its social and political composition—and then by examining the key mechanisms diffusing the occult into German culture. The sociological picture that emerges from this analysis suggests that the occult became the core of a mass movement in Germany not just because individual men and women found it efficacious but also because it adapted itself very quickly to the exigencies of modern consumer culture.

A Mass Movement

One sign of the occult movement's mass character was its size and geographical spread. Outside observers put the absolute number of Germans involved in some capacity in the occult movement in the tens of thousands. Theodor Traub, a Protestant minister who led a widely publicized attempt to unmask the medium Anna Rothe at the turn of the century, estimated that Berlin had at least six hundred mediums working in 1900.[2] Rothe, whose fame garnered her what were probably very large crowds for a mediumistic performance, reportedly drew one thousand people to one of the séances she staged for a meeting of a Berlin Theosophical club in 1901.[3] At the height of the Rothe scandal in 1902, a local newspaper stated that Berlin alone contained ten thousand spiritualists, four hundred mediums, and between fifteen and twenty spiritualist clubs.[4] Observers identified Munich, too, as a hotbed of occultism. A representative of the Roman Catholic Church there noted with concern in 1923 that in Munich alone more than ten thousand families had reportedly held séances.[5] Reports that hundreds of people flocked to occult groups also came in from Germany's smaller cities. A representative of a Protestant church in Chemnitz estimated that the local branch of the Gottesbund Tanatra (Tanatra association of God), an international group mixing spiritualist and Christian teachings, had 150 members.[6] Even well into the late 1930s, newspapers continued to report significant popular interest in occultism.

Another way to gauge the size and geographical spread of the German occult movement is to examine the evidence regarding the network of occult associations (summarized in table 3.1 and cataloged more fully in appendix A). More than two hundred clubs devoted to a wide variety of occult pursuits flourished from the last third of the nineteenth century until 1937, when the

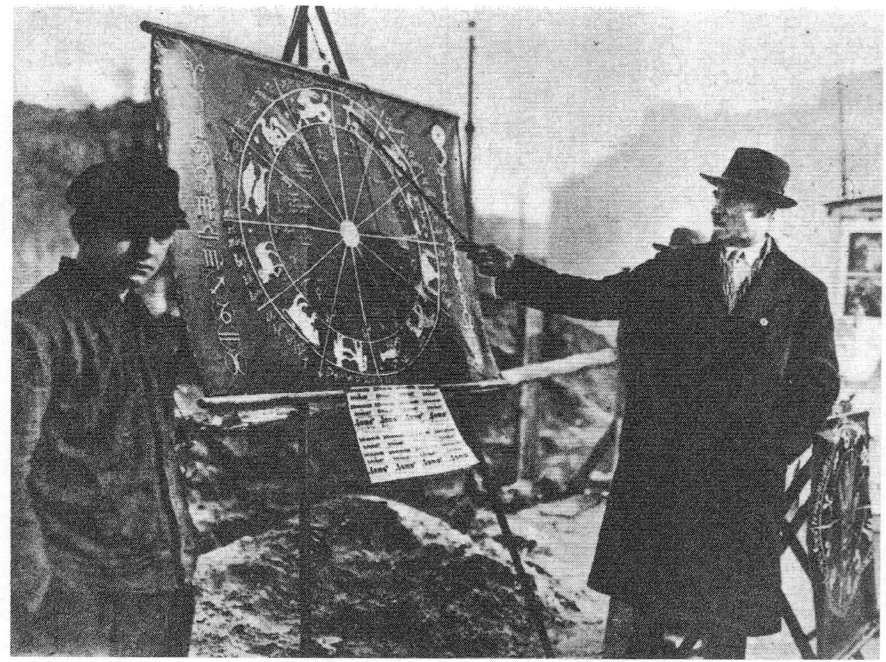

Figure 2. An enterprising astrologer casts horoscopes for customers on a busy city street. *Die Woche* 34 (24 September 1932): 1164.

Nazi regime officially banned all occult groups. Berlin and Munich together accounted for nearly eighty of these, with other large cities (e.g., Hamburg and Leipzig) housing ten or more each. Urban centers such as these proved hotbeds of occultism not just because of their educated and bohemian populations but also because their infrastructure allowed the curious masses ease of access to occult events. In Munich, for instance, lecturers often appeared in public places: local drinking establishments, train stations, and hotels. The writer Max Kemmerich spoke about astrology and its implications for human freedom to a meeting of the Uranus Gesellschaft für astrologische Forschung (Society for astrological research Uranus) in 1927 in the big hall of the Kreuzbräu.[7] Similarly, meetings of the Gesellschaft für psychische Forschung (Society for psychical research) and the Astrologische Gesellschaft (Astrological society) always drew a crowd to the restaurant at the Holzkirchener train station.[8]

Although table 3.1 might prompt the conclusion that modern occultism was

Table 3.1. Occult Clubs, 1869–1937

City	Total by City	Ariosophy	Astrology, Dowsing, Graphology, Palmistry, Pendulum	Occultism	Psychical Research, Parapsychology	Spiritualism, Magnetism, Mesmerism	Theosophy
Bad Schmiedeberg	2		1				1
Berlin	52	1	7	11	7	14	12
Breslau	4				2	1	1
Cologne	3			1	1	1	
Dresden	6			1	1		4
Düsseldorf	8	1		2	1	1	3
Frankfurt	3			1		1	1
Hamburg	13	1		4	1	4	3
Hannover	9		1			3	5
Leipzig	15		1	6		5	3
Munich	27		6	6	6	3	6
Stuttgart	4	2			1		1
Other	63	4	4	9		24	22
Total	209	9	20	41	20	57	62

Note: This table does not include the national umbrella groups, of which there were seventeen. One was devoted to Ariosophy, one to astrology, two to occultism, five to spiritualism, and eight to Theosophy. This table also excludes clubs dedicated to combating occultism, of which there were three. See Appendix A for a full list of occult clubs.

primarily a metropolitan phenomenon, a glance at appendix A will convince readers that such was not the case. Spiritualist circles flourished not just in Berlin and Munich but also in smaller towns. Oldenburg, Kunzendorf and Waldenburg (both in Silesia), and Limbach, Glauchau, and Mülsen St. Niklas (all in Saxony) had spiritualist clubs by 1900. In addition, an entire group of colonies incorporating occult beliefs and practices sprang up after the turn of the century, providing a rural retreat and, for some, a permanent home away from the bustle of the city. Most famous among these was Monte Verità, near Ascona in Switzerland, which had close ties to Munich's Schwabing subculture in the years before World War I. Other rural retreats flourished in the years after the war, including the Theosophically tinged Jungborn sanitarium in the Harz mountains.[9] The occult, in short, had an established presence in late-nineteenth- and early-twentieth-century Germany, representing a constant feature in the network of German voluntary organizations and enjoying a wide geographical spread.

Yet another sign of the occult movement's mass character was that it attracted Germans of widely divergent backgrounds, from the lowest to the highest echelons of the class hierarchy. A good proletarian representative was Joseph Weissenberg, who adroitly traded his occult talents to achieve both leadership and wealth. The son of day laborers in the small Silesian town of Fehebeutel, Weissenberg went to Berlin, where by 1907 he established a practice as a magnetist in a working-class slum. By 1926 he had become the leader of Friedensstadt, a spiritualist settlement that counted thousands of members, among them men and women from middle-class and aristocratic backgrounds.[10] Weissenberg was not alone in using his occult gifts to lift his class profile: the Viennese-born clairvoyant Erik Jan Hanussen (pseudonym of Hermann Steinschneider), who earned a good income as an occult lecturer and performer in Weimar Germany, was the son of poor traveling actors. His fame earned him the wrath of the Nazi regime, which murdered him in 1933, and the attention of the director István Szabó, who in 1989 produced a film about Hanussen's life.[11] Less famous Germans of proletarian background also embraced the occult. The writer Carl Zuckmayer, in fact, recalled a Westphalian miner who had been his comrade in the trenches of World War I. A dedicated spiritualist, this miner died on the front lines, but his wife continued to use spiritualist means to communicate with him as she struggled to make ends meet on the home front.[12]

Men and women of petty bourgeois origins also embraced the occult with enthusiasm. A case in point, Adolbert Haugg, was a postal worker turned "private scholar" who ran his own spiritualist club in Munich during World War I. The Verein Freibund, as it was called, met in local beer halls or hotels and featured Haugg's lectures and demonstrations on "the will." Typically drawing audiences of a few dozen people, these meetings often showcased one of the female audience members acting as a medium, while Haugg served as the hypnotist.[13] A policeman who attended a club meeting at a local hotel in 1917 noted that of the twenty-seven people present, sixteen were women. That evening, the audience listened to a lecture on the history of hypnotism by Haugg, then watched as he hypnotized a volunteer named Maria Schießl, a housewife married to a carter. To the amazement and delight of his audience, Haugg successfully took away Schießl's ability to count higher than five.[14]

Although Haugg did not seek to make a living by occult means, other Germans of his class background did. The Bavarian medium Claire Reichart, the daughter of a tailor, had worked as a salesgirl in her hometown of Hattenhofen, come to Munich as a dancer, and then set herself up as a fee-charging clairvoyant during the Weimar years.[15] Not all petty bourgeois mediums were women—a fact that did not escape notice by the state. In 1924, the Munich police department claimed to know of three hundred fortune-tellers working in the city, most of whom seemed to be either young women from the *Berufsklassen* (former waitresses, widows, and wives of civil servants) or men previously active as tailors and shoemakers.[16] This observation linking mediumship with class rather than merely the sex of the practitioners reflected a larger reality: men of petty bourgeois background (in marked contrast to their brothers from the higher classes) often worked as mediums. Rudi Schneider, who achieved fame as the investigative subject of Schrenck-Notzing's materialization experiments in the 1920s, was a good example of this pattern. Born into a lowly typesetter's family in a small Austrian town, in exchange for his mediumistic services to Schrenck-Notzing he was given training as a mechanic, which allowed him to achieve an independent economic existence in the big city.[17]

While proletarian and petty bourgeois Germans clustered heavily in spiritualist circles, the propertied and educated middle classes maintained a significant presence in a variety of occult sectors and dominated psychical research and Theosophy. As table 3.2 demonstrates, members in three key early psychical research and Theosophical clubs were drawn heavily from the bourgeois professions of law, medicine, business, and journalism. One sector of Germany's growing professional population noticeably absent from early occult circles was the academic professoriat. There were exceptions (among them Max Dessoir, a professor of philosophy at the University of Berlin and a founding member of Berlin's Gesellschaft für Experimentalpsychologie, and Theodor Lipps, a professor of philosophy at the University of Munich and the president of Munich's Psychologische Gesellschaft at the turn of the century), but this remained the case until the 1920s. Then, as a result of changes in academic psychology and philosophy (not least because of the work done in these fields outside of university circles), professors began to appear as members of occult groups and as authors or editors of occult publications. In 1927, for example, the Deutsche Kulturgemeinschaft zur Pflege der Astrologie (German cultural association for the promotion of astrology) counted among its members three professors: the University of Munich paleontologist Edgar Dacqué and the philosophers Johannes Maria Verweyen, of the University of Bonn, and Theodor Lessing, of the Technical University in Hannover.[18]

Table 3.2. Male Professionalism in Three Early Occult Clubs, 1884–1888

Group	Member	Occupation
Theosophische Societät Germania (Elberfeld, 1884)[1]	Gustav Gebhard	Business; cofounder Deutsche Bank
	Franz Gebhard	Business; private scholar
	C. W. Sellin	Education; Gymnasium teacher
	Wilhelm Hübbe-Schleiden	Law and international business; former colonial activist
	Ernst von Weber	Antivivisectionist; former colonial activist[2]
	Gabriel von Max	Fine arts; painter
	Carl du Prel	Philosopher (independent)
	Franz Hartmann	Medicine; physician and adventurer
	Bernhard Hubo	Business
	Hermann Urban	Medicine
	Franz Urban	Army officer
	Adolf von Spreti	Landowner; army officer
Psychologische Gesellschaft (Munich, 1886)[3]	Carl du Prel	Philosopher (independent)
	Albert von Schrenck-Notzing	Medicine; psychiatrist, hypnotist, parapsychologist
	Adolf Bayersdorfer	Art history; curator Alte Pinakothek (Munich)
	Albert von Keller	Fine arts; painter
	Gabriel von Max	Fine arts; painter
	Wilhelm Trübner	Fine arts; painter
	Alfred Mensi von Klarbach	Writer
Gesellschaft für Experimentalpsychologie (Berlin, 1888)[4]	Göler von Ravensburg	Art history; assistant director Nationalgalerie (Berlin) and lecturer at the Royal School of Art (Berlin)
	Albrecht W. Sellin	Farming; colonial activist
	Hans von Manteuffel	Police administration; eventually police commissioner of Berlin
	Hans Natge	Journalism
	Otto von Leixner	Writer; coeditor naturalist periodical *Gegenwart*[5]
	Julius Stinde	Writer
	Georg Voß	Art history
	Diederich Hahn	Banking; registrar at the Deutsche Bank; cofounder Verein Deutscher Studenten; member of German Reichstag[6]
	Karl Oswald Konstantin von Uechtritz-Steinkirch	Law; judge at Kammergericht (Berlin); member of Prussian parliament and German Reichstag[7]

Table 3.2. Continued

Group	Member	Occupation
	Max Dessoir	Student of medicine and philosophy; eventually professor of philosophy at the University of Berlin; editor *Zeitschrift für Ästhetik und allgemeine Kunstwissenschaft* (1906–)
	Albert Moll	Psychiatrist, hypnotist, and sexual reformer; prominent member Bund für Mutterschutz[8]

1. "Mitglieder Verzeichnis," Cod WH-S 812:2,1. Biographical information on most of these men can be found in Norbert Klatt, *Der Nachlaß von Wilhelm Hübbe-Schleiden in der Niedersächsischen Staats- und Universitätsbibliothek Göttingen* (Göttingen: Klatt, 1996).

2. Weber was the son of the composer Karl Maria von Weber. He founded the Verein zur Bekämpfung der Vivisektion (Society for the fight against vivisection) and converted Richard Wagner to the cause of anti-vivisectionism. Klaus J. Bade, *Friedrich Fabri und der Imperialismus in der Bismarckzeit. Revolution-Depression-Expansion* (Freiburg-im-Breisgaue: Atlantis Verlag, 1975), pp. 97–99. Winfried Schüler, *Der Bayreuther Kreis von seiner Entstehung bis zum Ausgang der Wilhelminischen Ära: Wagnerkult und Kulturreform im Geiste völkischer Weltanschauung* (Münster: Verlag Aschendorff, 1971), p. 145.

3. Albert von Schrenck-Notzing, "Albert von Keller als Malerpsychologe und Metapsychiker," *Psychische Studien* 48 (April–May 1921): 194–97. Rudolf Tischner, *Geschichte der okkultistischen (metaphysischen) Forschung von der Antike bis zur Gegenwart. II. Teil. Von der Mitte des 19. Jahrhunderts bis zur Gegenwart* (Pfullingen in Württemburg: Johannes Baum Verlag, 1924), pp. 224–25.

4. Albert Moll, *Ein Leben als Arzt der Seele: Erinnerungen* (Dresden: Carl Reissner Verlag, 1936), pp. 128–29. Max Dessoir, *Buch der Erinnerung*, 2nd ed. (Stuttgart: Ferdinand Enke, 1947), pp. 125–26. Dessoir contests some elements of Moll's account of the founding of this group. On minor details, both sources disagree with Klatt, *Der Nachlaß*. I have followed Klatt when such discrepancies occur.

5. "Otto Leixner (von Grünberg)," *Deutsches Literatur-Lexikon* (Bern: Francke, 1984), pp. 1192–93.

6. The Verein Deutscher Studenten was an influential nationalist student group. Hahn acted as the group's spokesperson at the 1881 celebration at the Kyffhäuser monument in Leipzig. At Deutsche Bank he worked for G. v. Siemens on the Baghdad train project. In 1893 he was elected to the Reichstag, where he remained in office, except for a four-year break in 1903–7, until 1918. "Diederich Christian Hahn," *Neue Deutsche Biographie* 7 (Berlin: Duncker & Humblot, 1965), p. 503. Hahn also served as the model for Diederich Hessling in Heinrich Mann's *Der Untertan*.

7. The Kammergericht was the highest civil court in Prussia. Biographical information comes from *Deutsches Biographisches Archiv/Neue Folge* (Munich: K. G. Saur, 1990–93).

8. Hannah S. Decker, *Freud in Germany: Revolution and Reaction in Science, 1893–1907* (New York: International University Press, 1977), p. 178. The Bund für Mutterschutz campaigned for sexual reform.

Long before university professors began to embrace the occult in significant numbers, however, bourgeois professionalism had become a marker of status in the occult milieu. One sign of this was that many occultists carrying professional titles had not earned them, but rather assumed them spontaneously. This reflected not just the performative aspects of occultism but also how "expertise" and "professional training" had become eagerly sought badges of legitimacy as Germans entered the period of high modernity. Hugo Vollrath, who acted as Franz Hartmann's secretary at the turn of the century and then went on to become a prominent Theosophical publisher, dubbed himself "Dr." Vollrath, although he had left the university without a degree.[19] Hartmann himself had practiced as a medical doctor, apparently without ever having earned the title. By the time his obituary appeared in 1912, he had also managed to assume the honorific "doctor of philosophy."[20] The trappings of professionalism were particularly sought after in the astrological and characterological sections of the occult revival, where special certification procedures, schools, and titles were set up to demarcate "scientific" astrologers and characterologists from their "amateur" competitors.[21]

Although the professional element in the German occult movement was largely male, neither maleness nor professionalism fully described the movement's bourgeois composition and character. Their names did not often appear on lists of occult authors or leaders, but nonetheless, middle-class women were present in large numbers in the occult movement. Early on, they played a key role in introducing and spreading occultism. Max Dessoir, in fact, recalled that he had begun his mediumistic forays in the company of several artistically inclined women before going on to help found the Gesellschaft für Experimental-psychologie.[22] The female membership of the Theosophische Societät Germania tells a similar story. Thirteen of the thirty-eight members were women, and one—Mary Gebhard, the oldest practitioner of Theosophy in Germany and a long-term student of modern occultism in all its forms— served as vice president.[23]

Bourgeois women also founded, led, and spoke at their own occult societies. One such woman was Hanna Vogt-Vilseck, a writer and singer who formed the spiritualist circle Die Sucher (The seekers) in Munich in 1918. Her group, which purported to combine the mental edification of its members with scientific research, featured lectures (mostly delivered by Vogt-Vilseck herself) on a wide range of topics: spiritualism, astrology, Theosophy, Anthroposophy, and even Goethe's theory of light.[24] By the late 1920s and early 1930s, female speakers appeared regularly at meetings of occult clubs. The lecture roster for the five Monday evening meetings of the Astrologische Gesellschaft München (Munich astrological society) in 1932, for instance, included two women.[25]

As audience members, women demanded—and received—presentations tailored to their interests and expertise. At a meeting of the Astrologische Gesellschaft München in 1927, one observer noted that the large audience consisted mostly of women, the majority of whom already seemed to possess a sophisticated understanding of astrology. Amazed, the reporter noted the dissonance between the women's appearance—he wrote that they looked like innocent knitters rather than Schwabing bohemians—and their astrological proficiency.[26] Similarly, a lecture delivered in Munich in 1930 by the astrologer (and lawyer) Hubert Korsch on the topic "Why Study Astrology?" drew 180 people, of whom two-thirds were women. Korsch pitched his lecture to the interests of his sexually mixed audience, stressing the importance of astrology to child rearing and getting married as well as to practicing law or medicine and choosing a profession.[27]

If bourgeois women showed up in significant majorities as audience members at many occult events, they also vastly outnumbered bourgeois men as mediums. Although it is difficult to learn much about these women as individuals, evidence that they practiced as mediums lies scattered in the texts of the German occult movement.[28] Madeleine Guipet, for instance, who first achieved fame in Munich as the "dream-dancer Madeleine G.," was the wife of a well-to-do French businessman; and the writer Hanns von Gumppenberg had his first convincing exposure to spiritualism through an unnamed woman from Munich's genteel society who had previously granted sittings to Schrenck-Notzing.[29]

As the membership lists presented in table 3.2 suggest, occult clubs also drew their membership from Germany's social upper crust. Albert von Schrenck-Notzing, for instance, was born with an aristocratic title, and his marriage to the heiress Gabriele Siegle gave him access to a large fortune and landed him on the board of directors at the chemical concern I. G. Farben.[30] Schrenck-Notzing used the wealth he thus acquired to fund his occult projects, hiring mediums like Rudi Schneider and building an elaborate research laboratory in his Munich villa. His money also helped him make his occult experiments a passion of Munich's high society. The elegant séances he staged at his home, which usually featured lower-class mediums, were thus both scientific experiments and social events for the city's economic and social elites.[31] Nor was Schrenck-Notzing by any means alone among German elites, as participants and observers alike regularly noted. The psychiatrist Albert Moll recalled the enthusiasm with which Eliza von Moltke, the wife of the famous general, had embraced spiritualism.[32] Similarly, when he first made contact with the Munich community of spiritualists, psychical researchers, and Theosophists in 1888, Max Dessoir marveled at the energy of the women helping to pioneer the new worldview locally. Among them were Albertine du Prel, Emma von Max, and the countess Caroline von Spreti.[33]

Occult activities even touched the social sphere of Kaiser Wilhelm II. Three members of the aristocratic Liebenberg Circle within which Wilhelm did so much of his socializing were heavily involved in spiritualism: Philipp zu Eulenburg, Axel von Varnbüler, and Kuno Moltke. Eulenburg, who sought spiritualist treatments for his neurasthenia, headed a family of devoted spiritualists and even used his spiritualist experiences to entertain the Kaiser. Wilhelm participated in at least one séance in 1888, but he did not share Eulenburg's passion for them.[34] The Kaiser, in fact, clearly feared that his friends' spiritualist interests might give political opponents a weapon against him. Thus he warned Eulenburg in 1903 to avoid revealing his occult predilections, explaining that such publicity might hand the Social Democrats a tool to use in their campaign to discredit the Kaiserreich.[35] Wilhelm also expressed disapproval over the involvement of civil servants in the occult movement. And if the newspapers were an accurate gauge, the occult had indeed spread into such circles. The periodical *Reichsbote,* for instance, blamed highly placed officers and civil servants for having introduced spiritualism to Potsdam just after the turn of the century.[36]

If the occult's appeal to Germans at all levels of the class hierarchy was yet one more indication that this was a truly mass movement, two final signs were the movement's cultural tenor, which was decisively syncretic, and its political valence, which was diverse. Germans eager to invigorate their spiritual lives looked to other parts of the world for inspiration, particularly to the East. In a revealing phrase, the writer and Schwabing resident Annie Francé-Harrar noted that in the 1890s her circle of bohemian friends had experienced a "spiritual wind blowing from East to West."[37] As her examples of Theosophy (inspired by the Russian medium Helena Petrovna Blavatsky) and Buddhism (whose importation from India was facilitated by Theosophy) indicated, *East* could mean from the European or Asian orient. Indeed, when Theosophy arrived in Germany in 1884, it had already been deeply affected by its founders' contact with Buddhism in India, where Blavatsky and her followers had moved earlier in the decade. Spiritual journeys eastward were also an important rite of passage for serious occultists. Franz Hartmann had lived in India in the early 1880s; Wilhelm Hübbe-Schleiden had been there for several years in the 1890s. Nor were such journeys limited to Theosophists, as the case of the astrologer Rudolf von Sebottendorf demonstrates. Sebottendorf, the son of a Saxon train driver, had quit his engineering studies at the Berlin polytechnic and spent several years in the late 1890s and early 1900s adventuring in Anatolia, where he also became a serious student of occultism.[38]

While many participants in the German movement thus embraced occultism flowing from Eastern sources, other Germans were not so ready to give up on Western traditions. These men and women experimented with joining the occult to a revamped Christianity, a pattern particularly visible in the spiritualist context. The cover of the spiritualist periodical *Zeitschrift für Seelenleben* (*Newspaper for spiritual life*), for instance, featured a logo arranged around the central figure of a Christian cross.[39] Nor was it uncommon for Christian elements to enter into the staging of occult events. In Munich in 1898, a Protestant minister from Berlin, Max Gubalke, chaired the congress held by the spiritualist Verband deutscher Okkultisten (Association of German occultists).[40] In 1929, the successor to this group, the Bund für Seelenkultur (Association for spiritual culture), opened its annual convention with a religious song.[41]

These Christian strains in the German occult movement pointed to an important Western dimension that coexisted with its orientalism. Franz Hartmann and Georg von Langsdorff, it is worth remembering, were both initially exposed to spiritualism in the United States, and many members of Germany's first Theosophical society had close contacts with American Theosophists. In addition, many of the professional mediums traveling the German occult circuit came from the United States, beginning with the infamous Henry Slade.[42] Germany also had important occult connections with its southern neighbors. From Italy came the famous medium Eusapia Paladino, a poor illiterate woman from Naples. Austria, too, sent many talented mediums northward. Their ranks included Willi and Rudi Schneider, Karl Weber, Erik Jan Hanussen, Rafael Schermann, and Maria Silbert.[43]

If participants jumbled Eastern and Western elements in their bid to integrate the occult with modern life, the movement as a whole also encompassed a wide variety of political orientations. One, of course, was völkisch. Ariosophical clubs in particular joined their occult pursuits to programs for racial purity and Germanic nationalism (see appendix A). Another was communitarian. The Oschm-Rahmah-Johjihjah Lodge, for instance, consisted of twenty-four members, nineteen women and five men, who lived together in a Theosophical commune in southeast Berlin just after the turn of the century. Shunning a leader as well as private property, lodge members understood their community as one dedicated not to social experimentation but rather to fostering the spiritual journey of each member toward enlightenment.[44] Indeed, despite the lodge's communal lifestyle, its focus on the spiritual journey of the individual was in keeping with the dominant bourgeois center of the movement, whose main project had less to do with wholesale political or social reform than *self*-reform. It should not surprise us, in any case, that the occult movement could encompass such widely divergent cultural and political inflections. Participants felt a deep alienation from the status quo and repeatedly showed their willingness to experiment widely to find a more satisfying alternative.

Texts as Tools, Presses as Patrons

Hans Fischer was an alienated office worker who often wondered if life held nothing more for him than the dull, daily routine of typing and filing in a small room shut off from the wider world. Obsessive reading on this question finally led him to a pamphlet on clothing reform that inspired him to produce a short piece of his own on the topic. Setting out to find a publisher, Hans chanced upon a man who agreed to bring out the pamphlet and invited him to join the staff at the press. In marked contrast to his previous job, Hans's new position at the press brought meaning to his life. It introduced him to the entire spectrum of reform movements—vegetarianism, naturopathy [*Naturheilkunde*], Theosophy, and nudism, to name only a few—and prompted him to join a nudist club. And it was on one of the club's outings that Hans finally encountered the occult in the figure of a certain Dr. Korn. With two nude female companions happily splashing in the water nearby, Hans and Dr. Korn lay unclothed in the open air and spoke about the world of immaterial spirits and occult medicine. Hans now resolved to study the occult sciences with Dr. Korn, whom he dubbed the "enlightener of the enlightened."[45]

This account of the making of a Lebensreformer first appeared in 1922 in an autobiographical novel written by an early leader of the German nudist movement named Egbert Falk (pseudonym for Georg Furhmann).[46] Although fictional, the story of Hans Fischer's education and reform captured important historical realities pertinent to the study of the German occult movement. Like Hans, many Germans found their way into the world of Lebensreform, including its occult variants, through texts published by the numerous small presses

Table 3.3. Occult Businesses, 1870–1937

			Number by Primary Specialty			
Type of Business	Total by Type	Ariosophy	Astrology, Dowsing, Graphology, Palmistry, Pendulum	Occultism, Lebensreform	Spiritualism, Psychical Research, Parapsychology	Theosophy
Bookstores, libraries	7			4	2	1
Health-related businesses	6			3	2	1
Institutes for advice and information	17		10	5	1	1
Lecture halls, schools	5		1	4		
Presses	61	3	11	20	8	19
Total by specialty	96	3	22	36	13	22

that proliferated from the imperial era onward. As table 3.3 shows, presses made up a particularly large sector of businesses that specialized in occult topics (see also appendixes B and C). Like Hans, moreover, many Germans found that the new small presses offered not just texts but many points of contact that involved them both as readers and as full-body participants in the burgeoning new occult movement. Hans Fischer's story, in short, reflected the important role played both by texts and presses in the diffusion of alternative German modernities, including an occult one.

How did texts function in the spread of occult beliefs and practices? To begin with, texts featured prominently in the conversion stories of many occultists. The modernist writer Gustav Meyrink, for instance, reported that he had been on the verge of suicide when an occult pamphlet shoved underneath his apartment door led him to embrace a Theosophical life instead.[47] Although Meyrink probably mixed fact and fiction to dramatize this story, text-facilitated conversions like his were widely reported by his contemporaries. The early German spiritualist Georg von Langsdorff had been an avowed atheist until 1859, when he chanced upon a newspaper article reporting the recent discovery of the spirit world.[48] Similarly, Gottfried Kratt recalled being a materialist, atheist, and socialist until his "conversion" to occultism in 1892. His conversion had occurred while browsing in a bookstore, where he had chanced upon a cheap edition of Carl du Prel's *Der Spiritismus,* which convinced him to trade in his former commitments for the new worldview of occultism.[49]

In addition to being stimuli to conversion, the many texts of the occult movement also functioned as informative billboards. Typically, occult texts came bundled with several pages of advertisements for related books or services that readers might find of interest. The advertisements accompanying E. Honold's spiritualist memoirs featured several volumes on dreams, life after death, somnambulism, and mind reading; manuals instructing readers on how to conduct their own séance or analyze their own handwriting; therapeutic cookbooks for those suffering from intestinal disorders or the diseases common to "mental workers" *(Kopfarbeiter);* self-help medical texts on understanding one's hemorrhoids and the disease-producing aspects of processed sugar; many books on human sexuality; and several inexpensive pamphlets directed to "everyman," whose titles—for example, "How Do I Become an Athlete?" and "How Do I Become Rich?"—indicated their contents.[50] Book covers became places to advertise not just further texts for readers to buy but also clubs they might join, bookstores they might patronize, and products they might sample. The front and back covers of a spiritualist pamphlet published in 1892, for instance, gave information about the Berlin spiritualist club Sphinx, directed aspirants to the spiritualist bookstore run by I. F. Conrad on Berlin's fashionable Friedrichstraße, and plugged the virtues of Himalayan "elephant tea" for mediums (available for purchase at a local store).[51]

The texts of the occult movement also provided important suggestions on how to stage an occult event. Many presses published manuals that provided simple, step-by-step instructions on how to cast one's own horoscope, conduct a family séance, or use a dowsing rod. Other occult texts could, on occasion, prompt occult acts. One particularly bizarre episode in this mode occurred in 1925, when the butcher Johannes Reichardt achieved fame as the "Alchemist of Gunzenhausen" for allegedly transmuting lead into gold with the help of powders and directions uncovered in his hometown of Gunzenhausen. Reichardt's discovery of these tools followed a prophecy Paracelsus had supposedly made in the sixteenth century. A small press with the catchy name Cloud Traveler had reissued the script of this prophecy in 1923, just in time to help Reichardt make his newsworthy alchemical discovery in 1925.[52]

Finally, while the numerous texts of the movement helped to publicize occult beliefs and practices broadly, they simultaneously helped create specialized niches in which occultists of differing persuasions could nest. Nowhere was this niche-creating function more visible than in the dozens of specialized periodicals that proliferated over the seven decades of the movement's existence (see appendix D). Those with a commitment to the scientific study of mediumism and allied psychic phenomena could consult *Psychische Studien* (f. 1874), which remained the preeminent journal of German psychical research until the 1930s and retained this position when it resumed publishing after World War II. In contrast, even by 1914 those interested in a more spiritualist approach to occult phenomena could choose from a dozen or so spiritualist journals. From the 1880s onward, readers eager to learn more about Theosophy had an equally large range of publications at their disposal. Preeminent among these were *Sphinx* (1886-96), edited by Wilhelm Hübbe-Schleiden and heavily influenced in its outlook by the psychical researcher Carl du Prel; *Lotusblüthen* (1892–1900), edited by Franz Hartmann; and *[Neue] Metaphysische Rundschau* (1896–1918), published and edited by Paul Zillmann. Following the establishment in 1909 of *Astrologische Rundschau*, Germany's first periodical exclusively devoted to astrology, over the next three decades more than two dozen German-language periodicals devoted to astrological topics appeared.

As this short survey suggests, occult texts were instrumental in precipitating conversions, advertising goods and services, educating novices and adepts, and creating specialized occult niches. Texts were able to serve these multiple functions, moreover, because behind them lay an extensive publishing system making occult reading matter cheaply and widely available. It was not just the more traditional system of German clubs, in other words, but the new small presses with their enthusiastic embrace of German consumer culture that helped organize, spread, and shape the German occult movement. These presses deserve our attention, moreover, because they helped connect the German occult to the larger context of German modernism.

One of the most obvious links between the occult and the wider modernist field was psychoanalysis, and Oswald Mutze, one of the earliest and most important presses of German spiritualism and psychical research, embodied this linkage particularly clearly. Founded in Leipzig in 1872 and active through the 1920s, this press had a list of several hundred titles whose diversity reflected the international dimensions of the occult movement.[53] The publication list included works by the Russian Alexander Aksakow, the Englishman William Crookes, the American Andrew Jackson Davis, and the Frenchman

Allan Kardec.[54] It also took the lead in publishing German authors and activities, bringing out several tracts either by or about Zöllner and his celebrated Leipzig experiments, works by prominent German occultists like Carl du Prel, and *Psychische Studien,* a leading journal of the occult sciences in Germany from the 1870s onward. Nor did Oswald Mutze publish occult texts exclusively; rather, the press pursued its interests in novel psychological trends more broadly, publishing authors and texts that quickly assumed canonical status within the field of psychological modernism. One was *On the Psychology and Psychopathology of So-Called Occult Phenomena,* by Carl Gustav Jung, who presented this study of the medium Hélène Preiswerk as his doctoral dissertation in 1902.[55] Another was *Memoirs of My Nervous Illness,* by Daniel Paul Schreber, whose autobiographical account of his institutionalization became famous in 1911 when Freud published a psychoanalytic interpretation of the case that quickly became a classic in the study of schizophrenia.[56]

While Oswald Mutze mixed occultism and psychological modernism, other presses linked the occult to German varieties of aesthetic modernism. The press of M. Poessl served the Munich naturalists in the 1880s and 1890s at the same time that it published the occult meanderings of the dramatist Hanns von Gumppenberg and Carl du Prel's reedited version of Immanuel Kant's *Dreams of a Spirit Seer.* The occult and the modern also overlapped at the press of Wilhelm Friedrich, one of the earliest and most important sponsors of Europe's literary avant-garde, whose authors during the 1880s and 1890s included Michael Georg Conrad, Karl Bleibtreu, Detlev Liliencron, Paul Heyse, Theodor Fontane, Lou Andreas-Salomé, Thomas Mann, Maximilian Harden, Henrik Ibsen, Friedrich Nietzsche, and Émile Zola.[57] During these same years, Friedrich also became one of the first to bring Theosophical texts to a German audience. These included works by Franz Hartmann, Karl Kiesewetter, and Carl du Prel, as well as the Theosophical periodical *Lotusblüthen.*[58]

If presses helped link the occult to aesthetic and psychological varieties of modernism, they could also function as sites for the mixing of the occult and Lebensreform, arguably the most important sector of popular modernism in Wilhelmine and Weimar Germany. Occultists and proponents of Lebensreform shared the common goal of easing Germans' accommodation to modernity, but differed in method. Whereas occultists emphasized spiritual means, proponents of Lebensreform emphasized more physical ones by embracing causes like the reform of clothing, diet, housing, and exercise. In practice, these two paths toward full accommodation with modernity were often embraced by the same people, and, unsurprisingly, many presses reflected this dual embrace.[59]

The Max Spohr Verlag embodied this reformist mixture particularly clearly. Founded in 1881, this press specialized in popular medicine but carried a book list of hundreds of volumes on a multitude of other topics, including many on the occult.[60] The press played an important role in the Lebensreform movement through its support for liberal crusaders like the sexologist Magnus Hirschfeld, who campaigned for women's rights, eugenically informed family planning, and sexual reform. The *Jahrbuch für sexuelle Zwischenstufen mit besonderer Berücksichtigung der Homosexualität* (1899-1923), edited by Hirschfeld and dedicated to the destigmatization of homosexuality, for instance, appeared at the Max Spohr Verlag alongside numerous occult texts.[61] These ranged from the rather scholarly overview by Karl Kiesewetter on the history of the occult to manuals like *Wie errichtet und leitet man spiritistische Zirkel in der Familie* (How to establish and lead a spiritualist circle in the family) (1894) that were targeted for a general audience.[62]

Other presses sat at the interface between the occult and völkisch strains of German modernism. One was the press of Max Altmann, who took over the German lead in Theosophical publishing after the initial work had been done by Wilhelm Friedrich.[63] Devoted primarily to occult and Theosophical topics, this Leipzig house also published a few völkisch tracts.[64] The press of Paul Zillmann also sponsored völkisch authors, particularly in its journal *[Neue] Metaphysische Rundschau,* which carried several articles by prominent Ariosophists like Lanz von Liebenfels and Guido von List in the first decade of the twentieth century.[65]

Whereas neither Altmann nor Zillmann made the link between the occult and völkisch modernism central to their publishing record, other presses did. These included all Ariosophical establishments and several astrological presses (see appendix B), which as a group exhibited several peculiar features. In the first place, they had very short publication lists. Whereas the houses run by Oswald Mutze, Max Spohr, and Max Altmann brought out hundreds of titles each, even the most active of these völkisch presses produced no more than a few dozen texts, and many published fewer than ten. Another peculiarity was that these presses shunned the eclectic and international approach taken by the occult mainstream. Instead, these presses tended to feature the works of a small group of German-speaking völkisch authors like Guido von List, Jörg Lanz von Liebenfels, Herbert Reichstein, A. M. Grimm, and E. Issberner-

Haldane. Völkisch-occult presses even seem to have shunned the wider world of occult publishing. Thus, in 1935 Herbert Reichstein published a list of recommendations for the reader dedicated to "the development of his character and his Nordic and Aryan world . . . view." The list began with Adolf Hitler's *Mein Kampf* and included Julius Langbehn's *Rembrandt als Erzieher,* several works by the "philosopher" of National Socialism Alfred Rosenberg, and a series of Ariosophical classics.[66] Standard works of the mainstream occult movement like du Prel's *Der Spiritismus* or Karl Kiesewetter's occult history did not appear on this list.

That occult and völkisch texts emanated in some cases from the same presses makes it tempting to overplay the importance of the occult-völkisch publishing enterprise.[67] It is important to realize, however, that presses focused exclusively on völkisch-occult texts belonged to a small and highly specialized sector of the overall market. Of a total of sixty-one presses, only twelve could be considered primarily völkisch. And the significance of this group shrinks further when we realize that, even combined, their publication lists were very small compared with those for a single mainstream press like Oswald Mutze or Wilhelm Friedrich. It should be clear by now, in any case, that the world of occult publishing had a structure whose complexity cannot be encompassed adequately in the *völkisch-occult* construct. A useful comparison here might be made to the press of Eugen Diederichs, which published on the new racial thinking, German mysticism, and the occult. Regularly tarred with the all-encompassing term *völkisch,* this press actually published books with neither a racialist nor a nationalist tinge, even in the 1930s.[68] Similarly, the Theosophical press of Paul Zillmann did more than just publish Ariosophical tracts. *[Neue] Metaphysische Rundschau,* for instance, published the racist essays of Guido von List alongside racially neutral pieces by such mainstream occult leaders as Annie Besant, H. P. Blavatsky, and Carl du Prel.[69]

We should not, in any case, be surprised that the publishing history of the occult in Germany consisted of a jumble of different political shadings, cultural styles, and social programs. This very variety reflected the ferment that accompanied modernist innovation as Germans struggled to accommodate themselves to the exigencies of the new age. Within this larger context, publishing houses acted as one of the crucibles in which new and experimental cultural forms were generated and fused. As previous historians have suggested, presses during this period were important not just because of their publication lists but also because they acted both as cultural patrons and as cultural entrepreneurs, nurturing carefully selected cultural currents while also selling and profiting from them.[70]

The Nirwana-Verlag für Lebensreform, founded before World War I, was a case in point. Plugging itself as not just a publishing house but as the biggest specialized business in Germany devoted to occult texts and items, the press claimed to offer customers a variety of valuable services: ease of access (located on the posh Wilhelmstraße, in the very heart of metropolitan Berlin), a regularly updated catalog that included hundreds of items, prompt and helpful service, and the advantage of buying from experts who had devoted years of study to the occult. Its catalog in 1922 consisted of 937 texts (most of them fully annotated) covering a wide variety of topics, including healthy living, human sexuality, nudism, occultism, spiritualism, magnetism, religion, Theosophy, occult novels, and astrology. Phrenological heads, scriptoscopes, and other occult props and instruments were also available for immediate sale.[71]

As this impressive catalog of goods suggests, the German occult belonged to the larger culture of consumption. "Buy this and you will be wiser, healthier, and happier" was a standard message that appeared in innovative ways. A poem printed in the 1922 catalog of the Nirwana-Verlag für Lebensreform exhorted consumers thus:

> There are many books, cheap and large,
> In this press for Lebensreform;
> To go to the source of wisdom
>
> .   .   .   .
>
> Study the catalog diligently,
> And quickly choose
> Many books, rare, ideal
> Solid works full of power,
> For every scientific branch,
> Especially for the occultist.
>
> .   .   .   .
>
> O, Friend of Wisdom, buy just one item
> And you will be royally satisfied.[72]

This poem captured the new consumerist ethos sweeping Germany in the late nineteenth and early twentieth centuries. It pitched goods not just in terms of price but in terms of consumer satisfaction, suggesting that the Nirwana-Verlag für Lebensreform had just the tools to help buyers achieve wisdom in this life (no need to wait until the next). In addition, the poem emphasized sheer convenience, informing readers that with a quick look at the catalog and easy mail order, they, too, could acquire real wisdom now.[73]

While institutions like the Nirwana-Verlag für Lebensreform were undoubtedly commercial businesses, finally, they were also more than this. The press ran a lending library well stocked with books on naturopathy, nudism, Theosophy, and occultism, sponsored lectures and demonstrations, and carried informational brochures about schools and services that customers might be interested in exploring.[74] As should by now be clear, presses like the Nirwana-Verlag für Lebensreform saw themselves as active agents in the vast movement for the reform of German life. They existed not only to make money but to promote a certain lifestyle whose modern character was striking. Hans Fischer's fictional experiences had a solid basis in fact.

Schools and Services

Readers picking up the Lebensreform book by Dr. Gustav Riedlin plugging the virtues of vegetarianism for self-development and world harmony would have quickly come upon an advertisement for an astrological advice service offered by the book's publisher Paul Lorenz. Prospective customers—civil servants, bankers, industrialists, merchants, speculators, lawyers, doctors, actors, students, housewives, and workers—were invited to write in for a personalized horoscope that could help them establish when it was advisable (or inadvisable) to take specific actions.[75] This advertisement pointed to a final area of economic activity in the occult mode, a sector devoted to occult schools and services. As the data summarized in table 3.3 and appendix C show, corporate bodies devoted to the occult included numerous schools, lecture halls, health-related centers, and institutes for advice and information, as well as presses, bookstores, and libraries. Although not reflected in this data, moreover, this sector of the occult economy also contained numerous independent practitioners who hawked their goods and services individually. Along with the traditional German club system and the new mass press, this network of corporate bodies and individual providers represented a third important channel for the mass diffusion of occult beliefs and practices into German culture.

Publicity and profit accrued to the numerous schools and institutes devoted to educating paying students about all aspects of modern occultism. Large cities typically had several such institutions. In Munich, the educational group Neuland brought members of Munich's psychical research community together with occultists dedicated to the construction of an occult worldview. During its short life, Neuland managed to sponsor several lecture courses on occult topics and to construct a well-equipped laboratory for mediumistic research.[76] Nor were educational ventures like this limited to specialized occult institutes. As one of Munich's major daily newspapers announced in 1930, the astrologer Heinz Artur Strauß was now offering a course on his specialty at the city's *Volkshochschule.*[77] For those too busy to take a class, occult institutes mounted educational exhibits that the curious could explore at their leisure. The occult information center Eclaros, for instance, planned in 1932 to sponsor a public exhibition on astrology, characterology, and graphology; the pendulum and the divining rod; Anthroposophy and Theosophy; spiritualism, hypnotism, and magnetism; and cabala, mysticism, and Buddhism.[78] Similar educational ventures appeared in Berlin and other large cities across Germany.

Whereas groups like Eclaros and Neuland targeted a general public, other institutes sought to reap profits from a more select clientele. This was particularly true in the astrological context, where institutes such as the Astrologische Zentralstelle (Astrological central office) flourished. In 1933, this office established an accreditation exam, for which aspiring astrologers could prepare by enrolling in one of the fee-based astrological training courses or by buying one of the exam-preparation booklets.[79] Already in the 1920s, astrologers certified and employed by such "professional" institutes were charging substantial fees for their services. Rudolf Sagittarius, an astrologer at the Institut für wissenschaftliche Astrologie und Graphologie (Institute for scientific astrology and graphology) in Kiel in 1929, for instance, offered paying customers a menu of options costing anywhere from three to fifty reichsmarks: the choices included the construction of a birth horoscope with an oral consultation, the construction of a birth horoscope with exact mathematical calculations, a graphological character analysis, or a graphological test for professional advice.[80]

Outside of Germany's network of astrological institutes, heavily dominated by men with pretensions to "professional" status, there was an older network of individual astrologers who gave lessons in astrology, set up astrological booths at local fairs, made house calls to cast horoscopes, and held office hours to give astrological advice to paying customers. Many of these more populist astrologers dabbled in other forms of occultism as well. They gave demonstrations of hypnosis and telepathy, occult character analysis, and occult techniques of healing.

One of the striking features of this part of the occult service economy was that, as noted above, it included many Germans of petty bourgeois background, both women and men. In Munich, for instance, the actress Josephine Zierer and the housekeeper Änna Zirngible had a business arrangement according to which Zierer gave lessons in astrology to pupils who then bought personal horoscopes cast by Zirngible. Zierer's pupils came to her primarily to receive these horoscopes, which were increasingly hard to obtain in Munich in the 1920s due to enhanced police surveillance. Zirngible cast the horoscopes according to astrological tables purchased from the "scientific" astrologer Ludwig Stenger, who also ran a small astrological book service.[81]

As the case of the bookseller Stenger suggests, men of petty bourgeois background also participated in this more populist niche of the occult service economy. A man in Leipzig, for instance, admitted to police that he had set himself up as an astrologer in 1928 after carefully studying a five-volume work addressed to lay people by the astrologer Karl Brandler-Pracht. He managed to earn a small income for himself by selling astrological pamphlets with titles like *Every Man His Own Astrologer* and providing a fee-based personal horoscope casting service.[82] Petty-bourgeois astrologers also seem in some cases to have had a distinct class consciousness. Thus, the young astrologer Christian Meier-Parm, a stringent critic of the elite astrology practiced at institutes like Korsch's astrological "central office," published an article on "The Horoscopes of Thirty-Five Women in Brothels" in order to make his point that astrology could also serve the masses.[83] Occultists were also adept at using the mail to find customers. The Munich astrologer Georg Schwab, the son of a shoemaker, admitted to the police in 1931 that he had culled national phone books for the names and addresses of three thousand people to whom he sent a flyer advertising his astrological service (1 mark per horoscope). His attempt to set up an astrological consultation service by mail was apparently one of the methods he resorted to in order to support his young daughter and pay off their 1,000-mark debt.[84]

That the "new worldview" movements, including the occult, proved remarkably adaptable to the modern marketplace did not escape contemporary notice. In a passage that might as well have applied to the occult movement, one critic lampooned Anthroposophy (a movement that broke off from the occult center in 1912–13) thus:

> What is Anthroposophy?
>
> It is the department store of all . . . disguised religions, for all social positions and professions, all sexes, all ages.
>
> You are a doctor? We carry four bodies and a few intermediate stages.
>
> You are a philosopher? Please, please, an infinitely rich stock, 253 world views. . . .
>
> You are a historical researcher? Please, go to the third floor: past and future times.
>
> You are an optimist? Please, check in with the woman dressed in white in our basement department for reincarnation.
>
> A pessimist? It's not so bad. Please, check in with the woman dressed in black in our unrivalled department for reincarnation, located in the basement. . . .
>
> A poor writer? Yes, yes, hard times for the press. Well, we always have quite a few newspapers and a book press; perhaps there is something to be done.
>
> But, of course, my lady. We have an especially carefully run department for new, inconsolable widows.
>
> You are a carpenter? . . . A noble profession . . . Christ's father . . . let's see what we can do for you. . . .
>
> Ah, honorable privy councillor, you are a politician and businessman? One moment please. Take a club chair and a Waldorf. You know, of course, about the director and the English minister of education . . . yes, really excellent international connections . . . there comes our department head for the tripartite division of the social organism.[85]

This satire captured an important facet of German high modernity: the new worldview movements whose proliferation was integral to the genesis of this modern age owed their success not least to their adherents' adaptability to the mass marketplace, symbolized here by the department store. In this, the occult was no exception. If the many clubs and rural retreats added up to an occult public, the many presses, mail-order businesses, department stores, schools, and individual providers catering to this public added up to a vibrant occult marketplace. Indeed, occultists' emphasis on achieving satisfaction in this world rather than the next was well suited to the offerings of the modern marketplace and its ability to cater to the ethic of "personal satisfaction."[86] With this highly public market as a backdrop, the chapters that follow will explore a few of the many other ways in which the German occult and the German modern fed each other, often in ways that no one person or group could directly control or predict.

Part II / The Occult in Action

CHAPTER FOUR

Varieties of Theosophical Experience

When thirty-eight men and women banded together in 1884 to found Germany's first major society of Theosophists, the Theosophische Societät Germania (TSG), they aimed at nothing less than the wholesale reform of German culture via occult means. This ambitious program hit a snag one year later, unfortunately, when evidence of fraud committed by Theosophy's international leader Helena Petrovna Blavatsky surfaced in the British press.[1] In the wake of this scandal, in December 1886 the TSG dissolved, but the group's members doggedly persevered in their original aim. Led by Wilhelm Hübbe-Schleiden, formerly president of the TSG, German Theosophists now threw their energy into making their newly founded occult journal *Sphinx* into a forum for cultural renewal in all its guises. As editor, Hübbe-Schleiden hoped to solicit contributions from such well-known occultists as Carl du Prel and a varied collection of public figures that included Ludwig Kuhlenbeck, Leo Tolstoi, Paul de Lagarde, and Kurt Eisner—very odd juxtapositions, to say the least.[2] What could Kuhlenbeck, a professor of law who soon became a vocal advocate of Germanic race purity, have had in common with the Russian writer Tolstoi, an ardent pacifist dedicated to updating Christian faith for modern times?[3] Similarly, what could Kurt Eisner, a social-democratic activist who eventually led the short-lived Bavarian republic of 1918–19, have had in common with Paul de Lagarde, an alienated cultural critic who located the causes of Germany's spiritual collapse with liberals, academics, and Jews?[4] Odd as Hübbe-Schleiden's list seems in retrospect, these juxtapositions pointed to a central fact about German Theosophy: from its earliest beginnings in the mid-1880s to its formal suppression by the Nazis in 1936–37, the Theosophical project of cultural renewal via occult means proved highly adaptable to a wide spectrum of reformist trends and political ends.

Theosophy's adaptability in the German context deserves our consideration for at least two reasons. First, we need to remove Theosophy from the teleological framework within which it has too often been placed. Discussion of the German occult movement has focused almost exclusively on the supposedly occult roots of National Socialism, and in their effort to locate these roots scholars have been particularly assiduous in investigating Ariosophy, a Theosophical offshoot. Although these studies have turned up a wealth of interesting information about Ariosophy, they have tended to obscure the history of mainstream German Theosophy—a much larger, at least equally influential, and certainly more sociopolitically diverse movement. To correct these biases, this chapter treats German Theosophy in all its variety, from the liberal to the proto-Nazi.

This, then, leads to the second reason that Theosophy's adaptability merits study. To put it bluntly, Theosophy complicates our view of fin-de-siècle reform culture in fruitful ways. Too often, historians have seen this reformist milieu in terms of what came later, trawling it continuously for signs of illiberalism and proto-Fascism. Valuable as this scholarship has been for our understanding of Nazism, it has often misread signs of a thriving reformist culture with political leanings that defy easy categorization. Theosophy was a case in point, for although it did produce Ariosophy, it was also an important site for reframing traditional liberal ideas around modern occult ones.[5]

These links between liberalism and German Theosophy deserve emphasis.[6] Understood as a political tradition not easily reducible to social or economic factors, liberalism in its classical form rested on a belief in the inevitability of progress, an emphasis on the sanctity and central importance of the individual, a hostility to any church claiming possession of an absolute truth, and a socially integrative vision of a coming classless society in which citizens would enjoy equal rights before the law. In late-nineteenth-century Germany, as industrialization and political unification proceeded apace, these classic liberal tenets had been called into question. Liberalism and progress ceased to be synonymous for many groups of Germans who had previously belonged to liberalism's constituency, and many transferred their allegiance to other social and political movements, including Theosophy, which recycled in spiritual terms old liberal notions of evolution, progress, social harmony, and the sanctity of the individual. The late-nineteenth-century German turn to Theosophy, in other words, may be read as an implicit critique of political liberalism and an attempt to carry elements of the liberal program forward in the broad field of modernist cultural experimentation.[7] In the crucible of fin-de-siècle modernism, however, the Theosophical program also became joined to decidedly nonliberal currents, as the example of Hübbe-Schleiden's oddly constructed list suggests. German Theosophy, indeed, presents an ideal example of the immense political flexibility and complexity of fin-de-siècle reform-mindedness, a case that this chapter makes by tracing three varieties of Theosophical activity and examining the very different political and cultural agendas to which the Theosophical project of cultural renewal via occult means was adapted.

In Pursuit of Universal Brotherhood

Adaptability, indeed, was a leitmotif of the international Theosophical movement more generally. Founded in 1875 in New York by the Russian adventuress Blavatsky and the American writer Henry Steel Olcott, the international Theosophical Society was based initially on a series of messages channeled through the mediumship of Blavatsky from a mysterious community of highly evolved beings known as Mahatmas, or Masters; collectively, they were called the Great White Brotherhood. Dedicated to humanity's spiritual enlightenment, these spiritual teachers sent messages that became the core of a growing intellectual system attempting to explain all of human history, religion, science, and philosophy in terms of a unitary and universal occult tradition. Within a decade, the society had established its headquarters in Adyar, India, and had branches operative across the Americas, Europe, Asia, and Australia. Drawing men and women from a wide variety of religious, social, and professional backgrounds, the Theosophical Society mixed mysticism and Westernized Buddhism with an intense attraction for the occult. It also provided a venue in which many of the reformist and experimental causes of the late nineteenth and early twentieth centuries flourished, among them women's rights, pacifism, clothing reform, prison reform, antivivisectionism, vegetarianism, and the Free India movement.[8] In Britain, where the Theosophical movement was particularly strong, Theosophists found a variety of political homes, from left-wing feminism and socialism in the late nineteenth century to right-wing fascism in the 1920s and 1930s.[9]

Early Theosophists understood themselves to belong to a spiritual vanguard dedicated to the cultural renewal of modern life on an occult basis. Critical of their era's rampant materialism and spiritual poverty, Theosophists sought to create a so-called "sixth root race," or universal brotherhood, that would live in full cognizance of humanity's spiritual nature and incorporate people from around the world without regard to religion, race, nationality, class, or sex.[10] Convinced that their movement would form the nucleus of this future "race," Theosophists made their commitment to universal brotherhood central to their self-understanding by specifying two courses of action. First, based on the assumption that precious pieces of knowledge about humanity's spiritual basis had been scattered among all the world's peoples, the society encouraged the comparative study of all the world's religions, philosophies, and sciences, with a view to uncovering the hidden, or "occult," truth thought to underlie them. Second, it promoted research on the "occult" powers slumbering within the souls of individual members. Taken together, Theosophists believed, these two methods would enlighten humanity about the true nature of reality and thus bind all people together in a harmonious community finally embarked on its cosmological journey back to reunion with pure spirit.[11]

One of the first Germans to feel the allure of this program was Wilhelm Hübbe-Schleiden, a founder and prominent leader of the early German Theosophical movement who made developing the occult sciences and strengthening universal brotherhood his main concerns. Hübbe-Schleiden's life, indeed, presents a historical puzzle typical of the political ambiguities embedded in fin-de-siècle reform culture, and thus makes an ideal starting point for our examination of German Theosophy.

Born to a Hamburg family that included various civil servants and a leading biologist, he received a law degree from the University of Leipzig in 1869 before going on to London, where he worked first for a large business and then for the German consul.[12] In 1875, he moved to Africa, where he and a partner opened a lucrative trade firm in Gabon. There, he witnessed and by some accounts participated in the punishment and brutal killings of two men who had robbed the firm, as a result of which, in 1877, he was tried, found guilty of murder, and deported. He successfully contested the charges and returned to Germany later that year. Quickly becoming involved in the growing movement to acquire German colonies, especially in Africa and Asia, he soon emerged as an excellent organizer and propagandist for Friedrich Fabri, one of the movement's key leaders.[13] For the next seven years, Hübbe-Schleiden threw his considerable skills and energies into this effort, which soon earned him national public renown.[14]

The seven years Hübbe-Schleiden spent as a colonial propagandist have earned him a standard place in histories of German illiberalism, a political tradition often invoked to explain the origins of National Socialism. The historian Hans-Ulrich Wehler, for instance, singles Hübbe-Schleiden out as a primary author of the ideology of "social imperialism," which cast Germany's quest for overseas empire as a reactionary solution to the sociopolitical problems that developed in the Kaiserreich after the economic downturn of 1873. For Wehler, social imperialism represented a "socially defensive" ideology, adopted by conservative elites as a calculated strategy to deflect attention away from Germany's need for domestic democratic reform.[15] Woodruff Smith, another historian of German imperialism, contests many of Wehler's conclusions, but persists in associating Hübbe-Schleiden with illiberal politics. Labeling him an early "radical conservative" and a "racist authoritarian," Smith sees Hübbe-Schleiden as one of the first of a new breed of conservatives who used colonial politics to fan the flames of German nationalism, anti-Semitism, and anti-industrialism.[16] Both Wehler and Smith, in short, place Hübbe-Schleiden in the pantheon of late-nineteenth-century proto-Nazis.

The problem with stopping the story about him there is that Hübbe-Schleiden's three decades as a Theosophist do not fit neatly under the banner of German illiberalism. Consider, for example, a letter Hübbe-Schleiden wrote in 1911, long after he had left colonial politics and had embraced Theosophy. Here, in what was hardly a ringing endorsement of the conservative political culture of the Kaiserreich, Hübbe-Schleiden berated German leaders, including Bismarck, as political eunuchs, German culture as a swamp of philistinism and pedantry, and German students as clever fools incapable of forming an independent thought.[17] A few years later, Hübbe-Schleiden once again made a statement that defied the illiberal label. This came just before the outbreak of World War I, when he gave a speech to German Theosophists imploring them to uphold now more than ever the liberal principle of tolerance set forth in Lessing's play *Nathan* by promoting the great cause of universal brotherhood among all the world's races.[18]

How are we to reconcile these two versions of Hübbe-Schleiden—the first a man of apparently deep conservatism, nationalism, and racism, the second a man who could plead for universal brotherhood on the eve of the war? A fuller consideration of Hübbe-Schleiden's activities as a Theosophist suggests that the truth may lie somewhere uncomfortably between. Hübbe-Schleiden emerges less as a proto-Nazi than as a politically ambiguous modernist engaged in a rather bizarre quest for both personal and national salvation.

Hübbe-Schleiden's conversion to Theosophy in 1884 had its roots in a deep personal change that began while he was still making his name as a colonialist. Whereas his public writings in the late 1870s and early 1880s made the case for Germany's need to expand abroad, his private journals reflected a man deeply conflicted about the direction his public life was taking. When his colonial activities brought him to the verge of settling in Paraguay to direct a project in 1883, a crisis with physical as well as spiritual dimensions overtook him. "Is there," he scribbled in his private diary, "any prospect of my finding spiritual relief from higher intelligences during my planned colonial activities in South America?" "How," he continued a few pages later, "is anyone to study the laws of nature . . . by what method is anyone to obtain . . . mastery of oneself? Where? India? South America?"

Desperate for release, he finally drafted a letter to Henry Steel Olcott, the president of the international Theosophical Society: "What do I have to do to become the Chela of one of the Tibet Brothers, to obtain a Mahatma guru. I mean the way in which I can apply, where and to whom whatever sacrifice may be required I am willing to undergo. I am not well off, but I will do anything if I am told how to do it, in order to obtain the wisdom of Eastern Occult Science and to gain a mastery over my own self. My animal nerve system is I am sorry to say perfectly out of order, but I trust this can easily be restored by occult power."[19] This passage—with its spiritual hunger for a guru, ready promise of personal sacrifice, and allusion to a neurasthenic breakdown—points to a strong religious urge driving Hübbe-Schleiden forward into a new life. In the grips of what his contemporary William James would have called "an acute fever" of the spirit, Hübbe-Schleiden followed this urge to its logical conclusion.[20] He joined the international Theosophical Society on 27 July 1884 and, that same day, assumed the presidency of the newly founded Theosophische Societät Germania.[21]

Following his conversion to Theosophy in 1884, Hübbe-Schleiden participated no more in colonial politics, but this did not mean that he forgot his colonial past.[22] In 1888, for instance, a German peasant woman's clairvoyant talents reminded him of visions that he had observed twenty years before among the inhabitants of equatorial Africa.[23] Hübbe-Schleiden himself, moreover, saw continuities between his colonial and Theosophical selves. As he wrote in a letter in 1915: "When I was young, thirty-five years ago, the Logos used me for German politics, in order to expand the economic and political horizon of the German people; five years later, [it used me] to introduce the Theosophical movement into the German cultural world."[24] Here, Hübbe-Schleiden betrayed his nationalist proclivities, proudly linking his life both before and after his conversion to promoting the development of the German nation.

This last comment also points to an underlying missionary zeal informing Hübbe-Schleiden's efforts on both the colonial and Theosophical fronts. If he had insisted as a colonial propagandist that Germany needed colonies to solve social ills like emigration and labor unrest, he now focused as a Theosophist on the spiritual ills plaguing the Kaiserreich. In 1884, for instance, he gave a speech on the "process of self-decomposition" in church circles. Germans, he noted, were "disgusted at the pathetic moralizing of [the] clergy, protestant or catholic [and to the] sensuous materialism and thoughtless pleasure hunting . . . [and] moral and spiritual decay" that had set in since unification. To all these spiritual ills, Hübbe-Schleiden announced, Theosophy offered the antidote of the so-called "transcendent world view."[25]

Hübbe-Schleiden's wholehearted embrace of the "transcendent world view," indeed, betrayed the links as well as breaks with his colonial past. The inaugural issue of the occult journal *Sphinx* in 1886, for example, carried Hübbe-Schleiden's statement on what this view entailed: "A true civilization must embrace the transcendent aspect of man. In order to do what they should, men must know what they are. The social tasks that become every day more pressing cannot be solved through legal requirements and police measures that are directed against the symptoms of seething movement. Instead, men must be given a complete worldview and brought to consciousness of the transcendent character of nature and of themselves."[26] As this passage suggests, Hübbe-

Schleiden aimed to give his readers a new worldview that would enable them to meet the social demands of modern times. Against the backdrop of the 1880s, a decade of widespread social unrest and political division, Hübbe-Schleiden offered the transcendent as a more effective antidote to Germany's ills than the "legal requirements and police measures" of the Bismarckian state.[27] His earlier advocacy of imperial expansion gave way to an embrace of a transcendent worldview. In other words, while his concern with addressing "the social problem" remained constant, his line of attack was new.

Although his methodology had shifted, Hübbe-Schleiden's understanding of the social problem after his Theosophical conversion continued to center on the problem of Germany's fragmentation. In his colonialist phase, he had been one of the first to recognize that German political life had to move beyond old dichotomies (e.g., Protestant versus Catholic, protection versus free trade) and instead embrace new causes like overseas expansion that could bring warring social groups together.[28] The quest for unity also informed his embrace of the transcendent worldview and the Theosophical goal of universal brotherhood, on the road to which he saw many allies in contemporary reformist causes such as socialism, female emancipation, vegetarianism, naturopathy, eugenics, and rational dress. But Theosophy, he believed, had something special to offer this reform milieu since its mode of operation was unique. Whereas a movement like socialism expected to reform the social order by forcing external relations among rich and poor, employers and workers, to change, Theosophists expected to reform society by first changing individuals from the inside—that is, by promoting their personal spiritual development through a deepened understanding of "the transcendent character of nature and . . . themselves."[29]

There were also important conceptual continuities before and after Hübbe-Schleiden's Theosophical conversion. An important one centered on the concept of race, which Hübbe-Schleiden had latched onto in the 1870s, when he became among the first to use Social Darwinian language to advocate German empire. Hübbe-Schleiden's embrace of Darwinian metaphors, however, did not mean that he saw imperial expansion as a death struggle between Germans or Aryans, on the one hand, and Mongols and Negroes on the other. Echoing the convoluted justifications offered by "new imperialists" all over Europe, for instance, Hübbe-Schleiden in 1883 had seen his colonial activities as part of a "civilizing mission."[30] Once he converted to Theosophy, moreover, he continued to invoke the concept of race, but he now used it in a Theosophical sense that emphasized the spiritual unity of all races.

Another conceptual continuity between Hübbe-Schleiden's brand of Theosophy and the colonialist milieu concerned his frequent invocation of *Weltpolitik* (world policy), which by 1914 was a buzzword in Germany. Popularized by Bernhard von Bülow in the late 1890s, Weltpolitik has usually been taken to be a foreign policy promoting German trade and industry abroad, a policy that had such concrete projects as building up the German navy and reducing tariffs to encourage trade.[31] Although Weltpolitik has most often been seen as an illiberal ploy to stall democratic reform on the home front, it was not only this.[32] Like most buzzwords, *Weltpolitik* meant different things to different people, and in a revealing speech Hübbe-Schleiden gave on the eve of World War I, he defined what the term meant for him. Calling Theosophy's cultural mission Weltpolitik, he explained that this was not a program of German economic expansion abroad but rather a project of human spiritual expansion that would result in the building of a new world culture, religion, and race. Weltpolitik, he promised, would bring about a new stage of human cultural evolution in which the shameful economic gap between rich and poor would disappear. Weltpolitik, he said, would bring about an age of universal brotherhood, in which all the living human races—the more evolved Aryan as well as the less-evolved Negro and Mongol races—would learn to work together in a much more united and spiritually sophisticated civilization.[33]

In his effort to promote the transcendent worldview, the Theosophical cause of universal brotherhood, and his own peculiar brand of Weltpolitik, Hübbe-Schleiden also believed that he had a special mission to fulfill, a mission that both linked him to and divided him from his colonial past. Reflecting back on his life in 1911, he noted that his major task had been to expand Germany's horizons: "[A] hundred times more important than the economic horizon is the expansion of the psychical horizon. Theosophy cannot help, however, unless people are given scientific evidence that their individual consciousness lives after death. This terribly dry task of scientific proof has fallen to me."[34] If the constant element in his activities as both colonialist and Theosophist had been the expansion of horizons, what was new after his conversion in 1884 was what kind of horizon he aimed to expand, and by what means.

As a colonialist, he had sought to expand Germany's economic horizon through propagandistic writing; now, as a Theosophist, he sought to expand what he called Germany's "psychical horizon" through the establishment of "scientific proof." Hübbe-Schleiden had received word of his special scientific mission just a few weeks after his conversion in 1884, in fact, when he had been contacted by a "Mahatma," or mysterious spiritual teacher, via an envelope that materialized out of thin air while he sat on a train bound for Dresden. The mysterious envelope turned out to contain a letter from a Mahatma named Koot Hoomi, who informed Hübbe-Schleiden that his life's task was to give the spiritual teachings of Theosophy a scientific grounding,[35] or as Hübbe-Schleiden put it in a public speech several years later, to convince Germans that "Theosophy is the scientific practice of religion."[36]

Making the transcendent worldview "scientific" and therefore acceptable to modern-minded Germans became Hübbe-Schleiden's obsession from this point in 1884 until his death in 1916. We can thank Rudolf Steiner, the founder and leader of the Anthroposophical Society, for a particularly vivid description of just what Hübbe-Schleiden's scientific mission turned out to mean in practice. When Steiner went to visit Hübbe-Schleiden in his home around 1900, he found his host's apartment full of elaborate wire contraptions. On closer inspection, it turned out that these contraptions were model chains of molecules in their physical and transcendent configurations. The wire models, in other words, were one of Hübbe-Schleiden's more graphic ways of offering scientific proof with which to persuade Germans to accept Theosophy and its message of transcendent reality and universal brotherhood.[37]

What are we to make of Hübbe-Schleiden's colorful life, first as a colonial propagandist and then as a Theosophical leader? How are we to understand his shift from advocating empire to advocating the transcendent, from producing savvy propaganda for overseas expansion to purportedly receiving letters out of thin air on trains and building elaborate molecular models on his apartment floor, from describing Africans as utterly uncivilized in 1875 to articulating his vision of a Theosophical Weltpolitik dedicated to bringing all the world's races together in a higher civilization in 1914?[38] The complexities of Hübbe-Schleiden's life and the lacunas of the historical record preclude easy answers, but certain conclusions seem clear. In the first place, Hübbe-Schleiden's life points to the larger context within which Germans embraced Theosophical occultism. His simultaneous advocacy of Theosophical Weltpolitik and universal brotherhood, indeed, suggest that he was neither a proto-Nazi nor an old-fashioned conservative dedicated to maintaining an undemocratic status quo at home and building a strong German presence abroad. He emerges, rather, as a politically ambiguous reformer repackaging traditional liberal themes, including a deep faith in progress and the underlying kinship of all the world's peoples, in spiritual terms.

What is particularly striking about his activities before and after 1884, moreover, is their modern-mindedness. Hübbe-Schleiden was particularly forward-looking in the tools he chose to accomplish his missions, whether colonialist or Theosophical, from his pioneering use of Darwinian language to his embrace of Theosophy and its peculiar brand of "scientific religion." This, then, suggests a final conclusion, which is that the best way to solve the historical puzzle of Hübbe-Schleiden is to invoke, once again, the concept of modernism. What other concept could possibly encompass Hübbe-Schleiden's crusading youth dedicated to addressing social and political questions in a new way, his lifelong embrace of a dizzying array of reformist causes and tools, his hopscotching from one knowledge realm to another, and finally, his turn to the pursuit of a "scientific religion" grounded on the investigation of occult phenomena? Seen in this way, Hübbe-Schleiden's life gives us insight into the politically complex byways through which the occult modernism of the fin de siècle emerged in Germany.

Cults of the Self

In June 1914, as nationalist sentiments presaging the outbreak of war rose across Europe, German Theosophists reaffirmed their commitment to internationalism by electing the Dutchman J. L. M. Lauweriks as their general secretary.[39] Even when war became official in August and the dream of universal brotherhood threatened to crumble into the realities of international strife, many Theosophists still made valiant attempts to salvage the original goal of their movement. Hübbe-Schleiden, for instance, hoped in November that the war would force Theosophists to pursue universal brotherhood in a new way. No longer able to work on the international stage, Hübbe-Schleiden speculated, German Theosophists would now have to find ways to induce their compatriots to reject petty nationalism and embrace "world civilization" *(Weltkultur)* instead.[40]

By 1914, however, the war was not the only force working against the original Theosophical goal of universal brotherhood. Yet another was what the popular German philosopher Hermann Keyserling called "the increasing tendency of all advanced people to be their own saviors."[41] Made in reference to the international Theosophical movement, Keyserling's shrewd insight into the *Zeitgeist* emphasized the fact that while Hübbe-Schleiden and other Theosophical leaders worked to realize the dream of universal brotherhood, others had flocked to Theosophy for quite different reasons. These men and women did not reject the original goal of universal brotherhood, at least not consciously or explicitly, but they did elevate the Theosophical directive to cultivate one's own occult powers into an end in itself. In the process, they gave the Theosophical movement in particular and the larger occult movement in general a novel emphasis on personal experience, an emphasis that amounted to a largely apolitical cult of the self.

The life of Franz Hartmann, an influential Theosophical leader with whom Hübbe-Schleiden worked closely, gives insight into the emergence of this form of self-focused Theosophy. Like many of his contemporaries, Hartmann had come to Theosophy after a youth dominated by restless seeking after spiritual goals that he could not define. For most of his childhood and youth in Bavaria, he recalled, the Roman Catholic Church had attracted him with its rituals and ceremonies but repelled him with its servile clergy, bigotry, and superstition. Science had offered an alternative pole for his allegiance and, although he found its blind materialism and loveless experts repellent, he had settled uneasily for its worldview nevertheless.[42] He carried this uncomfortable allegiance with him in 1865 to the United States, after a serendipitous encounter led him to assume the post of ship's physician on a vessel sailing for New York.[43]

In the United States, where he remained for the better part of two decades, Hartmann continued his restless spiritual search while indulging his oft-stated love of travel and adventure. Supporting himself as a doctor, he went first to various Christian sects, but found that they left him cold, concerned as they were with the literal word of the Bible or abstract theories of salvation that referred more to the egotistical desires of the individual supplicant than to any concern with humanity as a whole. A year he spent living with a Jewish rabbi and his family, followed by a stay with various Indian tribes that introduced him to a more communal and hospitable form of existence, did not entice him sufficiently to end his wanderings.[44] American spiritualism, the great religious awakening that joined Christian concern about the afterlife to a raw experiential element bringing the faithful into direct contact with dead spirits, provided Hartmann with his first tantalizing taste of nineteenth-century occultism.[45]

Perhaps it was his contradictory commitment to science, on the one hand, and his compulsion toward spiritual experimentation, on the other, that soon landed him at a life-changing public lecture in New Orleans. Combining rational discourse and professorial authority with a rejection of scientific materialism, this lecture was given by a Professor Peebles, whose sober explanations for the occult phenomena Hartmann had witnessed at a séance a few days before finally gave him the confidence to reject the materialistic teachings that he had so reluctantly accepted in his youth.[46] Hartmann now dedicated himself to experimenting with mediums and cultivating his own, limited, mediumistic talents.[47]

The reality of the occult world became an article of everyday knowledge for him, as his actions over the next few years testified. In Colorado, for instance, he lost a great deal of money by following the advice of clairvoyants who told him where to dig for gold. On the other hand, consultation with "a spiritual power" resulted in the alleviation of an unspecified problem he had acquired in his childhood through the "evil practice" of vaccination. Contact with a talented medium in Denver made materialized spirits a daily part of his existence and resulted in Hartmann himself levitating in air. Nevertheless, in spite of the fact that the occult had become a part of Hartmann's everyday world and informed his most important actions and significant experiences, he confessed to the feeling that something was still lacking. As he later described this situation: "I was, and am of course still, a believer in these phenomena, for I cannot 'unknow' that which I have actually experienced and known as well as any other fact in my daily life. . . . [B]ut my experience[s] . . . had already taught me that these phenomena were probably not always caused by the spirits of departed human beings, and that they surely often originated in occult but intelligent forces or powers at present unknown to us. My desire was to know the cause of such things."

Like many of his contemporaries, Hartmann felt pulled between two poles of knowledge: subjective knowledge based on personal experience, and objective knowledge based on the scientific elucidation of natural causes. Mediums presented him with his access point to that ultimate reality he had long desired to reach, but the spiritualist explanation that posited dead spirits as causal agents left him intellectually dissatisfied. In this state of skeptical crisis, a copy of the *Theosophist* fell into his hands. Edited by Blavatsky, this journal introduced him to the basic tenets of Theosophy, which came to him "like a revelation" and awoke in him a deep desire to make contact with Blavatsky and the spiritual masters whose pupil and messenger she claimed to be.[48] A letter expressing this desire was followed by an anxious wait, which soon ended with the arrival of a reply from Olcott and Blavatsky that, on behalf of the Masters, invited Hartmann to come to India to collaborate with them in the Theosophical project. He sailed for India soon thereafter.[49]

Initially at the Adyar headquarters and then in the Theosophical movement more generally, Hartmann finally found what he had long sought for in vain: personal spiritual experience ensconced in an intellectually satisfying framework. Sittings with Blavatsky became occasions not for communion with dead spirits from the beyond but for profoundly moving encounters with living teachers in the here and now. As he recalled in one of his many autobiographical publications, he had once sat with Blavatsky while she conversed with a Master. Although he himself was unable to see the Master and therefore had to rely on Blavatsky for full account of the conversation, Hartmann nevertheless experienced this mediated presence as a powerful stimulus to spiritual consciousness, recalling later that the Master's "influence pervaded my whole being and filled me with a sensation of indescribable bliss which lasted for several days."[50]

Hartmann's emphasis on the importance of personal occult experiences also showed up in his frequently expressed hostility to so-called spiritual authorities. Echoing Keyserling's astute observation about the spiritual anarchism of the modern age, Hartmann wrote in his memoirs that "[e]ach man has his guru and his savior in himself, and an external leader serves only to show the way by which to find this inner guru."[51] This strongly held opinion seemed contradictory, given his acceptance of Blavatsky and the spiritual message she claimed to channel, but in at least one important sense his insistence on individual salvation was itself an expression of Hartmann's attitude toward Blavatsky's importance within the movement. Admitting that Blavatsky may on occasion have produced occult phenomena not through her own mediumship but through conscious fraud, Hartmann nevertheless directed Theosophists to focus on her purpose, which was "to induce the people to study the higher laws of life, to raise them up to a higher conception of eternal truth, and teach them to do their own thinking."[52]

Nor did Hartmann ever shy away, as Hübbe-Schleiden did, from making his private occult experiences—no matter how strange—public. In numerous speeches given on the Theosophical lecture circuit, in countless books and articles, and as editor for the Theosophical periodical *Lotusblüthen* (Lotus blossoms, 1892–1900), Hartmann publicized his message of recovering occult reality and reawakening one's inner divinity. He also published numerous autobiographical works detailing his occult adventures around the world and several pieces of fantasy fiction featuring gnomes and other creatures from medieval fairy tales, all wielded to illustrate the complexities of Theosophical doctrine in simple narrative form.[53]

At times, Hartmann echoed Hübbe-Schleiden's laments about those Theosophists who forgot that the overarching goal of Theosophy was universal brotherhood. In a particularly scathing reference to this tendency of some Theosophists to dwell excessively on the subgoals of comparative study and occult research, for example, Hartmann dismissed those who pursued the former as grasping for mere "multitudes of facts" *(Vielwisserei)* and the latter after mere enthusiasm *(Schwärmerei)*.[54] But in the end, whatever his ideological commitments, Hartmann's brand of openly expressed and self-focused occultism soon became dominant in the German Theosophical movement.

Occurring at multiple levels of the movement, this shift was embodied especially clearly in the prewar life of Rudolf Steiner, who devoted most of his adult years to developing an occult system suitable for incorporation into modern life, a project that mediated between the two strains of Theosophical occultism practiced by Hübbe-Schleiden and Hartmann.[55] Steiner's commitment to scientific method echoed Hübbe-Schleiden, while his frank dedication to convincing others of the reality of the spiritual world by helping them experience it within themselves echoed Hartmann. Mediation, in fact, was an important theme of Steiner's life.

From earliest childhood, Steiner had been a person who delighted in intersections, geographical as well as intellectual and psychological, where normally separate spheres of modern life met and overlapped. Born in the small Austrian town of Mödling to a father who worked as a railway telegraphist and a mother about whom almost nothing is known, Steiner grew up in a home that provided a forum through which the world of the large city of Vienna paraded, profoundly impressing the young Steiner in the process. His first knowledge of German literature, a field he would later work in extensively, for instance, came from conversations he had with a well-read physician who used to come by train from Wiener-Neustadt every few days to treat patients in Mödling. After finishing his consultations, this doctor would visit with Steiner's family and often speak with the boy about his love of literature while waiting for a train back to the city. Just as the train connected Steiner to the larger world outside his home, his educational trajectory also reflected his status as a figure who moved comfortably between different worlds. His father, a freethinker, instilled in him the importance of independent thought and a technical-scientific education. Onto this Steiner from a very early age grafted an active interest in philosophy and the arts, particularly music. Sent by his parents to a vocational high school and then to the technical university in Vienna, where he enrolled in courses for mathematics, natural history, and chemistry, Steiner supplemented his scientific studies with philosophical ones. While still in high school, for instance, Steiner read Kant and Hegel. He continued such studies at the university in Vienna, where he attended lectures on philosophy given by Franz Clemens Brentano and others.[56]

His simultaneous pursuit of the natural sciences and philosophy, especially metaphysics, stemmed from Steiner's struggle to come to terms with what he later called "my perception of the spiritual world." His first exposure as a schoolboy to geometry proved immensely significant in this regard, since it legitimated, for the first time, his own experience of the reality of the unseen. Adept at the course of scientific studies into which his father guided him, Steiner nevertheless felt pulled first to philosophy and then to the arts because these disciplines seemed to offer him a bridge between his own experiences of the spiritual world and his academic knowledge of the natural one. Reflecting on this double pursuit at the technical university in Vienna, for instance, Steiner wrote:

> I had to study mathematics and natural science. I was convinced that I should find no relationship between these and myself unless I could place under them a solid foundation of philosophy. But I perceived a spiritual world, none the less, as a reality. In clear vision the spiritual individuality of every one revealed itself to me. This found in the physical body and in action in the physical world merely its manifestation. It united itself with that which came down as a physical germ from the spiritual world. Dead men I followed farther on their way in the spiritual world.

More forthright at other times and in other venues, Steiner hinted in this passage at his own faculty of clairvoyance, something he and his followers eventually came to accept as a fact.[57]

Steiner's evolving relationship with his own psychic faculties and the spiritual world did not prevent him from pursuing a varied intellectual career in the 1880s and 1890s, a career that helped him transform his private "perception of the spiritual world" into a public vocation. In Vienna in the 1880s, he developed contacts with various literary, progressive, and mystical groups. The circle of the feminist and Theosophist Marie Lang, for instance, which attracted artists, literati, and social reformers, also took in Steiner. It was here that Steiner first met Franz Hartmann, who had introduced Lang to Theosophy. Vienna also contained the mystical circle around Friedrich Eckstein, whose knowledge of ancient esoteric texts Steiner found impressive but whose insistence on keeping his knowledge secret Steiner found repellent. It was against Eckstein's emphasis on keeping esoteric texts esoteric, in fact, that Steiner began to articulate his vocation for "a public activity on behalf of spiritual knowledge" that would bring heretofore hidden knowledge of spiritual reality out into the public sphere. His first break into the intellectual milieu of Imperial Germany came in 1884 when, partially on the basis of Steiner's scientific training, Joseph Kürschner hired him as editor for a new printing of Goethe's scientific works that was to be included as part of Kürschner's series Deutsche-National-Literatur (German national literature). After completing this project, Steiner submitted a dissertation to Heinrich von Stein, a philosopher of Christian Platonism at the university in Rostock, and received a doctorate in philosophy. Moving to Berlin, Steiner continued to pursue his attempt to give voice to the inner life of the spirit and earned a living as editor of the Berlin literary journal *Magazin für Literatur,* which was then an organ of the Freie literarische Gesell-schaft (Free literary society). Powerfully attracted to artists like the Naturalist Otto Erich Hartleben, in whose literary circle he took part, Steiner was none-theless disappointed to find that artists' creative energies were not directed to the same ends as his spiritual strivings.[58]

Despite his misgivings about the literary milieu in which he now moved, Steiner managed to use his position as editor of *Magazin*—a post he assumed in 1897—to experiment with revealing his own occult experiences. One of these, an 1899 article on Goethe that gave "public expression" to "the esoteric from my own inner experience," resulted in an invitation to deliver a lecture on Nietzsche at the home of the famous Berlin Theosophists Cay and Sophie von Brockdorff. In a veiled reference to his penchant for expressing himself, either in written or spoken form, while in clairvoyant states, Steiner later wrote that this speech had great personal significance for him since it allowed him, per-haps for the first time, "to speak in words coined from the world of spirit."[59]

With this debut as a speaker on the Theosophical lecture circuit, Steiner quickly made a name for himself in German Theosophical circles. By 1902, he had become general secretary of the German section of the Theosophi-cal Society, an office he used as a forum for launching his effort to address the pressing spiritual needs of the modern age. As he explained in a 1904 book, these were intimately linked to the success of nineteenth-century science, which had raised profound questions of meaning answerable only by reference to the spiritual world. When individuals attained knowledge of this occult world, he promised, they would discover within themselves the capacity to function more effectively in the practical sphere of modern life.[60]

As the tenor of these comments suggests, Steiner's ultimate commitment was not to the brotherhood of humanity but the cultivation of individuals. An exchange between Steiner and his pupil Eliza von Moltke, the wife of a famous general, Helmuth von Moltke, gives a sense of how this worked in practice. In a 1904 letter, Moltke begged Steiner to send her instructions on how to work on herself in order to be able to help humanity. Leaving aside the question of how to help humanity, Steiner sent back a personalized exercise plan, with an accompanying note implying that these instructions came not from him but from higher powers (presumably the Great White Brotherhood) utilizing him as a vehicle of communication.[61]

The nature of these "exercises" was made clear in a letter Steiner sent to another pupil, a science teacher named Hans Wohlbold, to whom Steiner explained that the purpose of his exercises was to train the mind to perceive spiritual reality directly.[62] In order to sharpen and extend his pupil's imaginative capacities, Steiner recommended that each evening Wohlbold mentally replay his day, from the most recent moment first, then back to the preceding evening. He also suggested that Wohlbold practice concentrating mentally on a short phrase and then dropping the content of the phrase from consciousness while still maintaining the mental energy formerly concentrated on the thought.[63] Although modern readers may discern nothing particularly occult in these mental exercises, Steiner and his pupils did. To them, such exercises revealed the world of pure spirit that lay occluded behind the visible world of everyday life.

Steiner took this commitment to personal development via occult means and many of his Theosophical followers with him in 1912–13 when he finally broke with the group that had nurtured him. In its stead, he founded the Anthroposophical Society. Dedicated to cultivating knowledge of man's true being, the group focused not on "wisdom of God" but rather on "wisdom of man."[64] Committed above all to his project of bringing the occult knowledge of the spiritual world into modern everyday life, Steiner now explicitly rejected those who used their clairvoyant faculties while in an unconscious state. Perception of the spiritual world, he insisted, was something that modern men and women had to learn to integrate into waking consciousness. His desire to establish a seamless link between the occult and the everyday represented a decisive break with nineteenth-century spiritualism and its focus on the trance personality of mediums. It also broke with the original Theosophical program of bending the occult to the progressive enlightenment of humanity and the achievement of universal brotherhood. For Steiner, the occult was still a pathway to enlightenment, but its dominant tenor was individualist, not universalist. The occult now became a matter of personal will and conscious expression.

These trends away from an old emphasis on universalism to a new focus on individualism did not go unremarked or indeed uncriticized by other Theosophists. In a letter to a friend written in 1911, for instance, Hübbe-Schleiden bewailed Steiner's following among German Theosophists, implying that Steiner's teachings were nothing more than subjective occultism. Against this tendency, Hübbe-Schleiden reiterated his commitment to occultism based both on "authentic science and philosophy" and on public agreement among suitably trained researchers about the authenticity of the phenomena in question.[65] In a series of letters written to Steiner that same year, Hübbe-Schleiden stated (not quite honestly) that what had drawn him to the Theosophical Society in the first place in 1884 was not the occult but rather the project of universal brotherhood, implying that Steiner needed to return to Theosophical basics.[66]

Such complaints, however, did little to curtail the rising Theosophical tide of self-focused occultism. At a 1912 meeting hosted by the appropriately named Internationale Theosophische Verbrüderung (International Theosophical brotherhood), for instance, lectures featuring personal development dominated the program. These included talks with titles like "Barriers to Self-Knowledge" and "The Meaning of Art for the Life of the Spirit."[67] Businesses and commercial clearing houses also enthusiastically exploited the Theosophical cult of the self for profit. A good example of this was the Zentrale für praktischen Okkultismus (Center for practical occultism), which took "know thyself" (*"Erkenne dich selbst"*) as its slogan in the 1920s. Sporting the common Theosophical symbol of the sphinx, its promotional brochure offered advice about the occult path to self-enlightenment. Divided into departments of astrology, chiromancy, graphology, geomancy, dream interpretation, and so on, the flyer urged potential customers to send in their photos, samples of handwriting, dream descriptions, and questionnaires along with a fee ranging from 1 mark to 300 marks. In return, customers would receive an expert reading to help them on their way toward occult self-knowledge.[68] Self-development of the Theosophical variety also found a home, finally, in the many experimental colonies that sprang up in Central Europe at the fin de siècle. Most famous among these was Monte Verità, near Ascona, Switzerland, where such famous modernists as Hermann Hesse, Oskar Maria Graf, D. H. Lawrence, Franz Kafka, and Isadora Duncan rubbed shoulders with representatives of the German-speaking world, including the Theosophist Theodor Reuss, the anarchists Raphael Friedeberg and Ernst Frick, the feminist Franziska zu Reventlow, and the psychologist (and psychical researcher) Carl Gustav Jung.[69] Theosophy's cult of the self, in short, had become perfectly attuned to modern times.

Aryan Permutations

At a speech given in 1925, the Theosophical leader Hermann Rudolph took as his theme a phrase that captured the two facets of his movement's program. "The Theosophical brotherhood is the realization of divine self-knowledge," he announced.[70] Candidates for membership in the coming "sixth root race," he reminded his audience, were to be found among all the peoples of the world. Exhorting his listeners to weed out prejudice in all its forms, Rudolph warned that those who perpetuated acts of hate against others would be reborn as members of the group they had attacked. Those, in contrast, who worked in good conscience on the goal of universal brotherhood could look forward to the dawn of a new state, one in which individual freedoms would be guarded, political parties no longer needed, a constant peace assured, and the social welfare of all guaranteed.[71] Rudolph's ecumenical and utopian rendition of the Theosophical program contrasted sharply with the words of his contemporary Karl Kern, who insisted instead that "God is purified race!"[72] Coming from a member of the Theosophically influenced movement known as Ariosophy, Kern's statement neatly captured the völkisch variant of German Theosophical thinking.

At a basic level, there should be nothing surprising about such links between Theosophy and the völkisch milieu, given the similar conditions in which both movements were born. With roots in the 1880s, both belonged to the experimental field of fin-de-siècle modernism and overlapped significantly with the Lebensreform movement. Tapping the spiritual dissatisfactions of their age, both attracted followers hungry for a new kind of religiosity and proved adept at exploiting the new technologies of mass communication to spread their message. Both, finally, tapped the imaginative powers of the occult to articulate an "alternative modernity."[73]

And yet, just as it would be a mistake to ignore the overlap between Theosophy and the völkisch movement, one must also be careful not to stretch the links between these two movements too far. Only eight groups in Germany practiced the völkisch variant of Theosophical occultism known as Ariosophy, whereas more than fifty larger groups belonged to mainstream Theosophy.[74] Nor, despite their overlaps, were the two movements identical. Indeed, as the examples of Rudolph and Kern indicate, one of their most basic differences was ideological. Whereas Theosophy sought to build a new religion appropriate to all of humanity, the völkisch movement had no such universalist aim. It sought instead to fashion a race-specific religion that would speak to the spiritual needs of "Ario-Germans" exclusively. Racism and anti-Semitism, in other words, grounded the völkisch worldview in a way that had never applied to Theosophy.[75]

This is not to say that considerations of race played no role in German Theosophy: race did in fact matter to the movement. Theosophy aimed, after all, to bring the so-called "sixth root race" into existence, and its cosmology invoked a complicated hierarchy of racial development to explain the trajectory of human history. Drawing on the popularity of Social Darwinian thought, Theosophical doctrine mixed biological and spiritual notions of race in an often incoherent manner. Theosophists could insist that the race to which one belonged had primarily to do with one's degree of spiritual maturity, yet at the same time claim that such biologically understood "races" as the North Indian Aryans had achieved a particularly high degree of spiritual maturity.[76] Considerations of race, moreover, could enter the Theosophical milieu in other guises. Rudolf Steiner, for instance, often claimed that white Europeans had achieved a higher level of spiritual perfection than the African, Asian, or Jewish races. Sometimes, he even went so far as to claim that in the grand cycle of spiritual evolution, the Germanic race had advanced the furthest. At other times and with comparable frequency, however, Steiner reiterated the core spiritual unity of all the world's peoples.[77] Racism could even on occasion tinge the German Theosophical movement more directly. In a private letter that Hübbe-Schleiden wrote in 1902, for example, he dismissed an aspiring Theosophical leader as nothing more than a "Berlin Jew."[78] As unpalatable

as modern readers may find such anti-Semitic remarks, however, it is important to remember that this was a relatively mild statement for the times, and
one that Hübbe-Schleiden did not voice in public gatherings. Although concepts of race and certain forms of prejudice were undeniably to be found in the
mainstream German Theosophical movement, in no way, in short, were racism or anti-Semitism enshrined at the movement's ideological core.

Ariosophists, however, the most important exemplars of Theosophical occultism in the völkisch mode, exhibited no such ambivalence about race.
Ideologically, their movement rested on the thinking and writing of the Austrian Guido von List, who had made a name for himself in the 1870s as a writer
of fantasy novels about a glorious Teutonic past. In 1902, when his interests
turned toward mystical and occult topics, he began to read key Theosophical
works and study ancient Germanic runes and languages. Relying in part on a
series of clairvoyant visions received at the supposed ruins of ancient Teutonic
battles, he began to imagine an elaborate German past complete with an
ancient religion called Wotanism. By 1908, his fantasies extended backwards to
a Teutonic past in which an Aryan priesthood presided over a racially homoge-
neous society, and forwards to an ideal future in which Germans would live
once more in a state of total race purity. Through publications and the founding of the Guido von List Society in 1908, he drew a following among völkisch
groups all over German-speaking Europe. The writings of his followers may
have introduced Adolf Hitler to new varieties of political racism. Even more
significantly, List's mixture of occultism, racism, and nationalism informed
the ideology of the Germanenorden (f. 1912) and its successor the Thule Society (f. 1918), where the German Workers' Party, the precursor to the National
Socialist Party, emerged in 1919.[79]

Such links between the Ariosophical milieu and early National Socialism
bring up the important question of just what Ariosophy and Theosophy did
and did not share, beginning at the most superficial level with the movements'
names. Coined in 1915 by Jörg Lanz von Liebenfels, one of List's most important followers, *Ariosophy* played on the term *Theosophy*. The changed root,
however, indicated an important difference: rather than invoking the Theosophical goal of achieving "wisdom of God," the term indicated the quite
different goal of achieving the "wisdom of Aryans."[80]

Similar overlaps in form but differences in purpose also manifested themselves in the role each movement assigned to the occult. In the preface to the
Handbuch der Ariosophie (Handbook of Ariosophy, 1931–32), for instance,

the publisher Herbert Reichstein noted Ariosophists' support for such occult practices as mind reading, clairvoyant vision, and prophecy.[81] Like their Theosophical cousins, moreover, Ariosophists were not above exploiting their occult talents for profit. Reichstein was typical in offering readers reasonably priced "Kabbalograms" that used numerological techniques to analyze personal names. Ranging in price from 5 to 20 marks, these "Kabbalograms," he claimed, would help customers answer such weighty questions as whom to marry or whether and when to have a child.[82] Ariosophy and Theosophy were also united in invoking the occult knowledge of spiritual masters. According to Ariosophical lore, occult knowledge belonged exclusively to an elite priesthood, a clear echo of the Theosophical concept of a Great White Brotherhood. But behind these similarities lay an important difference based in Ariosophists' rejection of the Theosophical interpretation of occult knowledge. Ariosophists invoked occult knowledge, it was true, but for very different ends. Whereas Theosophists believed that the main purpose of the Great White Brotherhood was to share its occult knowledge with humanity so as to promote spiritual enlightenment—all without regard to race, religion, or sex—no such universalism informed the Ariosophists' invocation of occult knowledge.[83] For Ariosophists, occult knowledge was a tool for erecting a racially pure and sexually divided social order.

Social affiliations between the two movements tell a similarly complex story. Typical was the Theosophist Max Seiling, whose membership in the Guido von List Society in no way curtailed his propensity to forage for spiritual wisdom without regard to racial considerations. When he published a book titled *Was soll ich? Weise Lebensregeln, mit einem Anhang: Gesundheitsregeln* (What should I do? Wise rules to live by), he included excerpts from Mark Twain, Martin Luther, the Jewish Talmud, Marcus Aurelius, and Richard Wagner.[84] Theosophists and Ariosophists, moreover, on occasion sought out the same spiritual gurus. Seiling, for instance, patronized the mystic Alois Mailänder, whose other disciples included Franz Hartmann and Wilhelm Hübbe-Schleiden, neither of whom belonged to the Ariosophical milieu.[85] Clearly, Theosophists and Ariosophists could at times move in the same social circles without bothering too much about their movements' ideological differences.

Such complexity also informed the important realm of occult publishing, where Theosophists and Ariosophists took direct cognizance of each other. When List's *Die Bilderschrift der Ario-Germanen* (The picture-writing of the Ario-Germans) appeared in 1910, Franz Hartmann praised it in his Theosophical periodical *Neue Lotusblüthen.*[86] The Theosophical publishing world also gave Lanz von Liebenfels some of his first public exposure in Germany. This came in 1907, when the Theosophist Paul Zillmann began to carry Lanz von Liebenfels's essays in his journal *Neue Metaphysische Rundschau*. When Zillmann joined the List Society a year later, observant contemporaries might have been tempted to conclude that Theosophy and Ariosophy were headed toward unification. But such a conclusion would have been premature: Zillmann managed to juggle his Theosophical and Ariosophical commitments for years without ever finding it necessary to choose one over the other. Throughout the time he built bridges to the Ariosophical milieu, in fact, he also ran a Theosophical lodge whose by-laws admitted members without regard to sex or religious background, so long as candidates willingly pledged themselves to the laws of the spirit and the love of humanity.[87]

The significance of the Theosophy-Ariosophy publishing links pales somewhat, in any case, when we realize that of the many dozen essays that Lanz von Liebenfels published in German journals over the course of his career, only five ever appeared in a mainstream occult journal.[88] That is not to say that Lanz von Liebenfels did not know his occult sciences; in fact, he regularly reviewed occult publications for völkisch journals like *Stein der Weisen* and was an adept astrologer to boot.[89] But even as one of the most prolific of Ariosophical authors, Lanz von Liebenfels still devoted only a minority of his writings to occult topics. Of 22 books, only 3 dealt with occult topics and then only loosely.[90] Similarly, of the approximately 100 pieces he submitted to the völkisch journal *Ostara*, only 2 covered occult themes.[91] Finally, of the nearly 140 essays he wrote for other journals, only 5 appeared in a mainstream occult journal (Zillmann's *Neue Metaphysische Rundschau*), and even fewer touched on occult questions explicitly.[92] The occult, in other words, accounted for a relatively minor portion of his publication record.

Despite these multiple links between Ariosophy and Theosophy, dedicated Ariosophists were anything but neutral about Theosophy and mainstream occultism. The völkisch ideologue Richard Ungewitter, for instance, blasted Theosophy and Anthroposophy for promoting Germans' spiritual subjugation. The Theosophical doctrine of "world religion" particularly irritated him because it drew attention away from what he regarded as basic truth: every race had a unique religion that was an expression of its own blood.[93] As Ungewitter's comment suggests, what ultimately set Ariosophists apart was their emphasis on the primary importance of race and blood, an emphasis that marked them as full participants in the völkisch milieu of their era. The Ariosophist Werner von Bülow made this clear when he observed that because God had done nothing for German soldiers as they lay dying on the front lines of World War I, the masses had turned their backs on the churches and were now embracing the "original sources . . . from which the currents of our blood gush."[94] Echoing Bülow, the preface to the 1931–32 *Handbuch der Ariosophie* expressed the hope that the volume would become crucial to "the future of our race."[95]

The links between Theosophy, Ariosophy, and the early völkisch movement, in short, are difficult to generalize from, pointing less toward direct causal connections than toward the immense cultural and political flexibility of Theosophical thinking in early twentieth-century Germany. Perhaps of greatest significance is the fact that völkisch groups that did make use of Theosophical concepts did not absorb the Theosophical cult of the self or the quest for universal brotherhood to any great degree. Rather, they appropriated Theosophy's invocation of an idealized past and cosmic scheme of racial evolution in order to underpin their developing interest in imagining a new social order based on racist and nationalist grounds.

In many ways, Ariosophy provides an excellent example of just how far afield nineteenth-century ideologies and institutions like Theosophy could migrate in the twentieth century. A fruitful comparison here might be made with eugenics. Conceived of by its founder Francis Galton in the 1880s as a project for voluntarily improving one's genetic stock through a contracted marriage, eugenics became an international movement attracting individuals and groups from all parts of the political spectrum. In Nazi Germany, eugenic thought mixed with state-sponsored racism and resulted in a radical eugenic program consisting of involuntary sterilization and outright murder of genetic "undesirables." But early twentieth-century Germany also housed less-extreme manifestations of eugenic thought, many of which followed the lines of Galton's voluntary eugenic program.[96] In any case, given the broad popularity of eugenic thought in early-twentieth-century Germany, it would be remarkable had there not been connections between it and völkisch circles of the time. A similar point applies to Theosophy, which belonged to this same cauldron of reformist thinking. Theosophy's political flexibility, indeed, echoes a major theme of the next chapter: the immense aesthetic possibilities of occult phenomena, which modernists learned so quickly to exploit to their own ends.

CHAPTER FIVE

The Creative Unconscious

As the painter Wassily Kandinsky struggled to articulate his plan for the radical reconstruction of modern art, he immersed himself in the classics of German occult literature. These included Karl Friedrich Zöllner's study "Transcendental Physics," Carl du Prel's *Studien aus dem Gebiete der Geheimwissenschaften* (Studies in the occult sciences), Alexander Aksakow's *Animismus und Spiritismus* (Animism and spiritualism), and issues of the Theosophical journal *Sphinx.*[1] By late 1911, when he published his manifesto *Über das Geistige in der Kunst* (Concerning the spiritual in art), Kandinsky had had a conceptual breakthrough. The new art, he wrote, must conform to "the spirit of the times" by offering something "less suited to the eye than to the soul."[2] Firmly renouncing the Renaissance ideal of art as a representation of nature, Kandinsky here articulated the revolutionary notion that artworks should refer not to the objective world of the five senses but to the mental world of subjective experience.

Contemplating this new art a decade or so later, the German psychiatrist Hans Prinzhorn noted its affinities to the art of his mentally ill patients: both renounced the outside world, denigrated surface appearance, and made "a decisive turn inward upon the self." Far from implying any criticism, either of the new art or the productions of his patients, Prinzhorn used these affinities to postulate the existence of a universal creative urge binding the most accomplished of contemporary artists to the most seriously ill of schizophrenics. This creative urge, he went on to suggest, typified an age in which the "craving for direct intuitive experience [combines] with a mystical self-deification and . . . concern with metaphysics, from the genuine philosophical to the sectarian and Theosophical."[3]

These comments by Kandinsky and Prinzhorn underscore the degree to which occult beliefs and practices permeated the aesthetic culture of modernism. Authors of the caliber of Rainer Maria Rilke and Gustav Meyrink drew on occult ideas and experiences to fuel their creative processes; others, like Thomas Mann and Franziska zu Reventlow, eschewed occult acts but often took occult topics as their subjects.[4] Early German films also tapped the creative possibilities of the occult. Robert Wiene's *The Cabinet of Dr. Caligari* (1919) featured the adventures of the somnambulist Cesare and his mysterious handler Dr. Caligari; Paul Wegener's *The Golem: How He Came into the World* (1920) introduced filmgoers to the story of a rabbi learned in astrology and cabala who used his occult knowledge to bring a man of clay to life; the classic vampire movie *Nosferatu* (1922) included two devoted occultists on its production crew (the director Friedrich Wilhelm Murnau, who regularly consulted astrologers and avidly read Theosophical texts, and the designer Albin Grau, who was a spiritualist).[5] Painters, too, found creative inspiration in the occult. Their ranks included Max Ernst, Piet Mondrian, Kazimir Malevich, Hilma af Klint, Arthur Dove, Theo van Doesburg, Paul Klee, Hans Arp, Jackson Pollock, and, of course, Kandinsky.[6]

Although scholars have long noted the affinities these aesthetic pioneers felt for the occult, historians have been strangely reluctant to make this fact the focus of systematic investigation. How did these affinities develop and why did they persist? How deep did they reach, and what results did they yield? If Kandinsky's demand in 1911 that the new art speak to the soul drew heavily on fin-de-siècle German Theosophy and its deeply psychological understanding of a spiritual reality that lay beyond the reach of the five senses, Prinzhorn's observations a decade later made contemporary art, whether produced by Kandinsky in his studio or a schizophrenic in an asylum, an outgrowth of a Zeitgeist in which the psychological experiences and metaphysical concerns so common in occult circles occupied a dominant place. Taken together, these comments point to an underexplored process of exchange between art and the occult that reached well beyond the strict boundaries of the canonical modernists mentioned above. An examination of the forgotten history of the art-occult interface reveals that the occult sciences and the new aesthetic were but two facets of a single phenomenon: the emergence of a modernist sensibility defined by the primacy of—as Prinzhorn put it—"intuitive experience."

Munich Modern

The relationship between the occult and this modernist sensibility dated back at least to the mid-1880s and the founding of Germany's first major psychical research circle, the Psychologische Gesellschaft. Immediately linking art and the occult, the group's 1887 manifesto boldly announced that mediums would revolutionize the practice of art. Painters in particular would find that mediums made ideal models, for unlike traditional models who assumed their poses in a waking state, the mediums worked in a trance that artists could easily manipulate to produce gestures and expressions of unprecedented emotional depth and authenticity.[7] Artists, the manifesto implied, would find that the Psychologische Gesellschaft offered a unique venue in which to apply the new experimental psychology to the realistic treatment of psychological themes and topics in their work.

This promise proved immensely appealing to Munich's aesthetic vanguard, many of whose members joined the group.[8] One was the art curator Adolf Bayersdorfer, a founding member of the Psychologische Gesellschaft and a lifelong crusader against the city's conservative cultural forces. In the 1870s he had courageously supported a local exhibition of paintings by Gustave Courbet, a modernist forerunner whose vocal anticlericalism and suspected socialism made him a frequent target of criticism; Bayersdorfer went on to articulate the case for establishing the Munich Secession two decades later.[9] The Psychologische Gesellschaft's founding members also included the painters Gabriel von Max, who enjoyed recognition among fin-de-siècle art critics as an aesthetic pioneer equal in rank to Arnold Böcklin,[10] and Albert von Keller, who had won several prestigious art prizes and an honorary appointment to the Akademie der Bildenden Künste (Academy of fine arts) in Munich before joining the Munich Secession in 1892 and serving as its president from 1906 to 1920.[11] That these men epitomized the *Münchner Moderne* (Munich modern) was beyond doubt, for their interests, both aesthetic and occult, earned them the vocal wrath of local Roman Catholic authorities fulminating against the degenerative forces of modernity at work in their beloved city. Using their position in the Bavarian state legislature, these Catholic critics railed against Max and Keller as "decadent" and "pornographic" representatives of the modern spirit. The philosopher Theodor Lipps, who served as president of the Psychologische Gesellschaft at the turn of the century and whose aesthetic theories would soon influence Kandinsky, also came in for attack from these quarters as "irreligious" and "subversive."[12]

Just as the artistically oriented members of the Psychologische Gesellschaft embodied the modern spirit then beginning to permeate Munich, so, too, did their turn to psychical research sound emerging modernist themes. Take the case of the painter Gabriel von Max. Although brought up a Catholic, Max had little patience for contemporary Christian practice, which he once called "the purest swindle and fraud."[13] Not content to let his spiritual life slide, however, Max became a serious student of Buddhism, a founding member of Germany's first Theosophical group, and a participant in a wide variety of reformist causes, including pacifism.[14] A close friend of Ernst Haeckel, he embraced Darwinism and set himself up as an amateur anthropologist, going so far as to keep a troop of monkeys for companionship and observation in his home.[15] Disgusted with contemporary Christianity yet still a spiritual seeker, enamored of modern science yet critical of scientific materialism, Max shared the common ambivalence that occultists felt about science and spirituality. As an artist, he translated this ambivalence and its accompaniment, a fascination with the transcendent, into visual form by dedicating himself, as one contemporary put it, to painting "the foundation of the beyond, the overcoming of death, [and] the secrets of religious fanaticism displayed by female seers, the possessed, [and] martyrs."[16] Max, in other words, produced work after work featuring the psychology of extreme female spiritual experience: in 1875, he painted a dead girl being revived by Jesus;[17] in 1879, he portrayed a young woman being touched on the shoulder by a spirit from the beyond;[18] by the mid-1880s, he had rendered the ecstatic visions of the German nun Anna Katharina Emmerich[19] and the clairvoyant states of the seeress of Prevorst (Friederike Hauffe);[20] by the time he died, he had even painted a portrait of Kathie King, the control spirit of the English medium Florence Cook.[21] Not content merely to imagine what such scenes *might* have looked like, Max insisted on studying what they *had* looked like. Just as he had wheedled his way into the dissecting rooms of Viennese hospitals as an art student in order to examine corpses, as a mature artist he sought ways to bring a similarly realist eye to such topics as the

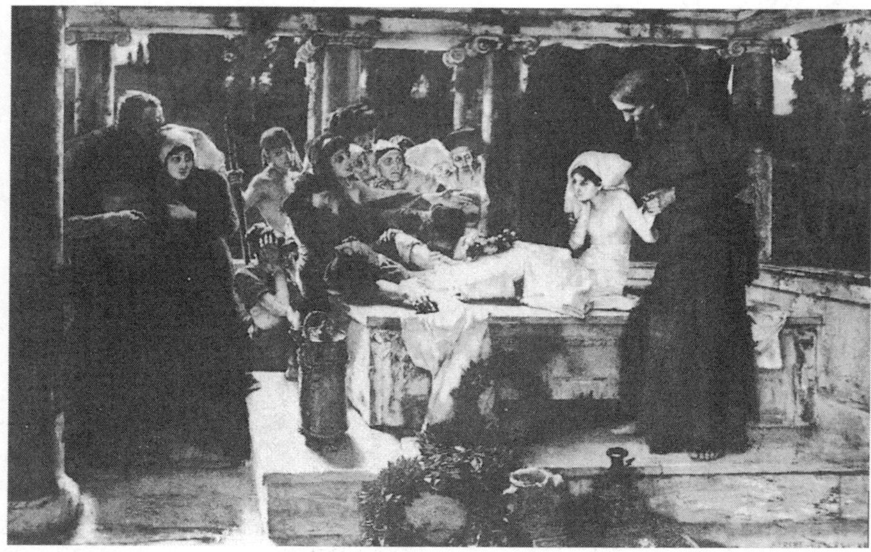

Figure 3. Albert von Keller, *Auferweckung der Tochter Jairi* (Revival of Jairus's daughter; 1886). Jesus brings a young woman back from death. Keller worked nearly a decade to get the facial expression and pose of the two central figures just right. His effort to portray this scene "realistically" precipitated his turn to the occult sciences in 1886. Keller's painting also featured in a famous psychical research experiment (see below). Oskar Müller, *Albert von Keller* (Munich: Karl Thiemig, 1981), p. 74. Owned by Staatsgemäldesammlungen (Munich).

experience of death and resurrection. The occult proved invaluable in this effort, for mediums, with whom he began to hold sittings in 1879, were nothing if not ideal models for the liminal experiences that so intrigued him.[22]

Max was by no means alone among the group's artists in seeking to exploit mediums for help in rendering extreme emotions and altered psychic states on his canvases. Although not a spiritual seeker like Max, Keller nonetheless shared Max's painterly interests in psychological realism. His first serious encounter with this challenge came while working on his painting *Auferweckung der Tochter Jairi* (Revival of Jairus's daughter, 1885; see fig. 3), which won a gold medal at the Berlin Jubilee Exhibition. The painting portrayed the resurrection of a young woman from death, while Christ the miracle worker stood on one side and an awe-struck crowd watched on the other. Numerous sketches and more than one hundred oil studies dating as far back as 1877 testified to how long and hard Keller had struggled to get the woman's facial expression just right.[23] Looking for ways to learn more about the human psyche and how it expressed such liminal experiences on the physical body, in 1886 Keller eagerly joined the Psychologische Gesellschaft.

As a key member of the group through the early twentieth century, Keller became deeply involved in exploring the interface of art and psychical research, hosting more than fifty séances in his home, using at least four mediums as models, and between 1885 and 1907 producing more than a dozen paintings involving scenes from psychical research.[24] One of his earliest experiments for the group took place in 1887, when he placed Lina Matzinger, the group's favorite medium, in front of a reproduction of his painting *Auferweckung* (see fig. 4). The idea behind these experiments was to use the painting as a suggestive object that would induce Matzinger to produce the facial

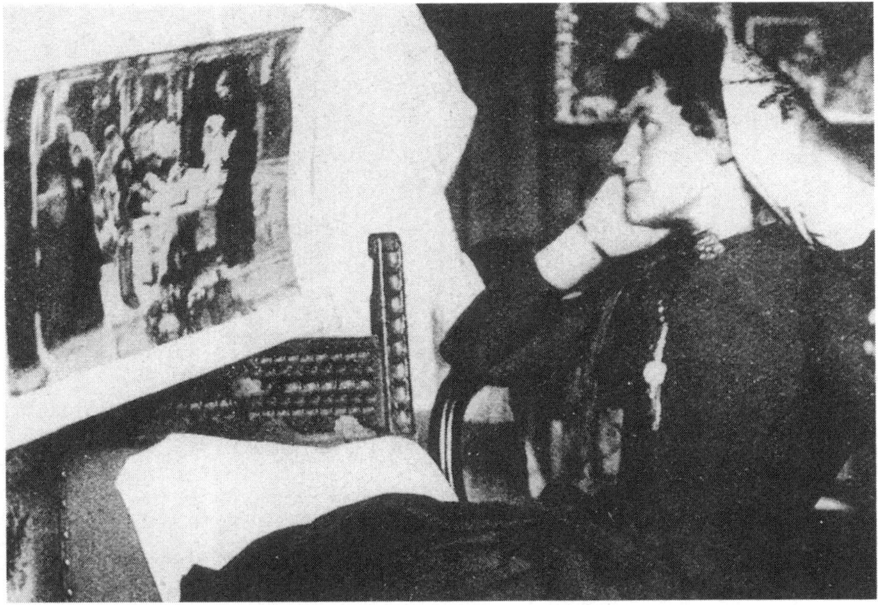

Figure 4. A psychical research experiment at Munich's Psychologische Gesellschaft (circa 1886). The hypnotized medium Lina Matzinger sits in front of Albert von Keller's painting of the revival of Jairus's daughter and reenacts the experiences of a woman returning from death. A camera mounted behind the canvas captures her pose and facial expression, which Keller then used as a basis for further artwork. Albert von Schrenck-Notzing, "Albert von Keller als Malerpsychologe und Metaphysiker," *Psychische Studien* 48 (April–May 1921): 199.

expressions and bodily gestures of a woman returning from death. A camera mounted just behind the copy of Keller's painting captured Matzinger's poses (a technique first invented by Max), and the resulting photograph then became the raw material for further paintings.[25]

These early experiments brought artistic results almost immediately. Keller's work *Die Somnambule* (The somnambulist) (1886–87) featured Matzinger in the pose of a cataleptic prophet. Another, *Spiritistischer Apport eines Bracelets* (Spiritualist transport of a bracelet) (1887), showed Matzinger dressed in Greek robes, pointing to bracelets she had mysteriously transported from elsewhere. Keller exhibited yet a third work, *Hexenverbrennung* (Witch burning), at Munich's Glass Palace in 1888 (see fig. 5).[26] Matzinger appeared in this painting as the model for a burning witch, and the smile on her face—an odd facial expression, given the fire at her feet—was the usual mysterious smile of a hypnotized medium. To produce this painting, Keller had translated the photographs taken of the hypnotized Matzinger, a woman suspended in that liminal state between waking and dreaming, into the painting of a burning witch, a woman suspended in the liminal state between life and death.

Keller and Max's interest in psychological liminality was a common theme among fin-de-siècle artists all over Central Europe. The most widely recognized explorer of this theme, Gustav Klimt, turned out work after work featuring females returning from the outer reaches of sexual ecstasy.[27] By the time Klimt began to go public with these interests in the 1890s, however, the artistic members of the Psychologische Gesellschaft had already been investigating psychological liminality for well over a decade. By conducting numerous experiments with occult phenomena, they had been among the first to tap an emerging modernist sensibility dedicated to exploring how the eruptions of unconscious drives, desires, and emotions played out on the surface of the human face and body.

Psychological liminality and its aesthetic potential, as it turned out, did not long remain the sole property of the group's male artists: female mediums soon threatened to burst their bounds as models and assume the mantle of aesthetic creativity for themselves. The most dramatic example of this inversion came in 1904, when the so-called "dream dancer" Madeleine Guipet arrived in Munich under the aegis of Albert von Schrenck-Notzing, then the motivating spirit of the Psychologische Gesellschaft. Schrenck-Notzing had invited the young bourgeois woman from Paris, where she was undergoing treatment for chronic headaches from the magnetist Emile Magnin. After

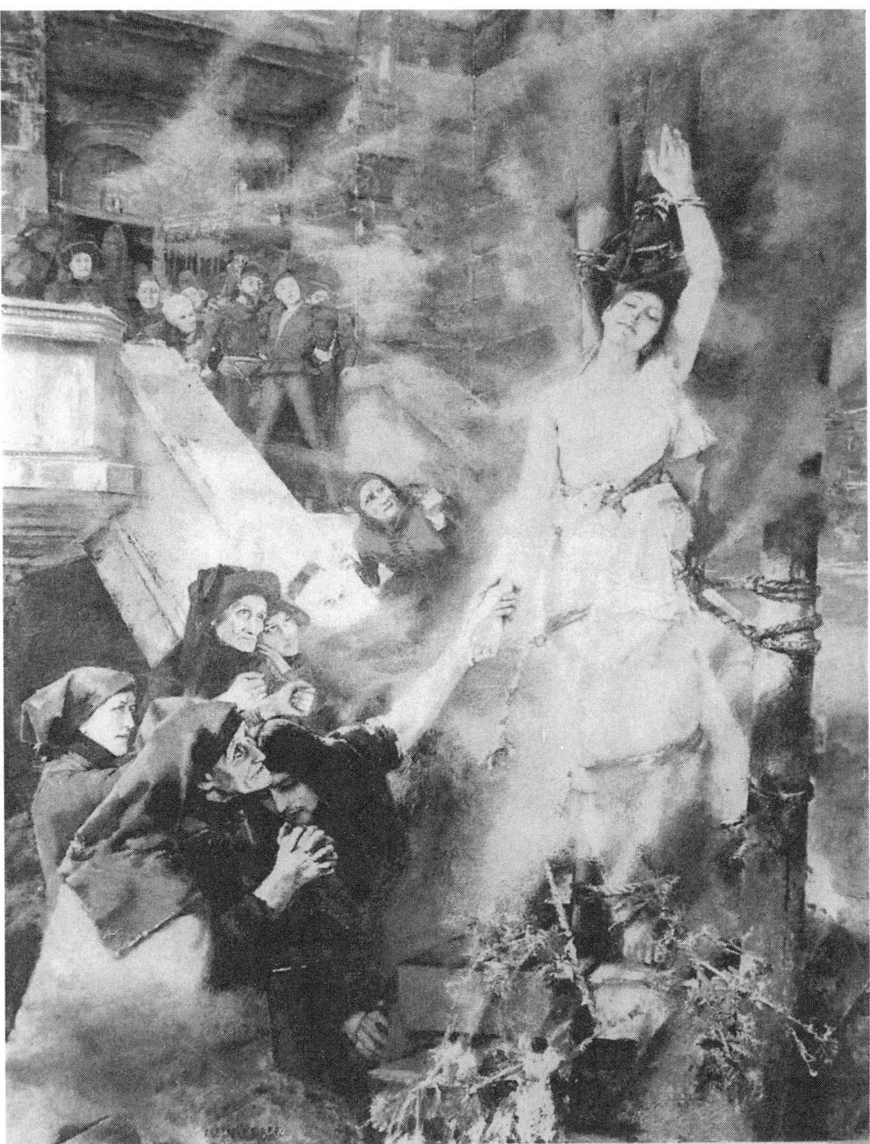

Figure 5. Albert von Keller, *Hexenverbrennung* (Witch burning) (1888).
Photographs taken of the hypnotized medium Lina Matzinger during psychical
research experiments at Munich's Psychologische Gesellschaft became the raw
material for this painting of a burning woman. Keller exhibited this painting at
Munich's Glaspalast in 1888. Oskar Müller, *Albert von Keller* (Munich: Karl Thiemig,
1981), p. 89. Destroyed during World War II.

quickly curing her complaint, Magnin discovered that by putting her under hypnosis and playing Chopin waltzes on the piano, he could induce Guipet to dance. This was a remarkable feat, for although Guipet came from a family of accomplished dancers, she herself had no formal dance training. Having speculated in 1902 that hypnosis might be used to facilitate artistic creativity, Schrenck-Notzing seized on the news of Magnin's discovery and eagerly invited Guipet to Munich for scientific investigation.[28]

Although she arrived as an object of scientific research, Guipet quickly became a public sensation. The first séance took place in Schrenck-Notzing's villa on the fashionable Max-Josef-Straße, where an audience of doctors, professors, and artists assembled. After introducing Guipet and her magnetist in a short preliminary lecture, Schrenck-Notzing put Guipet in a hypnotic state. Mozart sounded from the grand piano and, smiling the mysterious smile of a hypnotized medium, Guipet began to dance. A ruckus broke out immediately, as outraged audience members broke in to accuse Schrenck-Notzing of being a swindler. Guipet's dancing, they insisted, could only be the product of long study and practice and could not possibly be the dance of an unschooled, hypnotized woman. When these and similar charges appeared in the city papers, the uproar shifted into high gear.[29] As invitations poured in from clubs across Germany and Austria, Schrenck-Notzing and the men of the Psychologische Gesellschaft decided that the best course of action was to stage a series of public experiments featuring Guipet at a local theater. Although they were undoubtedly concerned to defend their scientific reputation, their decision to allow a full theatrical performance also showed just how permeable the boundaries between science and art, research and performance could be in an age of emerging mass culture. In the end, the Psychologische Gesellschaft procured Munich's Schauspielhaus, a newly built Jugendstil theater that then served as home to experimental theater in Germany, and to stage the production enlisted the help of several local cultural leaders, including Keller and the architect Gabriel von Seidl, who had just designed the Bavarian National Museum. Although hastily assembled, the three-day engagement was a huge success, with as many as five thousand people—among them three thousand doctors, artists, and scholars—flocking to see the show.[30]

A photograph of Guipet on stage at the Schauspielhaus documented just how far mediums had come since the 1887 manifesto extolling their virtues as models (see fig. 6). Whereas the manifesto had put mediums squarely at the service of artists, Guipet now put the investigators to work for herself, a power

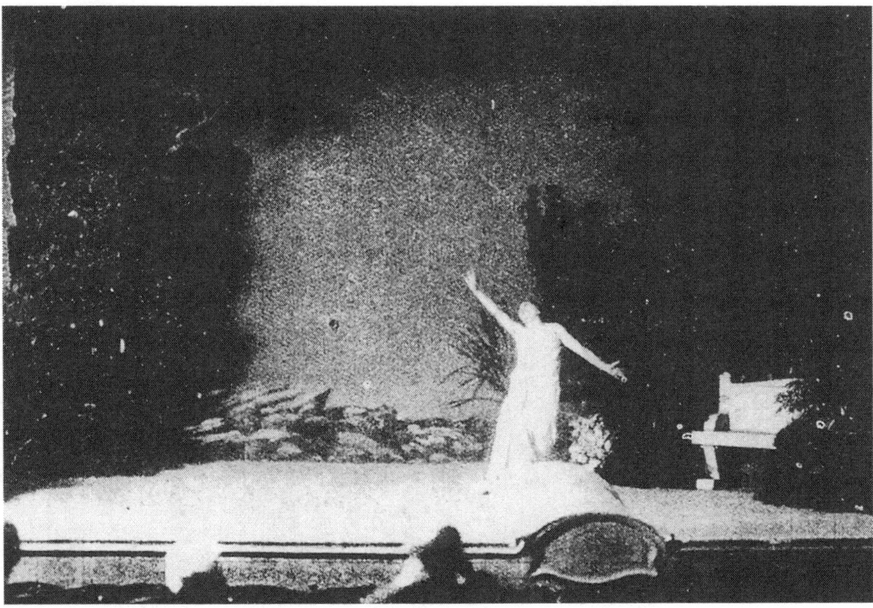

Figure 6. The dream dancer Madeleine Guipet (1904). After being hypnotized by the psychiatrist Albert von Schrenck-Notzing, Guipet dances on the stage of Munich's Schauspielhaus before a large audience of doctors, professors, artists, and lay people. Two of the people visible in the audience are Albert von Keller and Albert von Schrenck-Notzing, who were leading members of Munich's Psychologische Gesellschaft. Albert von Schrenck-Notzing, "Albert von Keller als Malerpsychologe und Metaphysiker," *Psychische Studien* 48 (April–May 1921): 209.

inversion between male researchers and female mediums that the photograph neatly captured. Two of the heads visible in the shadows just in front of the stage belonged to Schrenck-Notzing and Keller; Guipet herself dominated the stage, appearing at a moment of transformation, when mediums ceased to be passive experimental objects and instead emerged as active expressers of their own creative urges. Guipet's creative unconscious commanded the scene, and in the face of her talent the men of the Psychologische Gesellschaft had to be content to sit, literally at her feet, and watch the performance.[31]

Contemporaries experienced Guipet's dream dances as a defining cultural moment, one that gave them a glimpse into the mysterious sources of artistic inspiration in the modern world. Keller, for example, honored Guipet with a series of paintings featuring her as an artist in her own right. Unlike *Hexenverbrennung,* where Matzinger had acted only as the unnamed model, these works focused squarely on Guipet the dancer and betrayed the degree to which Keller's interest in the realistic portrayal of historical or biblical events with psychological dimensions had given way to a fascination with psychological experience.[32] Schrenck-Notzing, taking a slightly different tack, claimed Guipet as living proof that everyone had a creative urge in their psyche, an urge normally kept buried by social convention but occasionally liberated by techniques like hypnosis.[33] Echoing Schrenck-Notzing's universalization of the creative impulse, finally, the theater director Georg Fuchs paired Guipet with Isadora Duncan as co-creators of a thoroughly modern dance form—one that tapped the inner, "natural" rhythms of the human body.[34] Each in his own way had become aware of the creative unconscious and begun to sense the potential contributions that this creative unconscious might make to modern art.

This was quite a transformation, and one altogether unforeseen. The artists of the Psychologische Gesellschaft, of course, had never doubted the value of mediums to their work. Some had even gone so far as to draw an analogy between their own creative work and the trances of mediums. As Max had written in a series of autobiographical notes penned in 1882: "Painters are unconscious agents of spiritualism. Before the two-dimensional surface, on which they communicate their opinion of the third, they are medium and spirit."[35] But if Max had understood that trained artists could sometimes act like mediums, at least metaphorically, he had not dreamed that mediums with no artistic training could sometimes perform like full-blown artists. Nonetheless, this was precisely the conclusion to which the experiments of the Psychologische Gesellschaft had led. Mediums *had* revolutionized the practice of art, though not in the way the authors of the original manifesto had predicted. Mediums had ceased to be models, and instead had emerged as artists—albeit still unconscious ones—in their own right.

The Value of a Spirit Guide

How did other artists learn to create in the revolutionary new mode of modernism? How did they make the switch from a traditional aesthetic focused on an objective reality outside of themselves to a new aesthetic emphasizing the primacy of their own "intuitive experience"? Mirroring Guipet's trajectory, many fin-de-siècle artists made this switch by first breaking down in personal crisis and then breaking through to a new inner voice. Unlike Guipet, however, they tapped a novel occult tool known as a "spirit guide."

When the poet Rainer Maria Rilke finished work on *Malte Laurids Brigge* in 1910, for example, a crisis with aesthetic and personal dimensions quickly engulfed him. Unable to complete his new project *The Duino Elegies* he retreated in the fall of 1920 to spend time alone at a friend's castle near Zurich. There, Rilke found himself confronted one day with a mysterious text, one that he had penned in his own hand but not authored. The title page identified the work as having come from the personal papers of a mysterious Count C. W. Trying to explain this bizarre turn of events to a friend, Rilke recounted that he had merely written down what he heard from a male spirit during a recent nocturnal visit. To another friend, Rilke admitted that he had hatched the idea of discovering a volume of poems that would tell him something about the former inhabitants of the castle; three days later, he found the book lying before him. Unable to create, Rilke implied, he had to imagine a figure who could. Whatever their source, the mysterious poems in fact propelled Rilke out of his crisis, and shortly after finishing them, he finally concluded the long-delayed project of *The Duino Elegies*.[36]

Rilke's mysterious experiences resulted in an extraordinary piece of German literature, but the Count C. W. himself was profoundly ordinary, an example of what contemporaries called a "spirit guide." An occult tool widely employed for artistic experiments at the fin de siècle, spirit guides factored into the lives of such well-known contemporaries as W. B. Yeats, who wrote regularly with the help of a spirit named Leo, and André Breton, who considered automatic writing (writing under the control of spirits) the beginning of surrealism.[37] The widespread use of spirit guides, indeed, raises important questions for historians about the relationship between occult practices and new modes of artistic expression in the early twentieth century.[38] Why did artists work with spirit guides? Where did this practice originate? Who found it useful? And, perhaps most importantly, what was the significance of the spirit guide—a distinct alternative personality—to the creative process itself?

Foreshadowing Rilke's experiences, the case of the dramatist Hanns von Gumppenberg demonstrates in the first place that spirit guides could help struggling young artists through periods of professional and personal crisis. In the mid-1880s, Gumppenberg had found himself locked out of Munich's state-sponsored cultural circles and forced to turn to a variety of countercultural pursuits. He joined Michael Georg Conrad's *Gesellschaft für modernes Leben* (Society for modern life), home to German Naturalists and their novel claim that literature should treat subjects of contemporary import and present characters in all their natural truth. Simultaneously, Gumppenberg began to attend meetings of the Psychologische Gesellschaft and, having expected to encounter only hucksters and mystics, was surprised at the group's thoughtful and scholarly tone.[39] These countercultural activities came together in two plays: *Die Spiritisten* (The spiritualists) (1885), which demonstrated Gumppenberg's early knowledge of a local cultural phenomenon, and *Messias* (1890), which treated Jesus as an ordinary man forced to resort to charlatanry to promote his message of peace and justice. Both plays flopped, and the latter provoked the Catholic press to charge Gumppenberg—as it had Max and Keller—with blasphemy and atheism.[40] Feeling his dream of becoming a professional playwright slip away, Gumppenberg fell into ever greater isolation and depression.

In a pattern frequently reenacted among fin-de-siècle occult personalities, it was in this period of extreme duress that Gumppenberg joyfully discovered his spirit guide, who appeared at a private séance he staged in 1890 with a talented young woman previously employed by Schrenck-Notzing. Although Gumppenberg walked into the séance room a convinced materialist with no sympathy for the spiritualist explanation of occult phenomena, he left a believer. The critical point came when the tapping and turning of the séance table changed, signaling the presence of a new spirit who introduced herself by the name of Geben and announced that she had come to save him.[41] Feeling his frustration and isolation lifting, Gumppenberg now embarked on a period of intense research.[42] The results appeared in 1891, in *Das dritte Testament* (The third testament) and a supplement, when Gumppenberg sought to establish a new religion of personal conscience. "Each man must be his own savior," he announced, and he continued to pursue the implications of this spiritual anarchism—a hallmark of modernist religious practice reminiscent of the Theosophical cult of the self—for the rest of his life.[43] Having found his spiritual compass, moreover, Gumppenberg went on to become a prominent critic and extremely successful satirical writer for Munich's famous modernist cabaret *Elf Scharfrichter* (Eleven executioners).[44]

Spirit guides had helped Rilke and Gumppenberg (re)shape their voices as writers in ways that left a permanent mark on the literature of German modernism. Difficult as this transformation had been, since both authors were men, neither had had to contend with sex discrimination. Fin-de-siècle women with creative aspirations, in contrast, faced all the difficulties that men faced, but in addition had to deal with the extra burden of norms militating against women expressing and developing their artistic impulses. Although women had an increasing presence in the German art world, they still faced exclusion from most professional associations and the informal but important social networks of artists' communities. In addition, the culture of separate spheres worked to keep women as homemakers, rather than art creators. When, finally, women did create, they were usually limited to "minor" topics such as flowers, small animals, and children and found their creativity hampered by an "ideology of [male] genius" according to which men, not women, created great art.[45] Guipet had evaded these entrenched traditions by creating in a trance, a state in which she could not be held responsible for her acts. Other female contemporaries took a similar route by becoming mediums and getting in touch with their inner spirit guides. In the process, they evaded and at times even subverted the gendered norms of creative expression.

Take, for instance, the trance poet Clara Eysell-Kilburger. A Berlin journalist for the *Illustrierte Frauenzeitung* and *Modenwelt,* two of Germany's premier magazines for bourgeois women, by the late 1890s Eysell-Kilburger had become one of the most widely read female authors in Germany.[46] Despite this remarkable success, she turned away from journalism just after the century's end and began to experiment with poetry, drama, and fiction.[47] As Rilke would do a few years later, Eysell-Kilburger embraced the help of a spirit guide to conduct her literary experiments. Her first book of spirit poetry, written over the course of a short two weeks, appeared in 1902 with the title *Klänge aus dem Jenseits: Ein Mysterium* (Sounds from the other side: A mystery), and was followed six years later by the so-called *Trance-Dichtungen* (Trance poems) of 1908–9.[48] Her experiments with free-rhythm prose poetry and everyday language as well as the socially critical stance she took toward her topics, moreover, demonstrated her awareness of and participation in the up-to-date artistic trends that Gumppenberg had also tapped.[49]

Eysell-Kilburger's spirit guide helped her shift her focus as a writer, a transformation that bore the telltale marks of gender bending. As she explained in the preface to her first book of poetry, she had written the poems by relinquishing power over her ideas and becoming the helper of a masculine spirit named Otto Dalberg. She recalled feeling at times that she was in the grip of a foreign intelligence channeling his own creative impulses through her. At other times, she sensed instead that she herself was an important participant in the performance. Postulating either that she must have written the work under the influence of an inspirational power that had suppressed her own style or that she had changed so much as to renounce her own style, Eysell-Kilburger confessed her ignorance about the ultimate source of her poems.[50] But whatever their origin, it was clear that she had not been able to conceive of herself as a creator without resorting to a masculine element in herself. The spirit guide had allowed her to bypass the "ideology of [male] genius" and create a fresh aesthetic identity for herself, one centered on a newly discovered and masculine inner voice.

Eysell-Kilburger's simultaneous bow to and evasion of gender norms is an example of just how useful the device of the spirit guide could be. But Eysell-Kilburger had made her experiments from a situation of some security since she had already made her reputation as a writer before playing with a new style. Not so with Wilhelmine Aßmann, whose signature photograph portrayed a woman at the peak of her career as a trance painter (see fig. 7). Dressed in a costume typical of the Berlin Secession, she appeared in the photograph producing art "automatically"—that is, while in an unconscious state of mediumship. Displaying the luxuriant organic shapes typical of contemporary Jugendstil works, her trance drawings hung on the wall behind her. The photograph was remarkable, not just because of its obvious evocation of Berlin's avant-garde milieu but also because it portrayed a successful woman artist with absolutely no formal training. More surprising still, Aßmann had made her art, as much as her reputation, while in a trance.

Here again, the usefulness of spirit guides to evade and subvert gender norms about art was at work. Before discovering her talents as a trance painter, as it turned out, Wilhelmine Aßmann had been a very sick and unhappy woman. When the nearly simultaneous deaths of her son and sister sent her into a downward spiral of sorrow, her husband took her to various groups, looking for a cure. Since neither regular doctors nor Christian clerics seemed able to improve his wife's condition, Aßmann's husband turned in desperation to a spiritualist circle. His hope was that she might there contact the spirits of her loved ones and thus receive relief from grief. Although she never managed to communicate with the spirits of her son and sister, she did discover that she herself was a talented medium with a gift for automatic writing. Eventually, she made contact with her control spirit, a male entity by the name of Helize, and soon began to produce full-scale drawings evocative of flowers and plants. Refusing to see herself as the creative agent in these productions, she always insisted that she merely "served the paint" and, by extension, the creative impulse of her male spirit guide. Finally, on 4 August 1904, at age forty, she produced her first color picture. This new-found talent as a trance artist al-

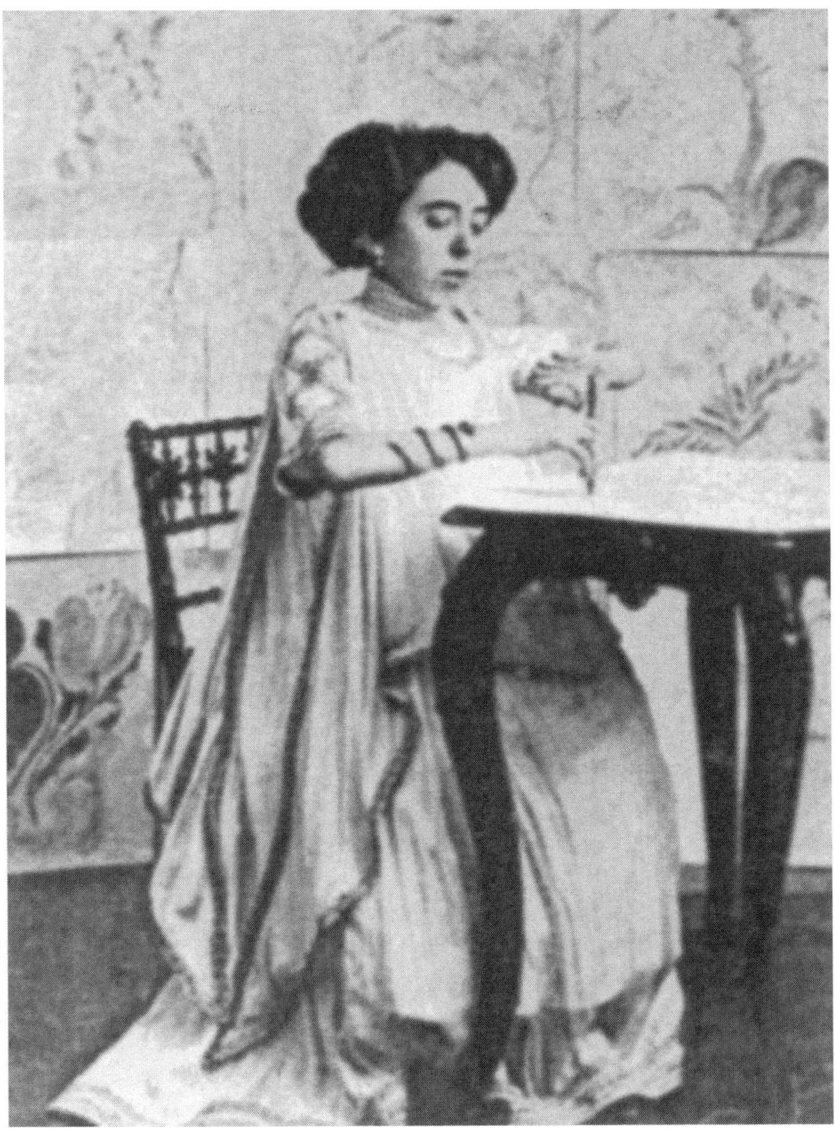

Figure 7. The Berlin trance-painter Wilhelmine Aßmann (1904). Surrounded by samples of her artwork and dressed in a Japanese kimono, Aßmann paints while in a trance. Aßmann's case exemplifies the potential of occult states of consciousness to subvert contemporary gender norms. Richard Baerwald, *Okkultismus und Spiritismus und ihre weltanschaulichen Folgerungen* (Berlin: Deutsche Buchgemeinschaft, 1926), illus. 6.

lowed Aßmann to build a completely new life for herself and become a proto-type "new woman." She began by changing her name to Frieda Genthes.[51] Then she created a market niche for herself with the help of a business that used her designs to decorate pillows, sold to the public under the slogan "flowers from another world." Eventually, Aßmann moved to Berlin, where she devoted herself to art and cultivating an exotic lifestyle that included dressing in kimonos and living in an apartment decorated in the then-popular Japanese style. All of this she accomplished by tapping the subversive potential of a spirit guide.[52]

The value of spirit guides, thus, lay in their multifaceted ability to offer release, particularly release from pain and the loneliness of personal crisis. Aßmann had lost a child and sibling; Gumppenberg had lost his professional compass and livelihood; Rilke had been unable for years to make headway on his *Duino Elegies* and was suffering in solitude with the burden of this un-finished project. All experienced the visitation of the spirit guide as a personal befriending. If spirit guides pointed the way out of personal crises, they also facilitated a breakthrough to another world, one beyond the reach of the five senses. Geben educated Gumppenberg about the world of the spirit; Helize helped Aßmann draw forms "from another world"; and the Count C. W. played to Rilke's long-term interest in the immaterial world of the spirit. Spirit guides, finally, seemed always to appear at moments of great aesthetic transfor-mation and, for female artists, gender transgression. Otto Dalberg contacted Eysell-Kilburger just as she began to experiment with the move from journal-ism to free-form poetry. Geben came to Gumppenberg just as he began to articulate a new and secular view of human spiritual evolution. Helize visited Aßmann just as she began to find a new vocation as an artist. And the Count C. W. appeared just in time to propel Rilke into a new language and understand-ing of poetry.[53] In all of these ways, spirit guides offered release, and the price of their service, it would seem, lay with the ambiguously authored works they left behind in their wake.

Theosophy and the Avant-Garde

Just as the spirit guides of the séance room acted as powerful tools for tuning in to one's inner voice, Theosophy offered yet another reservoir of equally powerful metaphors and techniques for creating art in keeping with the mod-ern spirit. Kandinsky, whose articulation of abstraction drew heavily on Theosophical tools, is undoubtedly the most famous example of what Theosophy offered the avant-garde. Born to a bourgeois family in Russia in 1866, Kandinsky abruptly gave up a promising career as an academic in 1895 and moved to Munich to pursue his dream of becoming a painter.[54] An international center of aesthetic as well as occult innovation, Munich quickly whirled the young man into its freewheeling culture of experimentation. Kandinsky began to move in the modern art circles of the Munich Secession, the Jugendstil movement, and the Phalanx group. At the same time, he immersed himself in occult studies. In addition to reading the works of such Theosophical leaders as Charles Leadbeater, Annie Besant, and Rudolf Steiner, he attended lectures given by Steiner, whose color theories intrigued him deeply, and practiced various mental exercises developed by Steiner to help aspirants access the occult world of pure spirit.[55] By the time Kandinsky sat down to write *Über das Geistige in der Kunst,* a milestone in the self-definition of modern art, Theosophy had permeated his plan for radical aesthetic change. Scientists working in fields as diverse as atomic physics and psychical research, he argued, had begun to study a reality behind the world of material appearances. Echoing Theosophical authors, he took this as a sign of the imminent "dissolution of matter" and demanded a new art to take account of the new reality.[56]

The art historian Sixten Ringbom has argued that Theosophy offered Kandinsky "a repertory of crude paradigms out of which the artist developed . . . his own pictorial idiom." In particular, Theosophy helped Kandinsky solve his so-called "information problem." How were painters dedicated to the depiction of an invisible spiritual reality to convince viewers that their artworks were not merely the products of a fantastic and highly private vision? Where were the immaterial objects, viewers might well ask, that no one could see but that artists now dared to paint in visual form? Kandinsky answered such questions by drawing on the Theosophical idea of the cosmos as resonating with the vibrations of immaterial entities. To paint the objects that made up this "sounding cosmos," artists had only to tune their souls to the cosmic waves and then let their ringing souls express themselves on the material canvas.[57] Artworks created in this way, moreover, would then play on the viewer in just the way that the cosmos had played on the artist. As Kandinsky explained in his 1911 manifesto: "Colour is the keyboard. The eye is the hammer. The soul is the piano, with its many strings. The artist is the hand that purposefully sets the soul vibrating by means of this or that key. Thus it is clear that the harmony of colors can only be based upon the principle of purposefully touching the human soul."[58] Artists and viewers, artworks and immaterial objects—all were bound together in a cosmic circle of resonance.

What Kandinsky made of this Theosophically inspired insight is, of course, well known. By renouncing the depiction of material objects, he freed himself to make the leap into pure abstraction. Whereas his canvases had previously depicted forms whose material origins remained recognizable as trees, houses, and human figures, he now began to produce works with no detectable roots in the world of visible appearances. The first of these, *Picture with a Circle*, came in 1911 (see fig. 8). For the next four years, Kandinsky mined the insights that he had gleaned from Theosophy to construct an art of pure abstraction.[59]

Full abstraction, however, was not the only endpoint for artists using Theosophical tools to develop their inner vision. Heinrich Nüßlein, for instance, found that Theosophical tools could overcome material barriers, though not of the kind that had plagued Kandinsky, and help him articulate an art of the fantastic. Born to a poor family and disabled by extreme nearsightedness from an early age, Nüßlein had found his painterly aspirations blocked on both the financial and physical fronts. When dedication and sheer luck turned him into a wealthy man by the mid-1920s, however, Nüßlein resolved to retire from business and pursue his long held passion for painting. As for so many before him, the occult sciences offered the road to self-reinvention. While meditating one day, he found himself writing automatically. Soon, this became a talent for automatic drawing, then an aptitude for clairaudience (hearing at a distance), and finally a gift for mesmeric healing and mummifying. His Theosophical studies taught him, most importantly, that not all objects worthy of being painted had a visible presence, and this insight gave him the courage to paint in spite of the visual handicap that had previously frustrated his artistic dreams. Referring to himself as an artisan and psychical picture-writer, Nüßlein began to produce prolifically.[60] An article in a 1928 art journal reported that he had produced two thousand paintings over the course of the previous three years; by 1935 Nüßlein was claiming to have produced eighteen thousand pictures in the preceding decade.[61] He also began to exhibit his art in galleries, both at home and abroad, including at his own castle (Schloß Kornburg) near Nuremberg and at galleries in Munich and London, where the devoted spiritualist Arthur Conan Doyle reportedly purchased one of his works.[62]

As they had for Kandinsky, Theosophical ideas and practices gave Nüßlein the tools he needed to translate inner vision into modern aesthetic acts. Like Kandinsky, Nüßlein believed that the proper content of art was spiritual, and

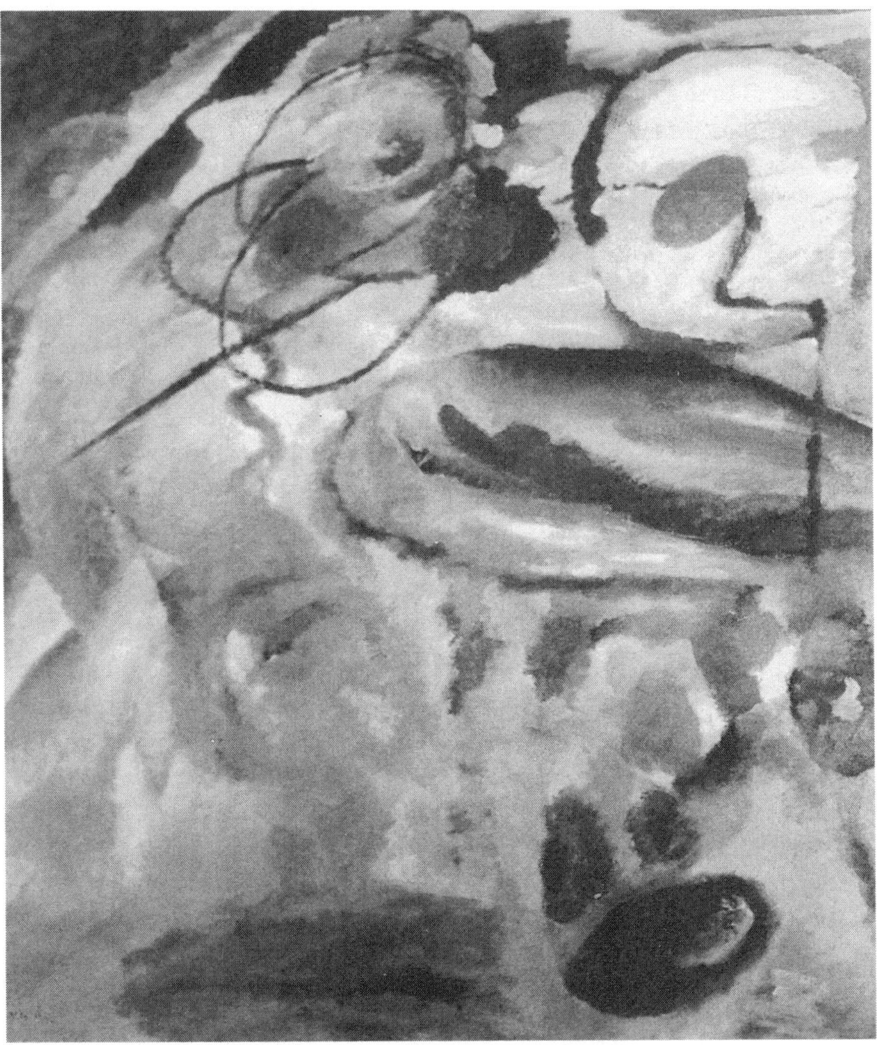

Figure 8. Wassily Kandinsky, *Picture with a Circle* (1911). Kandinsky considered this his first wholly abstract canvas. It portrays a spiritual reality beyond the reach of the five senses. Kandinsky produced it after immersing himself in a variety of alternative pursuits, including Theosophy. John Golding, *Paths to the Absolute* (Princeton, NJ: Princeton University Press, 2000), pp. 98 and 102. Owned by the State Museum of Art, Tbilisi, Republic of Georgia (Paris: ADAGP, 2000; London: DACS, 2000).

he drew on Theosophical ideas of cosmic vibrations to explain the source of his art. As his promotional literature put it, Nüßlein used his soul as an antenna to capture cosmic radiation that could then be translated into visual form. With his right hand moving the brush and his left hand opening and closing to catch the rays, Nüßlein's very posture at the easel suggested his function as a transceiver for the invisible waves of the cosmos.[63] Kandinsky and Nüßlein shared, in other words, a metaphysical conception about art and artistic creativity rooted in Theosophy. This did not mean, of course, that the works they painted bore much of a visual resemblance to one another. Although Nüßlein, like Kandinsky, eschewed the depiction of material objects, he never turned his back on form altogether. Paintings such as *Phantastische Landschaft* (Fantastic landscape) portrayed spiritual things that were fantastic permutations of material objects, without a doubt, but in no way abstract (see fig. 9).[64]

Theosophical tools, finally, could inspire artists to turn their inner vision into new forms of realism. No Theosophical figure did this more brazenly than Bô Yin Râ, a pseudonym for the painter Joseph Anton Schneiderfranken, who claimed to have used Theosophical techniques to paint Jesus from real life. Despite great financial difficulty, in the 1890s and early 1900s he had managed to pursue art studies in Frankfurt, Vienna, and Paris. By his mid thirties, he had become a successful professional painter exhibiting his characteristic landscapes in galleries around Germany.[65] Then, around 1912, just as Kandinsky began to pursue his Theosophically inspired vision of pure abstraction, Schneiderfranken had a rebirth, at once aesthetic and personal. He went to Greece, and when he returned to Germany in 1914 he had become Bô Yin Râ, a spiritual teacher whose philosophy would eventually influence a variety of contemporary artists, including Gustav Meyrink and the composer-conductor Felix Weingartner.[66]

Theosophy, Bô Yin Râ believed, gave him a fresh take on reality, "a totally new way of seeing and hearing," and his goal now became to translate his spiritual perceptions into visual form. If this quest had landed Kandinsky in abstraction and Nüßlein in fantasy, it deposited Bô Yin Râ in what might best be called occult realism. Invoking the slogan that nothing should stand between the eye and the soul—in marked contrast to Kandinsky's call for art that appealed less to the eye and more to the soul—Bô Yin Râ explained how artists in their creative moments receive the vibrations sent out by the original spiritual form and then enshrine these cosmic signatures in their artworks. The

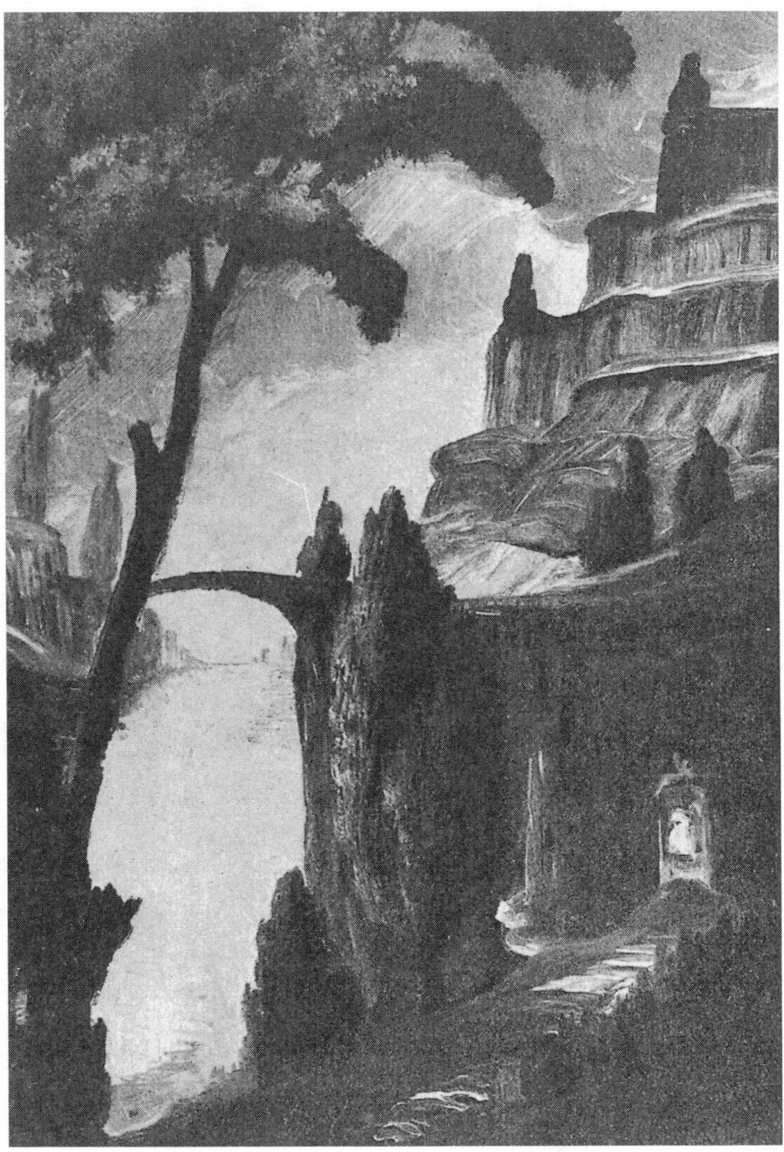

Figure 9. Heinrich Nüßlein, *Phantastische Landschaft* (Fantastic landscape; circa 1928). Nüßlein, a well-known Theosophical painter, stood at the easel with one hand on the brush and the other opening and closing so as to catch the waves of cosmic radiation surrounding him. He exhibited widely, and among those who bought his work were Arthur Conan Doyle, the creator of Sherlock Holmes. Georg Anschütz, "Phantasma und Kunst," *Schünemanns Monatshefte* 11 (November 1928): 1269.

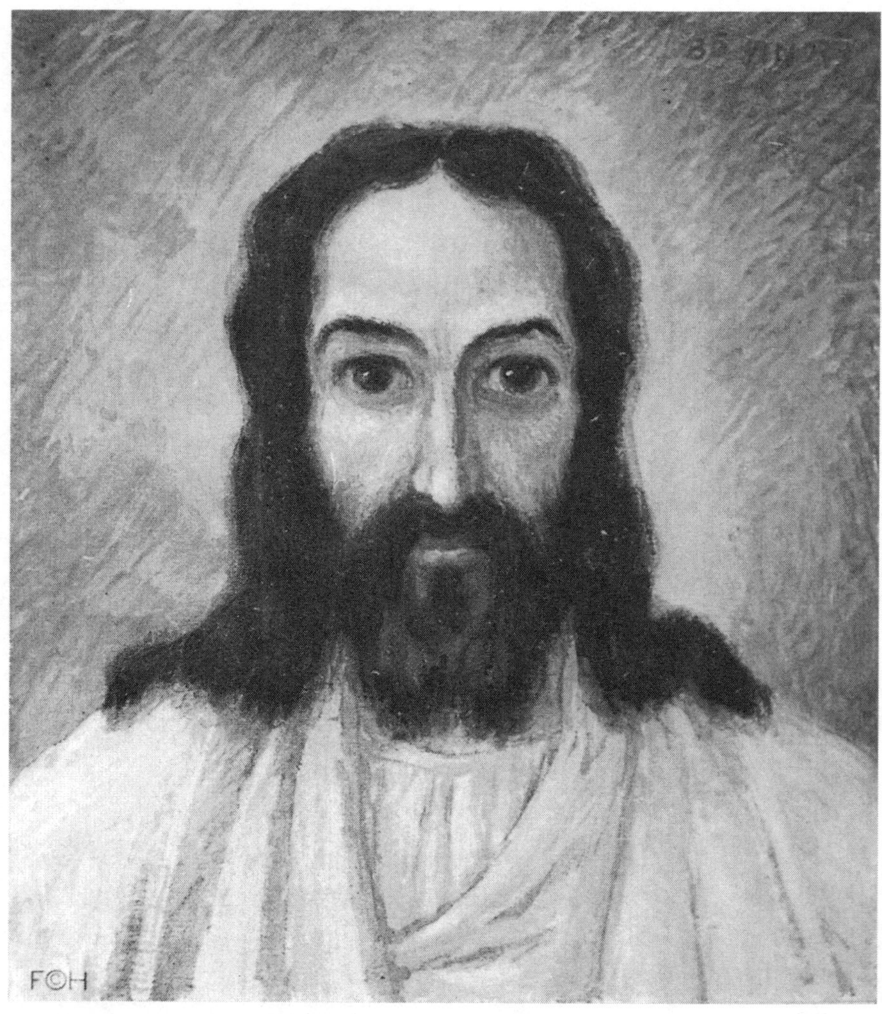

Figure 10. Bô Yin Râ, *Jesus* (circa 1932). A Theosophical guru whose followers included the writer Gustav Meyrink, Bô Yin Râ said he painted this portrait from real life. He claimed to have encountered Jesus in immaterial form during one of the many spiritual journeys he undertook according to Theosophical precepts. Rudolf Schott, *Der Maler Bô Yin Râ* (Munich: Franz Hanfstaengl, 1927), plate 19.

paintings themselves then become instruments radiating these waves from the world of the spirit into the viewer's soul. For viewers whose spiritual powers were sufficiently developed, Bô Yin Râ promised, his paintings were not simply a visual experience but a spiritual one as well.[67]

The most stunning product of Bô Yin Râ's Theosophical self-understanding was his portrait *Jesus* (see fig. 10). In a 1932 publication, he recounted how he had followed countless other artists in attempting to depict Jesus accurately through a variety of fantastic, conventional, and historical devices, only to find that none of these worked. Then, after years of training his mental powers, he had finally met the spirit of the former wandering teacher Jehoschuah. The portrait he painted as a result of this meeting was the product neither of a vision nor of an occult materialization; rather, he insisted, it represented the living Jesus as he had appeared to those who met him on earth two millennia earlier. Theosophically inspired spirit travel, so Bô Yin Râ claimed, had enabled him to paint this portrait of Jesus from "real" life.[68]

Examples of artists drawing on these and other Theosophical concepts and experiences could be multiplied. From Kandinsky's Blue Rider group came Franz Marc and Wilhelm Morgner.[69] Forgotten artists such as Oskar Reingruber, a transportation worker in Nuremberg, and Martin Friedrich Wegert, a professional illustrator in Munich, exhibited their Theosophically inspired works at a 1932 show in Munich on the "mysteries of inspiration."[70] And eurhythmy, a modern dance form pioneered by Rudolf Steiner, Else Klink, and others, also had Theosophical roots.[71] Whether in their psychical research, spiritualist, or Theosophical aspects, occult concepts as much as occult acts helped artists to turn away from nature and then—to use Prinzhorn's words once again—"inward upon the self." The occult clearly participated in the creation of the modernist aesthetic and ensured that no matter how visually esoteric it seemed to viewers, the new art would conform to the modern spirit.

CHAPTER SIX

Occult Sciences and Their Applied Doubles

Modernity inspired both optimism and despair.[1] At the start of the twentieth century, Germans lived in an increasingly bureaucratized mass culture pervaded by the hopeful faith that scientific knowledge and rational planning could solve pressing social issues efficiently and neutrally. Social hygienists, fatigue experts, and laboratory researchers, for instance, collaborated in the 1890s to create a new "science of work" that could address worker exhaustion and injury, thereby helping to alleviate a major cause of industrial unrest and political division.[2] Social modernists such as these sought new scientific tools to cure ills as diverse as crime, pollution, and disease, and in this quest they often turned to occult ideas and techniques. Germany's new experts— including its psychologists, doctors, policemen, engineers, lawyers, and architects—did so with some trepidation, of course, for the occult still carried an "unscientific" aura that was contrary to the cult of expertise. Optimism, nonetheless, often overrode ambivalence, and many of the new experts bent their talents to bringing a multitude of occult practices fully within the fold of the new socially relevant applied sciences.

But if modernity inspired hope, it also at times gave cause for despair, and Germans agonized in particular over the homogenizing pressures of the new order, pressures that threatened to strip them of their individuality. Enjoying the benefits of a state-sponsored medical system, for instance, they soon discovered that doctors could not always cure their sick bodies, and in any case usually turned them into nameless patients.[3] Confronted with modernity's darker side, Germans found that here, too, occult tools promised relief.

Eager to exploit modernity's potential while simultaneously rectifying its failures—to engage what the historian Detlev Peukert has called the "Janus face of modernity"—Germans infused the occult sciences with a sense of social relevance.[4] When the popular Berlin weekly *Die Woche* devoted an entire issue to the paranormal in 1932, for instance, the applicability of the occult to pressing social problems occupied pride of place. An article on the divining rod reported on "the city experiment" conducted by the Munich physician and amateur dowser Gustav Pohl: "Under strict official control, Pohl carefully investigated a town wholly unknown to him. On the city map he marked the pathogenic currents [*Reizstreifen;* the currents he discovered with his rod]. Then, the cancer cases for the last ten years were noted with a single cross by the city medical officer on the same map. The results were astonishing. All the crosses signaling a death from cancer lay along the pathogenic lines Pohl had marked."[5] As a result of Pohl's work, the article noted, doctors had begun to discover that patients suffering from cancer and other ailments such as asthma, sleep loss, and headaches could be restored to health simply by rearranging their lives—often simply by moving their beds—so as to evade the disease-causing currents streaming through the world around them.[6] Widely viewed as quintessential "diseases of modernity," cancer and these other chronic conditions here squared off against a powerful antidote: occult-inspired preventative medicine, duly certified by medical experts and public bureaucrats. So widespread did the applied science of dowsing become that even Hitler, notoriously hostile to the occult in general but fearful of becoming ill with cancer himself, hired Pohl in 1934 to dowse the Chancellery for harmful rays.[7]

At the same time that it offered practical tools for the alleviation of such social ills, the occult also promised to address one of modernity's most distressing concomitants: anonymity. It was to this issue that the astrologer Oscar A. H. Schmitz directed himself in a 1927 issue of the popular *Süddeutsche Monatshefte,* where he observed:

Everyone is asking themselves: Who am I? What is a self in general? A bare illusion of my material brain that will [eventually] vanish . . . or something transcendent that although embodied in matter . . . has its true basis elsewhere? The heart flees from the despair of the first answer to the consolation of the second. . . . That is why the churches are being filled once again. . . . Such emergency religion is of course often only an illusion that overlooks facts and proof. What distinguishes each new trend that leaves materialism behind, however, is the attempt to find new meaning that . . . offers the same path to salvation as religion, without coming into conflict with detailed scientific findings that must be accepted by modern men and women. . . . This is what all modern spiritual tendencies tend towards, including also astrology.[8]

Here, Schmitz highlighted an important goal of the modern occult program: scientifically grounded and self-focused salvation. Why this program proved so successful had as much to do with Germans' faith in the saving power of science as their despair over its spiritual poverty. If Schmitz's observation thus echoed the general modernist ambivalence tapped by the German occult movement, it also indicated something else. "Everyone is asking themselves: Who am I?": in this pithy phrase, Schmitz captured neatly a devilish dialectic set up by the pull of the new mass culture, on the one hand (*everyone* is asking themselves), and the push of individuals seeking self-knowledge, on the other (who am *I*). With its close attention to the subjectivity of psychological experience and its permeation of the consumer market, the occult easily adapted itself to this mass quest after private truth.

The occult sciences, in other words, seemed to offer valuable tools for many different facets of modern life. Despite the obvious problems, the new social experts found the occult's potential irresistible. And although they usually lacked the academic credentials that were quickly becoming a prerequisite for expertise, lay practitioners of the occult sciences insisted on their worth as rectifiers of modernity's failures. The age of social modernity had dawned, and with it flowered the occult sciences in all their practical glory.

Analyzing and Advising

At the close of the nineteenth century, the most apparently neutral of psychological claims often hid the sharpest of differences. When the American psychologist James McKeen Cattell reviewed work being done at Wilhelm Wundt's new psychology laboratory at Leipzig in January 1888, for instance, he observed that "the term *psychometry* can be confined to . . . the measurement of the duration of mental phenomena. Psychometry has received abundant attention from astronomers, physicists, physiologists and psychologists."[9] The manifest mildness of this observation belied a murky reality since the term *psychometry* by no means belonged only to laboratory psychologists like Cattell. Occult circles also had an avid and long-standing stake in the term, which they defined very differently. In March 1888, the Theosophist Wilhelm Hübbe-Schleiden used the term in its original sense in the occult journal *Sphinx*, where he reported on a series of psychometric experiments with a peasant woman from Kempten. During one particularly memorable experiment, he gave this woman a personal letter that he had just received but not yet had the chance to read. The woman had pressed the letter against her forehead, then described quickly and accurately the female letter writer and her actions at the time the letter was written.[10] As the juxtaposition of these articles suggests, two very different definitions of psychometry coexisted in Germany in 1888. Cattell's emphasized mental measurement; Hübbe-Schleiden's, in contrast, emphasized an intuitive faculty to sense something about the person who had handled an object (in this case, a letter) purely by making physical contact with it. Cattell's apparently neutral claim that the term *psychometry* could be "confined" to mental measurement, in other words, belied an unresolved issue: to whom did psychometry belong and what did it entail?

The muted tension over psychometry reflected in microcosm a problem that would plague both scientific psychology and the occult sciences well into the twentieth century. Now that human subjectivity had become an object of natural scientific research, investigators needed to establish by what means it should be studied and to what ends it should be put. While some investigators indulged Cattell's impulse to objectify and quantify subjectivity in pursuit of knowledge about the universal laws governing the human mind, others followed Hübbe-Schleiden in embracing the subjectivity of intuition as a method in itself—one that could deliver clairvoyant knowledge about the life of a particular person.[11] These psychometric tensions in 1888 presaged a demarcation battle that would rage for decades right in the gray area where the new psychology met the modern occult sciences. There, partisans of the intuitive approach to psychological phenomena butted heads with those who sought to render such phenomena amenable to "objective" investigation. At stake was the plum of scientific legitimation and all the prestige and earning power that went with it, not just for the new psychology but for the occult sciences as well.

Proponents of intuitive methods employed several strategies to solidify their scientific status. Followers of the "intuitive graphologist" Ludwig Aub, who climbed to fame in Munich in the 1890s for his remarkable ability to analyze a person's character and fate from a handwriting sample, spoke of his talent as both rational and intuitive.[12] The poet Max Halbe noted that Aub combined rigorous method with highly developed insight. Similarly, the graphologist Anja Mendelssohn praised Aub for pairing feminine devotion with a masculine love of experience, for being able to read character at once intuitively and rationally.[13] Nor were his followers shy about explicitly claiming scientific status for Aub. The doctor Johannes Dingfelder likened Aub to a mature chemist whose knowledge and experience enabled him to predict intuitively the outcome of a chemical reaction.[14] Other Aub enthusiasts embraced a metaphor comparing Aub to a piece of sensitive laboratory equipment. The engineer Adolf Würfl, for instance, called Aub a "microscope of the soul," and a Munich professor spoke of Aub as having "X-ray eyes."[15] Aub's status as both scientist and scientific instrument converged in the many obituaries written for him in 1926, when eulogists agreed that Aub's success had rested as much on his excellent grasp of graphology as a science as on his remarkable "ability for empathy." By combining the rational and the intuitive, his eulogists claimed, Aub had found a way to turn his body into a scientific instrument able to record the invisible "vibrations and rays" permeating the cosmos.[16]

While followers praising Aub's ability to be at once a clairvoyant, scientist, and scientific instrument thereby collapsed the distinction between subject and object, other researchers in the occult field struggled to maintain this separation, without which no claim to objectivity could stand. They did this by adhering to the measuring mania of brass-instrument psychologists like Cattell. To this end, the Berlin psychical researcher Fritz Grunewald (one of Schrenck-Notzing's many collaborators) developed "exceptionally efficient experimental outfits" in his home research laboratory in the 1920s. In a typical experiment reported in *Scientific American* in 1922, Grunewald placed his medium Ejner Nielsen near a special balance and magnetic needle that had been hooked up to a recording instrument, then instructed the medium to will a deflection of the balance and needle (see figs. 11 and 12). When the recording instrument released its ticker-tape display "proving" that the medium's effort of will had deflected the needle, the gloss of objectivity became complete: research object (Nielsen and his will), research subject (Grunewald), and instrument (balance, needle, and recording device) now stood fully distinct from one another.[17]

Psychometry's contested status raised a troublesome question. Were medi-

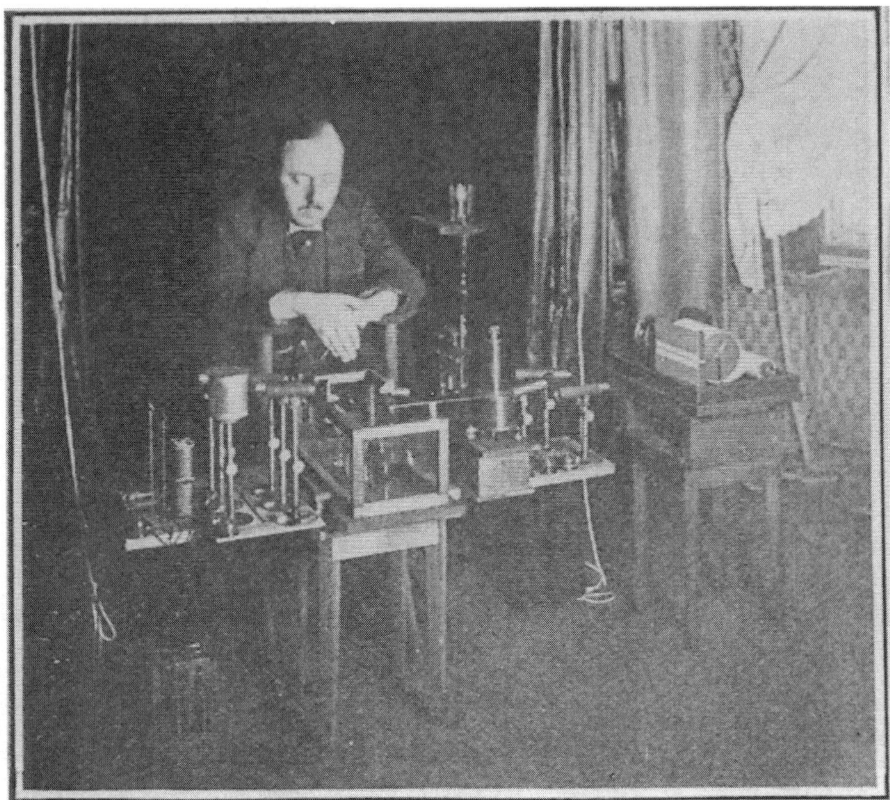

Figure 11. A parapsychological experiment, 1922. In the home research laboratory of
Fritz Grunewald, in Berlin, the medium Ejner Nielsen deflects a balance and a
magnetic needle by force of will. To the right, an instrument records the deflection,
giving the experiment the gloss of objectivity. Alfred Gradenwitz, "Investigating
Unknown Forces: The Unique Psychic Laboratory of Fritz Grunewald, at
Charlottenburg," *Scientific American* (July 1922): 30.

ums living instruments or experimental objects, astute analysts of character
or clever con artists? Social modernists who aspired to make the occult sciences respectable by making them objective attempted to bypass such issues
by jettisoning mediums. This approach emerged with particular clarity in
the scientific graphology movement, which had its roots in the Deutsche

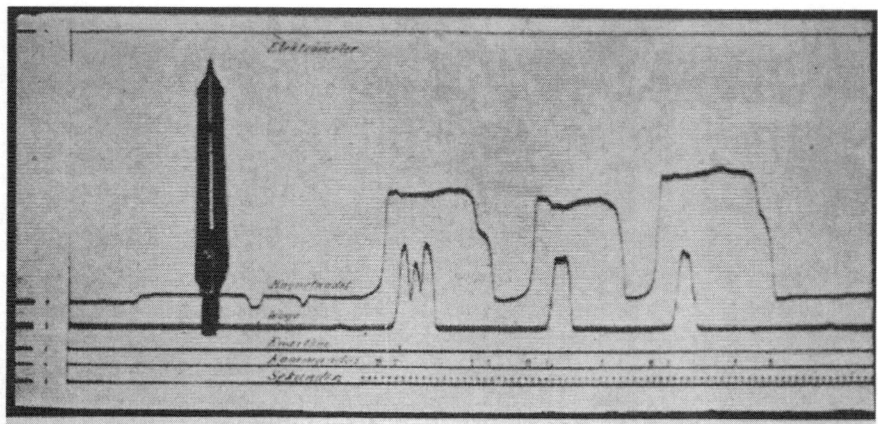

The medium, by exerting his will, causes a balance to deflect
and a magnetic needle to deviate; the records of the two phenomena are exactly parallel
A curve that records mediumistic processes

Figure 12. Making parapsychology objective, 1922. The readout from the
recording instrument visible in the experimental setup of figure 11 shows that
the parapsychological phenomena occurred simultaneously. Alfred Gradenwitz,
"Investigating Unknown Forces: The Unique Psychic Laboratory of Fritz Grunewald,
at Charlottenburg," *Scientific American* (July 1922), p. 30.

graphologische Gesellschaft (German graphological society), founded in Munich in 1896 by Ludwig Klages, Hans Busse, and Georg Meyer.[18] The group
aimed to investigate graphology scientifically and to break once and for all the
negative associations between graphology and the occult. Theorizing that
handwriting expressed personality, scientific graphologists sought to develop
an analytic system that would correlate personality types with such factors as
the size, shape, and angle of a person's script. Although mediums had no place
in this scheme, thus obviating one of the major stumbling blocks on the way
to an apparently objective understanding of human personality, scientific
graphologists nonetheless found it by no means easy to shake the occult
stigma. Busse's 1898 article "Graphologie und Okkultismus: Die Entwicklung
der Graphologie zur exacten Wissenschaft" (Graphology and occultism: The
development of graphology into an exact science), for instance, appeared in a
new periodical titled *Wissenschaftliche Zeitschrift für "Okkultismus"* (Scientific
journal for "occultism").[19] The word *Okkultismus,* encircled by quotation

marks, indicated the journal's slick attempt to claim the occult for science, but this was surely not the decisive break for which Busse and his colleagues had hoped.

Three decades later, scientific graphologists had still not won the demarcation battle against their "intuitive" counterparts, although they had secured a firm foothold in the burgeoning new field of scientifically informed police work. At the first congress of a new joint forensics-graphology association in Leipzig in 1924, for instance (the *Deutscher Bund der gerichtlichen Schrift-anverständigen und Berufsgraphologen* [German association of forensic writing experts and professional graphologists]), drew a mixed crowd of police officials and graphologists. After a representative of the Leipzig police department delivered a welcome speech, the participants hotly debated the topic of how to combat the abuse of graphology, a tacit reference to intuitive practitioners like Ludwig Aub. In addition, attendees discussed how to supervise the training of graphologists, the publication of a professional journal, and the setting of fees, all topics geared toward drawing professional boundaries around their group.[20] By the end of the decade, the journalist Walter Benjamin could laud scientific graphology as a unique "German achievement" but still bemoan the popularity of vulgar graphology that catered "to the philistines' curiosity and passion for gossip by offering to reveal the 'truth' about Tom, Dick, and Harry, and a whole gallery of revelations about everyone from their ancestors to the housewife."[21]

Despite the continuing turf wars, the success that scientific graphologists had begun to enjoy by the 1920s derived in large part from graphology's adaptability to the burgeoning new culture of professional advice-giving known as "applied psychology." By the early twentieth century, applied psychology had superseded experimental psychology as the hot new area of study as social modernists, practitioners of this new field, sought to demonstrate the practical worth of their expertise to the solution of contemporary problems. Books with titles such as *On the Psychology of Amputees and Their Prostheses* (1921), *The Problem of Work Hours* (1924), *Psychotechnics in the Service of the German Railway* (1925), *New Contributions to the Theory and Practice of Intelligence Testing* (1925), *Psychotechnics of Sales* (1926), and *Psychotechnics of Airplane Pilots* (1928) proliferated as psychologists scrambled to prove their worth at matching individuals to social roles efficiently and accurately.[22] Eager to achieve professional status and solidify their niche in the large new bureaucratic institutions of mass society, applied psychologists concentrated their efforts mainly on industry, business, and the armed forces, dividing themselves into various subspecialties. Psychotechnicians, for instance, labored to assign individuals to specific tasks by assessing their technical abilities. Expression psychologists and characterologists, in contrast, built on the theoretical insights first articulated by Klages in his 1916 book *Handschrift und Charakter* (Handwriting and character) (reprinted fifteen times by 1932) and sought to assess something more intangible: the individual's character and will. While psychotechnicians proved their worth in selecting workers for simple tasks such as typing or driving a street car, expression psychologists and characterologists devoted themselves to selecting leaders, particularly managers for industry and officers for the armed forces.[23]

As much as applied psychologists may have wanted to distance themselves from occult enthusiasts, the proximity of their fields often prevented this. For one thing, Klages, a pioneer of applied psychology, was also a vocal proponent of scientific graphology, a field that had not yet shaken its occult roots. For another, "intuitive" practitioners of the occult sciences, including graphology, could and did make the case that they, too, offered applied psychological services. Aub, for instance, counted many satisfied patient-customers among his followers, including a theologian in Augsburg who recommended a consultation with Aub to all who had lost their inner spiritual equilibrium. Germany's leading scientific graphologists, finally, did not always shun the work of intuitive graphologists. Anja Mendelssohn, whose 1928 book *Der Mensch in der Handschrift* (Man in his handwriting) Walter Benjamin lauded as "the science of graphology at its very best," wrote approvingly of Aub and his alternative graphological style.[24]

"Intuitive" and "scientific" practitioners of astrology found that the new fashion for applied psychology offered similar prizes and pitfalls. Like its graphological cousin, scientific astrology flourished in interwar Germany and attracted such illustrious backers as the biologist Hans Driesch, the philosopher Johannes Verweyen, the paleontologist Edgar Daqué, and the writer Theodor Lessing.[25] Driesch spoke for many of his professional scientific colleagues when he defended his interest in astrology by noting that "one should never cut off the path to possible knowledge."[26] Herbert von Klöckler, a retired military officer who supported himself as a freelance astrologer in the 1920s, echoed this sentiment in his 1926 *Astrologie als Erfahrungswissenschaft* (Astrology as an empirical science), part of the "metaphysics and worldview" series edited by Driesch. There, Klöckler urged investigators to take a strictly objective approach to the phenomena in question by shunning the intuitive methods favored by occultists and Theosophists and instead embracing scientific methods such as statistical analysis. Was there a statistically significant correlation, Klöckler asked, between particular constellations of stars and certain earthly events such as childhood death, suicide, accidents, fraud, theft, murder, or divorce? Did the heavens conform in some way to the choices made by individuals to pursue professional paths as diverse as painting, writing, medicine, law, mathematics, physics, astronomy, or the clergy? Concluding on the basis of more than seven thousand cases that statistical analysis did support some astrological principles, Klöckler called for further study.[27] Other scientific astrologers seconded Klöckler's claims in a 1927 issue of *Süddeutsche Monatshefte* devoted entirely to astrology. Heinz Artur Strauß, for instance, urged readers to think of astrology as an extension of the science of heredity, explaining that the arrangement of the heavens could affect one's fate and character in the same way as one's hereditary material. Echoing Strauß a few pages later, Werner Achelis made the links between scientific astrology and the new field of applied social sciences explicit, placing astrology squarely under the rubric of anthropology *(Menschenkunde)*, grouping it with physiognamy, graphology, psychoanalysis, and clinical psychology as a practical science dedicated to the objective study of human subjectivity.[28]

Although scientific astrologers labored mightily to render their field "objective" and join it to the new science of psychology, they never succeeded in completely dissociating themselves from intuitive astrologers, who continued to enjoy immense popularity well into the 1930s. As one astute Catholic observer noted in 1935, Germans suspicious of the hard sciences and their perceived hostility to life seemed to find this kind of astrology particularly enticing because it offered technical analyses carried out according to intuitive methods.[29] If intuitive astrologers could thus offer the best of both worlds—logical rigor and emotional warmth—they also offered services geared specifically to the psychic needs of private individuals. As a leading representative of this astrological sector, Karl Brandler-Pracht published numerous self-help manuals with such appealing titles as *Successful, Happy Living through Attention to . . . Astral Influences: A Guide to the Practical Application of . . . Cosmic Waves by which Any Man Can Become the Master of His Own Destiny* (in German: *Erfolgreiches, glückliches Leben durch Beachtung der Tattwischen, und Astralen Einflüsse: Ein Schlüssel zur praktischen Verwendung der mit dem menschlichen Leben engverbundenen kosmischen Schwingungen, wodurch jedermann zum Herrn seines Geschickes werden kann*) (1920).[30] Here and in other works, Brandler-Pracht emphasized the populist and practical side of astrology, continually reminding readers that astrology aimed not to predict the future but to help them discover their inner selves; this quest, moreover, should not be left in the hands of experts but rather returned to individual aspirants, who could be coached to develop their own powers of logic and psychic intuition.[31]

No matter of which persuasion, the scientific or the intuitive, character analysts working in the fields of graphology and astrology aimed—like their counterparts in mainstream psychology—to analyze subjectivity, to pin down the individualizing features of a specific person, and to offer advice based on this analysis. Such lofty goals soon foundered on paradoxes endemic to the new mass culture. Although character assessments were designed to discover individuality, for instance, individuals often received their analysis on a standardized form. The writer Michael Georg Conrad confronted this irony in 1901 when he signed up for a scientific analysis of his handwriting by Paul Jury, an employee of the Graphologisches Institut in Hannover. The analysis came back to Conrad on a four-page printed document. Following a first page with a generic explanatory letter on the merits and limitations of graphology as a tool of character analysis came a five-part form, each part corresponding to one of five standardized personality sectors: intelligence, force of will, temperament and instinct, inner life, and general character. In the first category (intelligence), Jury's analysis identified Conrad's very high logical and imaginative abilities and his weak business acumen; in the third category (temperament and instinct), Conrad scored high on sincerity but only average on warmth of feeling; in the fourth (inner life), Conrad received high marks for his prudence and was rated as not particularly irritable or sensitive.[32]

Analysts working with intuitive methods encountered similar paradoxes. Those who solicited customers through regular columns in periodicals, for example, furnished "individual" advice in a highly impersonal and public venue. Those seeking self-analysis sent in pertinent samples and information—of handwriting and birth time and date, say—and then read a usually anonymous analyst's reply in the next issue of the periodical. These replies typically mixed the naming of character traits with recommendations for future personal development. A 1918 column in the *Zentralblatt für Okkultismus* (Journal for occultism), thus, informed one advice seeker that handwriting analysis had shown him to have a simple but sensitive personality, a desire for intensification and contemplation, doubts about his career choice, and no detectable magical abilities. It informed another that his handwriting showed a marked predilection for graphology, whose study was highly recommended, and referred him to a Berlin magnetist for treatment.[33]

Examples such as these suggest that the modernist goal of individuation often clashed with the standardized forms and long-distance methods by which these analyses were generated. Whether practicing intuitive or scientific forms of character analysis, it would seem, Germans found it very difficult to evade the depersonalizing effects of delivering and receiving advice in a mass culture.

Seeking and Siting

After visiting a sugar-beet estate near Magdeburg in June 1930, an official with the U.S. Department of Agriculture, C. A. Browne, submitted a report on dowsing in contemporary Germany to *Science* magazine. Initially amazed that this ancient occult practice still persisted, Browne soon came to understand why:

> With the growing population of Europe there has been a constantly increasing need of new supplies of water for agricultural, industrial and municipal purposes and this want is reflected in the increasing number of dowsers . . . who are ready to supply the demand for their services. Even those who scoff at the rod as a relic of superstition do not hesitate to employ it should the occasion arise. In this respect they are following the attitude of Sir Herbert Maxwell, who once remarked, "I don't believe in the divining rod, but I don't deny that its virtues are genuine; and were I in straits to find water, I would employ without hesitation a professional water finder—rod and all."[34]

Five years later, when the biologist Fanny Moser published a critical overview of the modern occult sciences, she, too, pointed to the practical demands that led even skeptics to overlook the stigma of the occult label:

> "Criminal clairvoyants" and "criminal telepaths" to the side of Justice! An odd sight! The postwar era blessed us with it more and more, especially in Germany: lawyers, police workers, public prosecutors, judges, and other authorities used these "mediums with special abilities" officially and unofficially to expose crimes, solve robberies, find missing persons and so on. . . . The other side: "criminal telepaths" and "criminal clairvoyants" as defrauders in court! Some are found guilty, others innocent.

All of this, Moser observed, was but the "newest phenomenon of modern judicial administration."[35] Taken together, these comments underscore the relevance of occult techniques to the problem of detection in interwar Germany, whether of water or missing objects and people. Dowsing and criminal mediumism proved appealing as well as appalling to social experts in fields as diverse as police work, engineering, architecture, and agriculture. And because these experts enjoyed no monopoly in the open market for services, they sometimes found themselves collaborating with and at other times butting heads with lay practitioners of the same occult techniques. This section considers the reasons for and results of this two-way traffic so typical of interwar modernism.

Criminal mediumism found its official application in the field of forensic science, which evolved as part of the European judicial process in the nineteenth century and became a recognizable discipline in the early twentieth century. An early and dramatic application of forensic concepts and techniques to legal problems came in 1888 in connection with the Jack the Ripper murders in London, when doctors examined victims' wound patterns in an effort to glean useful knowledge about the assailant. Earlier in the decade, the foundations for the new practice of fingerprinting had been laid and, by the end of the 1890s, the practice was being championed by people like Francis Galton, better known for his activities on behalf of British eugenic reform. Fingerprinting soon became but one of a battery of forensic techniques, including blood testing and ballistics analysis, that emerged as a standard part of police procedure in the early twentieth century. These new practices found their codifier in the Austrian magistrate Hans Gross, whose 1893 *Handbuch für Untersuchungsrichter als System der Kriminalistik* (Handbook for investigating magistrates) became a classic of modern forensic science,[36] and their popularizer in Arthur Conan Doyle (also an ardent spiritualist), whose Sherlock Holmes stories brought them into popular awareness.[37]

As early as 1890, the Berlin spiritualist Egbert Müller had advocated the use of mediums for criminal investigations, and by the 1920s the practice enjoyed widespread recognition in Germany.[38] Table 6.1 summarizes information about twelve of the most famous cases of criminal mediumism during this period. Police departments in Leipzig, Hannover, Braunschweig, Insterburg, and Berlin employed criminal telepaths and clairvoyants for help in solving robberies, murders, and missing-persons cases. In 1928, moreover, teams of legal experts in Iserlohn and Dortmund conducted careful experiments to determine the reliability and efficacy of mediums for criminal investigations.

Table 6.1. Criminal Mediumism in Germany, 1911–1930

Mediums	Hypnotists	Forensic Activities	Court Proceedings
Else (Marie) Günther-Geffers	None (self-hypnotized)	Worked privately and for the police in several robbery-murder cases; featured in police experiments (Iserlohn, Dortmund, Berlin, and elsewhere 1920s)	Found innocent of fraud (Insterburg 1927–28)[1]
Mrs. Gerber-Wieghardt		Featured in police experiments (Iserlohn and Dortmund 1928)[2]	
Erich Möckel	Paul Hildebrecht	Worked privately	Both found guilty of fraud (Bernburg 1924)[3]
Mrs. Diederich	Mrs. Hessel	Featured in police experiments (Leipzig 1921)[4]	
Various	August Christian Drost		Drost found innocent of fraud (Bernburg 1924–25)[5]
Mrs. "G"	Mr. "G"	Worked privately (Laublingen 1919–25)	Mr. "G" found guilty of fraud (Balingen 1925–26)[6]
Kara Iki		Solved robbery-murder for the police (Leipzig 1920)[7]	
Mr. Savary		Worked for police (Hannover, Braunschweig, Saxony)	Found guilty of fraud (Stendal)[8]
Mr. Migge		Worked for police on missing-persons case (Insterburg)[9]	
Mrs. Roth-Karoly	Mr. Roth-Karoly	Worked privately (Leipzig 1924)[10]	
Mr. Petzold		Worked privately	Found innocent of fraud (Munich 1911)[11]
Erik Jan Hanussen	None (self-hypnotized)	Worked privately and for army and police	Found innocent of fraud (Leitmeritz 1928–30)[12]

1. "Die Hellseherin bei der Mordaufklärung," *Kriminalistische Monatshefte* 8 (August 1928): 182–83. Hermann, "Die Iserlohner Hellseher-Experimente," *Kriminalistische Monatshefte* 10 (October 1928): 221–24. Carl Pelz, *Das Hellsehen: Ein Kriminalfall* (Munich: Ludendorffs Verlag, 1937), p. 5. Fanny Moser, *Der Okkultismus: Täuschungen und Tatsachen*, vol. 2 (Munich: Ernst Reinhardt, 1935), pp. 610–11. For a useful bibliography for all aspects of criminal telepathy, see Albert Hellwig, *Okkultismus und Verbrechen: Eine Einführung in die kriminalistischen Probleme des Okkultismus für Polizeibeamte, Richter, Staatsanwälte, Psychiater, und Sachverständige* (Berlin: P. Langenscheidt, 1929).

2. Hermann, "Die Iserlohner Hellseher-Experimente," pp. 221–24.

3. Hellwig, *Okkultismus und Verbrechen*, pp. 37–86.

4. Albert Hellwig, "Gibt es nachweisbar echte Fälle von Kriminaltelepathie? Eine Betrachtung zum Insterburger Okkultistenprozeß," *Kriminalistische Monatshefte* 6 (June 1928): 122. See also *Ist Hellsehen möglich? Der Insterburger "Hexen"-Prozeß gegen das kriminal-telepathische Medium Frau Günther-Geffers, mit 20 Abbildungen* (Königsberg: Königsberger Allgemeine Zeitung, 1928).

5. Hellwig, *Okkultismus und Verbrechen*, pp. 88–246. Moser, *Der Okkultismus*, pp. 609–10.

6. Hellwig, *Okkultismus und Verbrechen*, pp. 247–326.

7. "Der Telepath als Detektiv," *Zentralblatt für Okkultismus* 13, no. 11 (May 1920): 521–22.

8. Albert Hellwig, "Abschrift: Kriminaltelepath Savary," 9 January 1928, PDM 7107, StArMü.

9. Hellwig, *Okkultismus und Verbrechen*, pp. 31–32.

10. Reports by Dr. Schulz (24 May 1924) and Dr. Marloth (7 May 1924) in PDM 7107, StArMü.

11. "Der Hellseher Petzold vor Gericht," *Zentralblatt für Okkultismus* 5, no. 4 (1911): 248–50.

12. Moser, *Der Okkultismus*, pp. 611–16. For Hanussen's account, see Hermann Steinschneider, *Der Leitmeritzer Hellseher-Prozess Hanussen: Ausführliche Wiedergabe der sensationellen Gerichts-Verhandlung mit zahlreichen bisher unveröffentlichten Dokumenten* (Teplitz-Schönau: Selbstverlag, c. 1930).

Although the results of this and other studies were far from encouraging, detectives continued the occult practice, prompting the Munich police department to circulate an internal memo in 1929 explaining why it was forbidden to use criminal telepaths for police work. Because the results of police investigations could affect the reputation, honor, economic standing, and freedom of citizens, the memo observed, police employees should strive to use only those investigative methods proved reliable according to contemporary scientific standards. These did not yet include criminal telepathy and clairvoyance.[39] But police detectives were under immense pressure from private parties eager to recover lost jewelry or missing relatives by whatever means worked. When the legal system could not address their problems or they could not persuade the police to employ mediums officially, individuals often employed the mediums directly.

Else Günther-Geffers counted as among the best known and most successful of these mediums. She began as a palmist in 1912, then worked as a clairvoyant during World War I in a recovery camp for soldiers. When her husband lost his job as a school director during the hyperinflation of 1923, Günther-Geffers discovered that she could support her five-person family with her earnings as a criminal clairvoyant catering to both private customers and police detectives. Simple but dramatic, her technique as well as her success quickly vaulted her to national fame. Typically, Günther-Geffers's employer would bring her to the scene of a crime; once there, she would hypnotize herself, then with eyes closed and head thrust forward "like a bloodhound" would follow the trail of invisible clues supposedly left behind by the malefactor (see fig. 13). A companion would then ask her questions to clarify the case: What is the criminal's name? How was the victim murdered? Where did the killing take place? What happened to the body? Günther-Geffers clarified many mysteries in this fashion, several for official customers. Her success brought her not only public visibility but also negative scrutiny from certain quarters in the legal system; when, however, in 1928 she faced more than thirty counts of fraud in court, testimony from more than one hundred witnesses resulted in her acquittal, and the extensive coverage the trial received in Germany's major mass-circulation periodicals enhanced her fame all the more.[40]

Clearly, criminal mediumism had both its advocates and critics among law-enforcement officials, whose disagreements helped ensure that questions concerning the validity, reliability, and applicability of occult techniques would remain open. Cautious advocates of the practice included Vienna's chief of

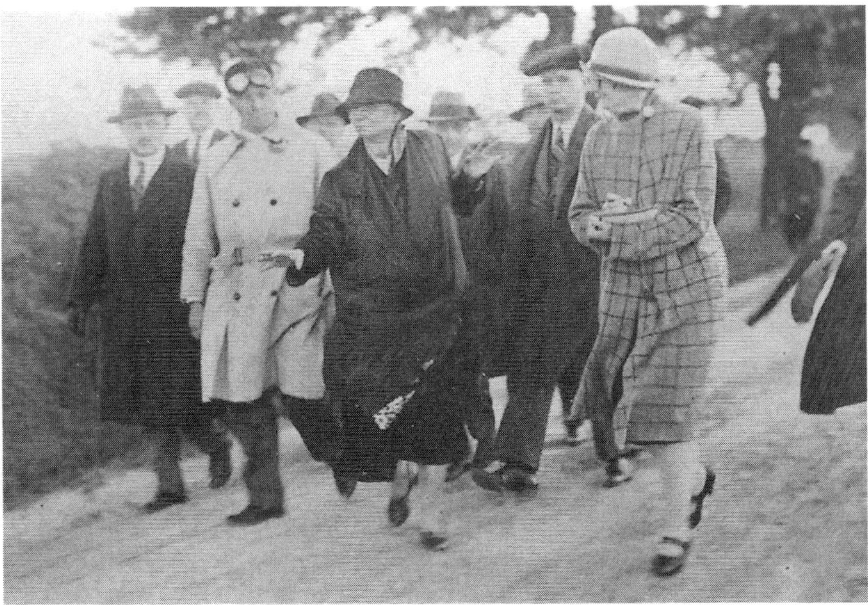

Figure 13. Crime search, 1929. The telepath Marie Günther-Geffers working with policemen and scientific researchers on a robbery-murder case. Officials enlisted Günther-Geffers's occult abilities to follow a trail of extrasensory clues. She was one of several mediums active in police work in the 1920s. Albert Hellwig, *Okkultismus und Verbrechen* (Berlin: P. Langenscheidt, 1929), illus. 5.

police and prominent psychical researcher Ubald Tartaruga. Tartaruga dismissed the notion that mediums could solve crimes single-handedly, but conceded that mediums might serve to reconstruct the way a crime unfolded. Using a metaphor that put legal experts solidly in control of the process, he noted that a medium was nothing more than a "lantern" that would shed light wherever its wielder directed.[41] Other police workers echoed Tartaruga's caution, as did the Dortmund detective who observed in the trade journal *Kriminalistische Monatshefte* that "clairvoyant experiments are valid only when conducted under perfect investigative circumstances by unquestionably expert men of science."[42] Still other officials bemoaned Germany's backwardness in its acceptance of criminal mediums as part of professional law-enforcement teams.[43] But despite some professional support, criminal telepathy also had its professional critics. Among the most prominent was the head of the district court *(Landgerichtsdirektor)* of Potsdam, Albert Hellwig, who did not reject criminal mediumism out of hand, but refused to grant it scientific status in its current form.[44]

While legal experts struggled to determine whether or not criminal mediumism constituted a legitimate investigative practice, the courts began to engage with a different aspect of the problem. Unable and unwilling to rule on the scientific question, they sought to determine whether or not specific criminal mediums and their hypnotists had practiced in good faith, an issue that came to the fore in a nationally publicized trial involving the hypnotist August Christian Drost, who had participated in several official criminal investigations in the early 1920s. Born to a farmer and his wife near Göttingen in 1873, Drost had been a model citizen. After earning a degree as a teacher and then working at a series of Catholic schools, he moved in 1901 to Dessau, where he attended his first lecture-demonstration on hypnotism. Hooked, he began to study hypnotism with a local healer who was also teaching the practice to three other men: a bailiff, a dentist, and a bank employee. By 1908, Drost had married and moved to Bernburg with his family for another teaching job; there, he began to conduct experiments as a hypnotist under the aegis of the local natural healing club where he also practiced psychotherapeutics. During the war, he used his hypnotic skills to treat his comrades and, after the war, he gave lecture-demonstrations on hypnotism in order to raise money for various charitable ends, including war memorials. It was as a result of these many experiences that Drost encountered several mediums with pronounced psychometric skills. Fascinated, he began to experiment with applying their skills to criminal investigations.[45]

By 1924, Drost's activities had landed him in court, where 135 witnesses answered questions about forty-five instances of criminal mediumism. When expert witnesses could not agree on the scientific validity of the practice—the physician and psychical researcher Rudolf Tischner claimed that mediums could be used much like police dogs, while Albert Hellwig remained steadfastly skeptical of the entire practice—the court fell back on the question of Drost's moral character. Here, even skeptics like Hellwig concurred with Tischner that Drost and his mediums believed in their own abilities and thus had practiced their art in good faith. Drost's acquittal in 1925 succeeded on precisely these grounds.[46]

Good faith and scientific validity may have been central in the courtroom, but in the all-important battle for public opinion only one question really mattered: Did mediumism work? The court had hoped that the case would dissuade citizens from consulting criminal mediums once and for all; instead, the case helped promote the technique all the more, not least because of the detailed testimony given by a variety of witnesses in official positions:

- A local police commissioner recounted that Drost and his medium had helped his family locate a key in a room that had been thoroughly searched beforehand.

- The Nordhausen public prosecutor directed police to Drost after their official investigation of a local murder proved inconclusive. Drost's medium had related many details of the case correctly. However, under questioning, the witness admitted that the medium had also gotten other details wrong.

- A senior criminal detective of Dessau testified that he had used Drost's services many times. He described one robbery case in which Drost's medium had managed to determine how a thief entered the crime scene. The medium even named the thief, who was in fact apprehended six months later according to evidence obtained by other means.

- A train inspector recounted how he had turned to Drost and his medium for help in solving the case of a murdered railway official. The team named the murder weapon, specified the direction taken by the murderers, identified them as two brothers named Braß who were at that very moment in Duisberg eating on the promenade, and gave detailed descriptions of the men. The train official had used these clues to track down two gangsters wanted for other crimes, including twenty murders. When he finally caught up with his suspects, both were dead, but the one whose corpse he inspected in the morgue had indeed been wearing the suit described by Drost's medium.[47]

To the question "Did it work?" testimony such as this gave a resounding "Yes!" And because such dramatic success made excellent copy, the mass press quickly turned Drost into a national sensation. He was besieged daily by invitations and letters. Police officials reported that victims of robbery now regularly insisted that their cases be referred to Drost and not to an internal police detective. A major Berlin publishing firm courted Drost for the rights to his written works, and a major film company asked him to do telepathic and clairvoyant trials in front of a camera.[48] Scientific validity and good faith may have been important issues in the legal realm, but in an age dominated by mass enthusiasm for quick solutions to problems, what counted was what, apparently, worked.

A much less complicated sense of excitement surrounded dowsing, a second science of detection. Consider, for example, the young woman portrayed in figure 14. Everything about her suggested modern times. Her bobbed hair, loose top, and short skirt marked her as a "new woman," while her raised hands grasping a metal rod betrayed her as a participant in the new dowsing craze. Contorted by the invisible waves running from an underground water supply through the rod to her nervous system, her face and pose gave graphic illustration to the intimate connections between the modern body and the modern environment. As this photograph suggests, the new craze for dowsing belonged to the new ecological holism, a sensibility linking individuals to their total environment, at once social, economic, and physical.[49]

First mentioned during the Renaissance, the divining rod had featured in an illustration for an early edition of *De re metallica* (1556), a classic humanist text by Georgius Agricola, who noted the instrument's popularity among German miners.[50] Interest in dowsing continued into the modern period in some parts of Europe, but had virtually died out in German-speaking regions by the 1850s. In the 1870s and 1880s, brief notices on the practice appeared in various journals, including the occult *Psychische Studien* and *Sphinx*, the bourgeois *Schorers Familienblatt*, and the avant-garde *Zukunft*, but scientific interest did not resurface again until the 1890s, when the Dublin physicist and psychical researcher Sir William F. Barrett made the links between mediumism and the rod a focus of intensive study. Barrett's studies excited much attention in Germany, and by the eve of World War I, a host of technical experts, whose ranks included engineers, physicists, and geologists, had taken up the practice.[51]

In Germany, the new craze for scientific dowsing exploded into public awareness just after century's turn. It began in 1903, when *Prometheus*, a weekly paper devoted to "progress in trade, industry, and science," carried a favorable report by Cai von Bülow-Bothkamp, accompanied by a series of articles debating the pros and cons of Bülow-Bothkamp's trials.[52] The *Zentralblatt für die Bauverwaltung* (Central journal for building administration) followed this in 1905 with a glowing account by Georg Franzius, a highly placed naval engineer with the admiralty in Kiel, once again followed by commentary, both supportive and critical.[53] The spectacle of military and technical elites disagreeing so hotly over the validity and applicability of an occult practice proved too much for the mass press to resist. Periodicals (e.g., *Daheim* and *Die Gartenlaube*) picked up the story, as did technical supplements to major daily papers (e.g.,

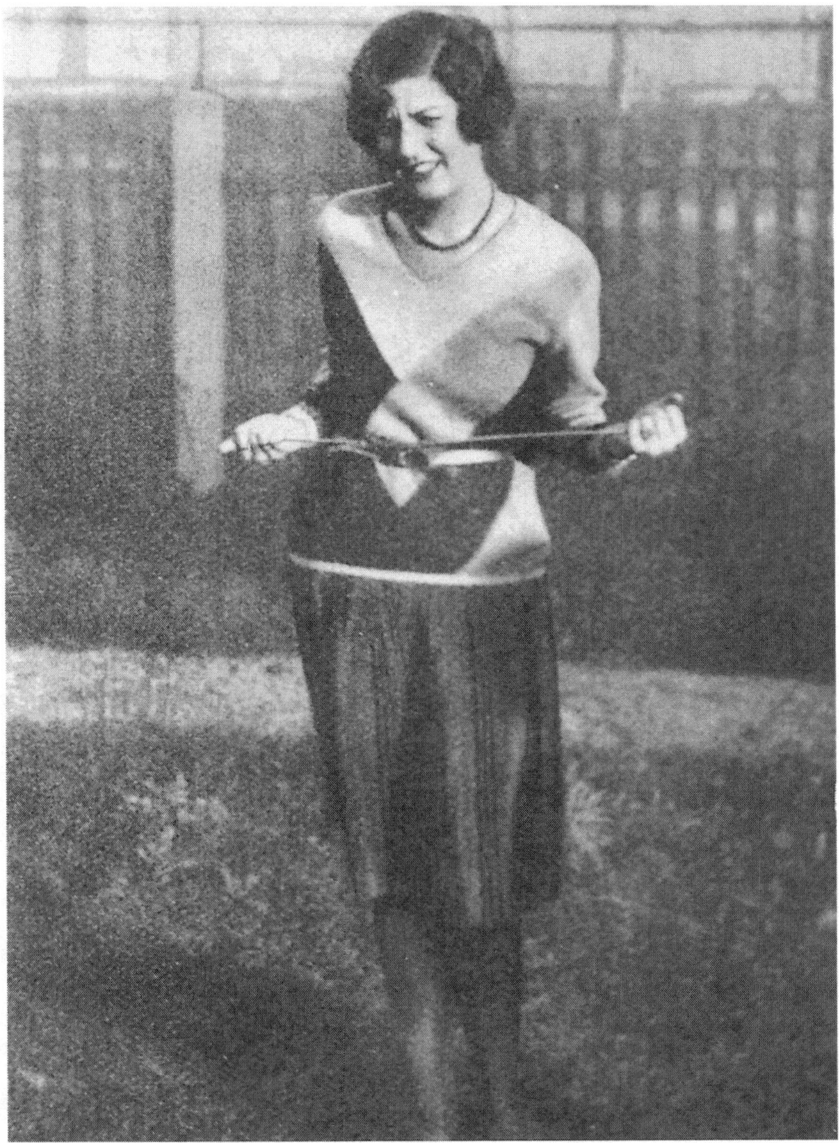

Figure 14. A young woman (identified in the source only as Mrs. Wildhagen) gripping a dowsing rod, 1931. The contortions of her body and face signal that she is crossing an underground water passage whose emanations have been picked up by the rod. Note the urban setting and her modern dress and bobbed hair. Dowsing became very popular in Germany in the 1920s and 1930s. Carl von Klinckowstroem and Rudolf von Maltzahn, *Handbuch der Wünschelrute: Geschichte, Wissenschaft, und Anwendung* (Munich: R. Oldenbourg, 1931).

Berliner Tageblatt) and regional journals for folklore and local history. Trade journals for building administration, pump and drill technology, pharmaceuticals, social medicine, gas lighting, urban water management, and industrial patents entered the fray, with contributions to both sides of the debate. And those with both scientific credentials and long experience in the occult milieu published their own comments in the popular press, as did Max Dessoir in his favorable essay on dowsing that appeared in *Die Woche* in 1906.[54] The highpoint of the prewar dowsing mania came when the state dispatched an official to German Southwest Africa to conduct dowsing experiments on behalf of the Reich.[55]

Like scientific graphologists and astrologers, scientific dowsers quickly organized themselves into a social movement with a pronounced professional following. Declaring themselves a nonpartisan group for the collection of statistical data on dowsing, several dozen men and women banded together in 1911 to establish the Verband zur Klärung der Wünschelrutenfrage (Association for the elucidation of the dowsing question). In addition to Franzius, the group's leaders included Robert Weyrauch, a professor of engineering at the Technical University in Stuttgart, and the Munich physician Eduard Aigner.[56] By 1912, the group had 299 members, including 40 from building professions, 32 from engineering, and at least 10 each from medicine, law, banking, and manufacturing. Corporate groups such as the Apenrade Power Station, Hamburg's Architecture and Engineering Club, the Department of Building Inspections for the Königsberg Ministry of Agriculture, the Bavarian Mining and Iron Works, and Munich's Psychologische Gesellschaft also joined.[57]

After the war, experts' interest in dowsing continued unabated. Founded in 1921, for instance, Hannover's Internationaler Verein der Wünschelrutenforscher (International club of dowsing researchers) attracted numerous professionals, including the geologist Kurt Osswald, the engineer Nikolaus Kremer, and the physician Paul Beyer. The group promoted dowsers and research on the divining rod, especially as it related to drilling for water, minerals, and metallic ores, and published a journal.[58] Institutes with comparable expert profiles also proliferated. A conference held in Munich at the Institut für Wünschelruten-und Pendelforschung (Institute for research on the dowsing rod and pendulum) in 1933, for instance, included speeches by a radiologist and a physicist who presented scientific evidence for the existence of a "divining effect"—that is, the ability of the rod to register radiation emitted by underground formations.[59] As late as 1937, favorable reports on dowsing continued to appear in professional medical journals.[60]

In contrast to the frictions that surrounded criminal mediumism, not to mention both scientific graphology and astrology, the relative success of scientific dowsing raises many questions. Why were modernity's new social experts more willing to embrace dowsing than scientific graphology or astrology? And why, given the significant issues, both legal and scientific, surrounding criminal mediumism did dowsing remain relatively free of such entanglements?

For one thing, scientific dowsers succeeded in fulfilling both intellectual and practical needs more effectively than their counterparts in other occult sciences had ever done. Two of dowsing's most visible enthusiasts, in fact, had also been among Germany's most public critics of popular occultism. Aigner had been a vocal opponent of the Munich spiritualist Adam Rambacher,[61] while the writer Karl von Klinckowstroem had published and lectured widely on "mediumistic tricks."[62] What made scientific dowsing acceptable to these sharp-minded critics was its amenability to explanations at once materialist and holist. As early as 1913, Aigner had estimated that between 5 and 10 percent of the general population possessed dowsing abilities resulting from physiological peculiarities in the human organism.[63] The problematic psychological claims that informed both intuitive and scientific forms of graphology and astrology had no place here. Dowsing, moreover, suited the new vogue for a scientifically grounded ecological holism very well. Klinckowstroem and his collaborator Rudolf von Maltzahn provided an excellent example of this mentality in their 1931 dowsing textbook, where they presented the divining rod as an instrument ideally suited to preventative measures in the emerging field of environmental health. For those who became sick under special weather conditions such as the Föhn (known to induce migraines) or in particular locales such as a poorly situated house (known in some cases to induce cancer), dowsing offered proven relief. Locating the cause of sickness with the land and water formations under and around these human habitats, the authors argued forcefully for the usefulness of the divining rod in preventing such tragedies. Never again should an Alpine sanitarium, for instance, be sited in a place where the Föhn was a regular occurrence; nor should new human settlements be built in places where dowsing had established the local presence of non-hygienic terrestrial influences. As these last comments suggest, finally, dowsing appealed to social experts because it fulfilled clear practical needs, medical and economic. In their 1931 textbook, Klinckowstroem and Maltzahn had made this very clear, citing the proven usefulness of the divining rod for geology, hydrology, dam technology, medicine, and the science of siting homes (*Lagerstättenkunde*).[64]

If dowsing flourished in part because it proved so well suited to the prevailing vogue for practical and holistic applications, its success may also have rested on less tangible negative reasons as well. Unlike criminal telepaths, dowsers practiced their science at a safe distance from the German judicial system. When applied, their skills treated matters not of legal but rather of industrial, economic, or medical import. This related to another factor in dowsing's German success: degrees of professionalization. By and large, dowsers came from established if changing professions such as engineering and architecture.[65] Enthusiasts of criminal mediumism, in contrast, coexisted with modern detectives and legal experts in a new forensic terrain that had as yet no clearly established boundaries, accreditation procedures, or corporate identity. Ironically, perhaps, what made the new social experts in architecture, engineering, and related fields more willing than their law-enforcement counterparts to embrace occult practices was their relatively established professional position. This may also have been an important factor in explaining the relative success of the occult sciences with professional physicians, a topic taken up in the next section.

Healing and Harming

Health—understood as both a spiritual and physical state—had been a major focus of interest in the German occult movement from its inception. The early spiritualist Georg von Langsdorff subscribed to such natural healing practices as magnetic therapy, the light cure, and special diets.[66] Similarly, Wilhelm Hübbe-Schleiden, Germany's first Theosophical leader, always made sure to order vegetarian meals for himself before traveling on society business.[67] This concern for healthfulness extended well beyond the circle of leadership. Aspiring occultists who, for instance, studied with the Berlin magnetist and Theosophical publisher Paul Zillmann learned to maintain purity of both spirit and flesh by opening their day with a snort of cold water through the nose, doing their occult exercises while taking deep breaths of fresh air, and sharply limiting their intake of such spirit-disturbing substances as alcohol, strong spices, and caffeinated drinks.[68] And almost all occult journals carried regular columns with titles like *Dietetic Corner* that recommended the healthful benefits of cool, early-morning baths followed by a morning dew rinse, and barefoot runs through freshly turned fields, supplemented by quick sun baths.[69]

With its heavy emphasis on the intimate connections between the health of the body and the health of the mind, the occult movement offered Germans a multitude of tools for coming to terms with the massive changes convulsing their medical system from the late nineteenth century onward. For hundreds of years, medical theories of disease etiology had stressed the "constitution" of patients: their temperament, physique, and peculiar life story. The ability to discern the medical individuality of each patient quickly and accurately had been the hallmark of the good healer. By the eve of the twentieth century, however, scientific theories had begun to emphasize the specificity of disease, locating the origins of sickness not in the patient's constitution but in such material causes as germs and other pathogens. With specialization on the rise, the hallmark of the good physician now became the ability to exploit the insights of the modern laboratory for the rational diagnosis and treatment of specific diseases. These changes, coupled with the development of the new social-insurance system in the 1880s and its dramatic expansion in the 1920s, prompted doctors and patients alike to complain of the depersonalizing and alienating effects of the new order.[70] And although diseases such as smallpox, tuberculosis, and cholera had largely been eliminated by the 1920s, the persistence of cancer, heart ailments, and other chronic conditions confronted Germans with the therapeutic limitations of even the most scientifically informed and rationally organized medical system.[71]

The changes roiling conventional medicine in late-nineteenth- and early-twentieth-century Germany had their counterpart in the reformist impulses informing the thriving culture of Lebensreform, in which the occult played a major role.[72] Proponents of Lebensreform criticized the autocratic and impersonal doctor-patient relationship of conventional medical practice.[73] They held, moreover, that industrial society created its own health problems and argued that these could be solved only by returning to nature. Accordingly, they extolled the more personal, "natural," and healthful benefits of homeopathy, mesmerism, spirit healing, hydropathy, vegetarianism, therapeutic gymnastics, massage, nudism, and naturopathy. Aided by an 1873 law that effectively deregulated medical practice throughout the new German empire and made it possible for healers of all orientations to practice medicine without a license, lay healers offering these "natural" cures proliferated and found many of their patients in the Lebensreform milieu.[74] Ultimately, enthusiasts of Lebensreform quested after a multifaceted holism. For them, getting back to nature meant not only reharmonizing their mind and body but also reunifying a modern society atomized by rampant individualism. Paradoxically, given their goal, they believed that the path back to this natural state of harmony lay with the individual. The reform of life, they preached, necessitated that each individual reform him- or herself. To the endemic social and economic harms of modern existence, Lebensreform activists thus urged a very private cure.[75]

Despite the uneasy coexistence in which practitioners of conventional and alternative medicine now found themselves, healers of all orientations experimented freely with the therapeutic potential of the novel occult practices, beginning with mediumism. One particularly enterprising lay healer named Adam Rambacher, a Munich spiritualist, claimed in 1908 to be able to use his skills as a medium to channel the healing powers of Lourdes directly, thus saving his German patients the expense and hassle of the long pilgrimage to the holy site in France.[76] Doctors with orthodox credentials also sought to tap the potential of mediumism. In 1914, for example, the Munich physician Johannes Dingfelder predicted the future medical use of psychometric individuals like Aub. Unlike physicians, who often required instruments that caused pain to examine patients and who had in any case gleaned their knowledge by the cruel practice of vivisection, Dingfelder speculated that mediums might well make such invasive medical practices obsolete.[77] By the mid-1920s, the Berlin physician Walter Kröner had begun to investigate such possibilities with his medium, a Mrs. F., who also happened to be a medical student at the University of Berlin. While in a trance, Mrs. F. could sense a patient's sickness intuitively (whether or not the patient was in the room) and then, using technical knowledge gained in her medical studies, identify the disease with a higher than 50 percent rate of accuracy.[78]

Occult practices that drew on characterological techniques appealed to a similarly diverse group of healers. In 1923, the lay practitioner G. W. Surya, for instance, published an entire series on occult medicine, the fifth volume of which treated the topic "occult diagnosis and prognosis." Recommendations included techniques for reading the eye, facial expression, palm, nails, and handwriting, as well as information on the use of the divining rod, the sidereal pendulum, astrology, psychometry, and clairvoyance.[79] Professionally accredited psychiatrists like Karl-Günther Heimsoth, moreover, praised the usefulness of astrology to doctors struggling to achieve insight into a patient's peculiar constitution.[80] Occasionally, the eclecticism of occult medical practice could also result in the most fantastic of claims. Calling himself a psychoanalyst, magnetist, and pendulum researcher, the lay healer Balthasar Wehdanner, for example, advertised himself on a flyer featuring a picture entitled "Christ as Magnetist," with a caption informing potential customers that Wehdanner and Christ used one and the same force to bring the dead back to life.[81]

Whether in the more sober assessments of Heimsoth or the more sensationalist claims of Wehdanner, occult medicine clearly enticed German healers of both conventional and alternative orientations. Although this appeal undoubtedly had many sources, one in particular took on special importance in the interwar years. This was the so-called crisis of medicine that began to fracture the German medical profession in the mid-1920s and received its most effective spokesperson in the Danzig surgeon Erwin Liek, who began in 1925 to reflect publicly on what was wrong with conventional practice. In a 1932 contribution to *Süddeutsche Monatshefte,* Liek observed:

> We doctors have had a surprising experience as servants of social insurance. The insurance system was set up during a time in which the materialist worldview ruled. Man seemed to be an elaborate but knowable machine. Experts—that is, doctors—were supposed to be able to eliminate mistakes in construction and operation. . . . But what did daily experience teach us? The best medicine, the most successful operation, the most careful physical-dietary treatment remained useless, so long as the most important factor on the part of the insured was lacking: the will to recover. In other words, besides the progress of modern medicine the most important thing since the beginning of the century has been the rediscovery of the soul.

Here, Liek criticized the reductionist, materialist, and mechanist thinking that had come to characterize orthodox medical practice. Being a good doctor, he suggested, involved more than just being a highly accomplished scientific expert. Healing also had a psychological dimension: the patient had to have the will to heal and the doctor had to have the ability to inspire trust. Noting that Germans continued to flock to alternative lay healers, although conventionally trained physicians outnumbered them by almost four to one, Liek observed simply that "lay healers are often better psychologists than are doctors."[82] All of this added up to a "crisis of trust," and when Georg Honigmann began the journal *Hippokrates* to overcome this multifaceted crisis in 1928, Liek became a founding member, and he was joined by Rudolf Tischner, the Munich eye doctor, homeopath, and psychical researcher.[83]

Although Liek himself never dabbled in the paranormal, other orthodox physicians did. Such doctors sought to address the "crisis of trust" that Liek and others were identifying by broadening the scope of their practice and making common cause, at least partially, with occult healers. Such was the case with Erich Hartung, a physician with a university medical degree who began to explore occult medicine in the 1920s to find a cure for his profession's crisis. In 1925, just as Liek was beginning to go public with his famous critique, Hartung made an eloquent case for the merits of occult medicine.

The transcendent worldview constituted one of the primary appeals of occult medicine, Hartung explained. Whereas conventional doctors worked in a materialist framework, occult practitioners explicitly rejected materialism, and this rejection translated into major differences of practice.[84] Trained to use a variety of invasive diagnostic procedures and expensive technologies, orthodox physicians identified maladies quickly, without thereby gaining any insight into illnesses' true origins or ultimate cures. In contrast, occult practitioners used a variety of inexpensive and noninvasive techniques (e.g., clairvoyance, the sidereal pendulum, physiognomy, graphology, iridology, consultation with séance spirits, and astrology) to achieve an intuitive and fuller understanding of a sickness. Whereas orthodox physicians generally avoided making predictions about the course of an illness, occult practitioners had intuitive techniques for making such predictions and even determining the proper timing of treatment.[85]

Echoing Liek's criticisms about the preponderance of reductionist thinking in a medical system too heavily dominated by the natural sciences, Hartung also extolled occult healers for not forgetting the medical uniqueness of each patient. This was another way of formulating the widespread feeling that state-sponsored care forgot the individual in an effort to rationalize and standardize disease and health for the masses. As Hartung pointed out, despite its generalizable features, illness was always individual. Doctors, he insisted, must treat not the generalized sickness but the sick individual.[86]

If the transcendent worldview and the individualist orientation of occult medicine lured patients, Hartung observed, there was in any case a growing area of overlap in therapeutic practice. Conventional medicine, he pointed out by way of example, now recognized the efficacy of diet control and hypnosis, two therapeutic elements to which occult healers had long paid close attention. Despite the fact that lay practitioners still relied primarily on homeopathic remedies, while orthodox doctors used mostly allopathic drugs, Hartung noted that some practitioners in both areas were beginning to experiment with the remedies of the other side. Certain therapies, of course, remained contested.

Academic physicians, for instance, were not likely to experiment with spiritualist therapies or faith healing, nor were occultists for their part likely to abandon such effective techniques.[87]

Hartung's comments, designed to identify a middle ground between conventional and alternative medicine, had their echo among lay healers with occult commitments, and some capitalized on the emerging potential for reconciliation. Herbert Fritsche, for example, a Theosophical writer and disciple of Gustav Meyrink, urged healers to master scientific medicine first and then round out their studies by immersing themselves in the work of living occult masters such as G. W. Surya, Peryt Shou, and August Strindberg and classical authors such as Samuel Hahnemann, Jakob Böhme, and Paracelsus. Fritsche promised that by combining technical and spiritual expertise, modern healers would then be able to treat the whole patient—body and mind.[88]

Although this hybrid form of healing drew enthusiasts from all parts of the political spectrum, historians have devoted by far the most attention to its völkisch associations. They have traced, for example, the links between such early völkisch ideologues as Richard Ungewitter, a leader of the German nudist movement, and such völkisch occultists as the Ariosophist Lanz von Liebenfels.[89] Others have detailed the way in which magnetists such as Joseph Weissenberg secured fame in the interwar years for joining spirit healing to German nationalism. Those eager to hear mediums channel such Germanic icons as Martin Luther and Otto von Bismarck while simultaneously seeking relief for their agonized bodies flocked to Weissenberg's meetings. One enthusiastic devotee even compared Weissenberg to Adolf Hitler in 1934, noting approvingly that while Hitler set about reorganizing human society, Weissenberg would do the complementary job of reorganizing humanity's inner life.[90] Still other historians have examined the enthusiasm that many top Nazis, including Rudolf Hess, Heinrich Himmler, and Julius Streicher, had for natural healing, including especially in the case of Hess its occult variants.[91]

Although such data is impressive, it must be treated with caution since the alternative culture that boomed in Germany from the 1890s through the 1930s encompassed many different orientations. Reformism appealed to the far Right as much as the center and far Left. Just because völkisch and Nazi ideologues read occult medical texts and even practiced occult medicine by no means meant that the entire field of occult medicine belonged to their camp.[92] Indeed, against every instance of völkisch or Nazi enthusiasm for alternative medicine, including occult medicine, one could proffer a counterexample. In his 1930 book *Kosmische und irdische Strahlen als Erreger der Krankheiten* (Cosmic and earthly rays as disease pathogens), for instance, the lay healer Alexander Müller applied occult concepts to human health and closed by pleading for the end of xenophobic nationalism and the dawn of the age of true human unity.[93] More often than not, however, occult medical practitioners simply had no overt political orientation. For the most part, their works were not marked by völkisch calls for race purity or national rebirth but with a desire to minister to patients fed up with the therapeutic status quo.

Occult healers quickly discovered, indeed, that one of their main selling points was the promise to rectify a major drawback of the conventional medical system: its tendency to treat patients as anonymous bodies rather than as individual sufferers. Shortly before war broke out in 1914, for example, the Psychomagnetisches-suggestives Heilinstitut (Psychomagnetic-and-suggestive institute of healing) opened its doors in Munich on the posh Prinzregentenstraße, offering a range of services stretching from mesmeric to telepathic healing. Its slogan—"Individual medical treatment: Healing even in serious cases"—indicated the degree of confidence its proprietors had in their brand of treatment and their attention to "personal" needs.[94] The Zentrale für praktischen Okultismus (Center for practical occultism) offered a similarly individualized form of treatment. With "know thyself" as its official slogan, the center boasted a department of astrological medicine that would cast a personal horoscope to discover the cosmic origins of a patient's peculiar ailment, then prescribe and even dispense the appropriate medication tailored to one's individual requirements.[95]

If occult healers thus proved savvy in exploiting the perceived weaknesses of conventional medicine in their advertising, what they were able to deliver in reality often turned out to be a completely different matter, for in the end occult healers had to contend with the same socioeconomic forces squeezing conventional medicine in the 1920s. Occult healers *promised* to provide the sick with just the kind of personalized medical care denied them by the modern health bureaucracy. But because occult healers solicited patients on the open market, the reality was that occult care often reproduced the medical evils its practitioners sought to rectify. The Zentrale für praktischen Okultismus was a case in point. Prospective patients sent in a standardized questionnaire asking for astrological, medical, and religious information. Working through the mail, medical consultants would then return a diagnosis and recommend a course of treatment, never having physically met with the patient. The center, in short, lured patients with the carrot of personalized service, but cured them without personal contact.

The depersonalizing effects of the mass market showed themselves most visibly in columns devoted to medical advice, which were a regular feature in occult journals and a major forum for soliciting and delivering occult medical care. A doctor in Bremen, for example, offered diagnoses by mail to readers of the *Zentralblatt für Okkultismus*. Prospective customers sent a photograph or a good print of the hand, along with a description of symptoms. In return, these mail-order patients received a "personalized" medical profile in a special column entitled "psychological diagnoses." There, one woman found out not only that she had a strong, willful character, a disposition to fantasy, and a rather masculine demeanor, but also that her left lung was weak and her heart slightly agitated. The doctor's advice? That she put her neck in a lukewarm wrap every evening for thirty minutes, take a five-minute bath at twenty-six degrees Celsius three times per week, and not mull matters over too deeply.[96] Medical advice such as this came in a thoroughly anonymous manner. Never having met her doctor, this patient accessed her "personalized" diagnosis through the anonymity of the mass press. What, critics might well have asked, enabled her caregiver to speak with such authority on the ills of a patient never physically examined? Both healer and patient would have pointed to occult medicine in their answer, for occult methods supposedly worked as well with a patient a day's train ride away from the practitioner as they did in a doctor's office. The occult was thus perfectly suited, at least in occultists' minds, to personalizing care in the new world of mass culture.

The irony of claiming that long-distance care could be rendered personal by occult means returns us, finally, to the theme of modernism and its multiple faces. As the American intellectual historian David Hollinger has astutely noted, the study of modernism often feels like "a walk through a multisided room of mirrors. Each wall is said to be 'modernist,' yet each reflects light differently and makes it difficult to get a clear view of any object in the room, including the walls themselves."[97] This chapter has examined the reflections between two of these walls: the social modernism embraced by experts seeking applied solutions to practical problems and the psychological modernism embraced by Germans eager to shore up their individuality against the encroachments of mass society. Between these two mirrored walls sat the occult sciences, which offered tools not just to construct the new social modernity but also to rectify what many perceived as its deepest failures.

Part III / Policing the Occult

CHAPTER SEVEN

The Crimes of Anna Rothe

In March 1902, two officers on the Berlin police force interrupted the medium Anna Rothe in the act of plucking first a hyacinth and then a narcissus flower out of thin air. They grabbed Rothe's hands, wrestled her to the ground, and whistled to bring several more policemen pouring into the room. As the other séance participants watched in horror, a female police assistant subjected Rothe to a physical examination that revealed 157 flowers as well as several oranges and lemons tucked under her petticoat. Placed under arrest and charged with fraud, Rothe spent most of the next year in jail awaiting trial.[1]

Rothe quickly became a cause célèbre. Her story was rehearsed repeatedly on the pages of Germany's major periodicals, where her authenticity as a medium was hotly debated. Two of Berlin's most famous lawyers were assigned to her defense; the prosecution, in contrast, hired three of Berlin's most prominent doctors as expert witnesses. Weeks before her court date, all tickets to the proceedings had been snapped up by a public eager to witness the coming spectacle with their own eyes.[2] By the time her case came to trial in the spring of 1903, Rothe's fame was such that the magician Harry Houdini made sure to attend the proceedings, and the *New York Times* sent a reporter to cover a trial that held the attention of the "world of culture" for an entire week.[3] When the court returned a guilty verdict and sentenced Rothe to eighteen months in jail, the attention continued: for days, weeks, and even years afterward, the case of Anna Rothe continued to elicit passionate commentary and debate.

For historians, Rothe's story raises many questions. How are we to understand the discrepancy between, on the one hand, the crassness of Rothe's acts and, on the other, the harshness of the state's response and the intensity of public interest? What are we to make of the fact that so many policemen went to capture this frail, middle-aged woman who could have posed no physical threat to any one of them? And, given that Rothe's followers were perfectly content with their medium and considered her phenomena to be wholly authentic, how are we to explain the state's intervention in this mutually satisfactory private arrangement? Why, we might ask further, did two prominent defense attorneys agree to take on her case, three medical experts testify against her, and most major German newspapers carry extensive coverage of her arrest and trial? And why did her case continue to cause unrest and controversy even after her sentencing? How, in short, are we to interpret the fact that Anna Rothe was treated and punished as if she were a serious public threat, when all she had done was pull two flowers out of nowhere?

The answer, I propose, is that Anna Rothe was indeed a serious public menace—that she and her followers threatened to erase a boundary fundamental to the cultural stability of fin-de-siècle Berlin. This was the boundary between science and the public, between those who produced new knowledge and stoked the engines of socioeconomic and cultural progress and those who enjoyed its fruits but did not participate in its production. Rothe had transgressed against this epistemological order; even worse, she had provided opportunities for others, too, to transgress. When Rothe and her followers took it upon themselves to found a science of the spirit aimed at the general enlightenment of humanity, they committed an act of epistemological anarchism that challenged the cultural authority of official German science.[4]

Rothe's case is of historical interest because it exposes the volatility and contested nature of the boundary between science and its public in Berlin at the turn of the century.[5] On the one hand, her story reveals the extent to which a modern scientific ethos had permeated the Berlin public, for her followers as well as her critics all claimed to hold "scientific" positions. On the other hand, it exposes an important tension in Berlin's liberal vision of itself as a metropolis of science and progress; it was, after all, a core tenet of liberal thought that truth and freedom should evolve in tandem—that scientific growth and social progress were interdependent. What, then, to make of this uneducated woman and her devoted followers who claimed to have discovered a truth so basic that human enlightenment and well-being could not continue without assimilating it? If science was basic to the enlightenment of the Berlin public, what role was allotted to the public to participate in the scientific enterprise and, thus, in its own enlightenment? The case of Anna Rothe derived its significance from the fact that it not only posed these questions, but showed that they had no clear answers.

In exposing the complex relationship between science and the public in fin-de-siècle Berlin, Rothe's case also allows us to observe some of the basic dynamics and contradictions of Germany's growing liberal culture. This assertion may come as a surprise to anyone accustomed to thinking of the Wilhelmine period as an era of embattled German liberalism. There is, of course, much to recommend this view. In the 1890s and the early years of the twentieth century, Germany's liberal parties had lost their electoral base and were receding to the political fringes. With the *Kulturkampf* of the 1870s and the antisocialist laws of the 1880s, the German state had acquired a well-deserved reputation for disregarding individual rights and not tolerating differences of religious and political opinion. All of this is true, but a view based solely on those facts fails to acknowledge the signs of a liberal culture thriving outside the confines of high politics. Most importantly, it neglects the wide limits of public debate that occurred outside the German state, in local clubs, civic associations, and mass-circulation newspapers, where Germans sought to reformulate traditional liberal values for contemporary needs.[6] These traditional liberal values included a belief in the possibility of human progress, a faith in the improving power of science and technology, a commitment to constitutional government, and the ideal of autonomous individuals acting freely according to reason. Rothe's story exposes a fault line that opened up at the fin de siècle over the question of how science related to progress. Whereas Rothe's defenders sought to make spiritualism a populist science of the spirit with ethical implications for everyday life, many of her detractors sought to absorb the novel psychological phenomena into a more secular project for human improvement under the control of scientific professionals.

One of the telltale signs that Rothe's story belongs to the history of German liberalism is contemporaries' recurrent use of the term *civilization* to define the issues at stake in the case. As one participant put it at the time: "The Rothe case is not simply a problem of criminal psychology, but more broadly one concerning the history of civilization."[7] This chapter seeks to make sense of comments such as these by considering four different stages in the drama. The first section lays out the background to the Rothe case, describing her rise to fame and the controversy that broke out over her skills as a medium long before her arrest in 1902. It shows that Rothe was an object of contention partly because her followers and critics shared a similar intellectual framework. The second section examines the strength of the popular occult movement in fin-de-siècle Berlin and the anxieties it aroused among local scientific and re-ligious authorities, who perceived popular occultism as a threat to the episte-mological order in which they had a significant stake. The third section offers an anatomy of Rothe's trial in 1903. Here, the attention is on the confrontation between the personal testimony offered by Rothe's followers and the opinions offered by expert witnesses—between the confrontation of two different kinds of modern truth. The fourth section examines the discussion of the verdict by the liberal press in Berlin and explains why so many contemporaries agreed that Rothe's case was a significant and highly unsettling episode in the cul-tural history of their era. A concluding section weaves the various strands of the argument together and offers some remarks on the tensions surrounding knowledge and its control in fin-de-siècle Germany.

The Controversy over "the German Eusapia"

Rothe's fame—and notoriety—rested on her claim to materialize physical objects during her séances. Whereas most individuals who styled themselves "mediums" were known for such mental feats as clairvoyance and telepathy, only a few possessed Rothe's apparent gift of materializing objects, such as flowers. The dearth of German mediums sufficiently gifted to produce such physical phenomena, in fact, had rankled German spiritualists for years. They had been forced to content themselves with short visits from foreign mediums or to travel abroad to conduct such high-level séances.

It was in this state of national deprivation that Anna Rothe rose to fame as "the German Eusapia," a name that referred both to her German birth and her ability to produce physical phenomena rivaling those of the world-renowned Italian medium Eusapia Paladino.[8] Like the Italian medium, Rothe came from the working class. Born in Altenburg, Saxony, on 8 September 1850 to a foreman bricklayer and his wife, Rothe lost her parents and two sisters to cholera while still a minor. To support her remaining siblings, she was forced to go to work as a household servant. She married at eighteen and soon produced a daughter. When her daughter's fiancé died in 1890, Rothe began to see the dead man in her home. She had been prone to visions from an early age, but these were so powerful that her husband took her to a healer in Zwickau, who "cured" Rothe by informing her that the visions were not the sign of an illness but of her strong powers as a medium.[9]

Rothe then began to conduct séances and by the middle of the 1890s had garnered an enthusiastic following among German spiritualists. Her talent for spirit-knocking developed first; soon thereafter, her ability to perform complex materialization phenomena had emerged as well. This, more than anything else, enabled her to move beyond the spiritualist circles in Saxony to which she had previously been limited and become a medium of national renown. Eventually, her successes attracted the attention of a former cognac merchant and journalist named Max Jentsch, who became her impresario in 1896. Jentsch managed her séances as well as her public relations and helped Rothe vault into the international community of psychical researchers and spiritualists. Invited to give sittings with occult circles around Europe, she traveled to places as far-flung as Berlin, Breslau, Chemnitz, Leipzig, Dresden, Vienna, Düsseldorf, Munich, Hamburg, Schwarzenberg, Breitenbrunn, Zwickau, Paris, and Zurich. By the late 1890s, she was well known both at home and abroad and ready to move from her base in Chemnitz to pursue fame and fortune in the beckoning metropolis of Berlin.[10]

Rothe's séances, the cornerstone of her success, followed a set pattern. After paying a few marks to gain admission to the proceedings, participants were seated around a table or in rows around the room. Rothe would present herself for investigation by a female member of the audience in order to establish that she had not concealed any objects on her person. After a short introduction by Jentsch, her impresario, Rothe would lead a prayer and promptly fall into a trance. Various phenomena, both mental and physical, would then unfold. Typically, the medium began by manifesting different personalities. These would bring news from the beyond, dispense personal advice, and diagnose and prescribe for the ailments of the assembled. These personalities included famous historical figures—Luther, Zwingli, Frederick III, and King Ludwig of Bavaria—as well as the deceased friends and relatives of séance participants. Sometimes Rothe's own control spirit, a girl named Friedchen, also spoke.

Spirit communications were usually followed by stunning physical phenomena. Flowers and other objects—fruits, religious statues, gold dust, amulets, and gloves—often materialized, apparently out of thin air. Books with blank pages suddenly acquired spirit-writing. Occasionally, spirits appeared. When Rothe's trance came to an end, after a short prayer the séance would be over.[11]

From the beginning, Rothe's feats of physical mediumship were intensely controversial, and it was not uncommon for participants at a single séance to draw vastly different conclusions about the significance of what they had witnessed. Ardent spiritualists saw the medium's productions as direct communications from the spirits of the dead. In contrast, spiritualists and psychical researchers of a more cautious temperament, while considering many of the phenomena to be authentic, kept an open mind about their origins and causes. They usually accepted the mental phenomena as unproblematic, but professed a cautious skepticism toward the physical ones. A final group, including some spiritualists and many psychical researchers, saw—or at least suspected—that Rothe "produced" all of her phenomena through trickery, and they did not hesitate to take their accusations of fraudulence before the German public.

What made Rothe's séances wholly believable to some but dangerously fraudulent to others? All sides gave the same answer: because of "evidence." To ardent spiritualists, Rothe's séances provided compelling personal evidence for the reality of life after death. Rothe, they claimed, put them in communication with séance spirits who were their deceased family members and friends. Spiritualists' certainty stemmed from the fact that séance spirits identified themselves by name and confirmed their identity by reciting personal information that could not be known by anyone in the room except close living relatives and friends. Once a spirit had established its identity, séance participants were ready—with the help of Rothe's astonishing materialization phenomena—to receive "gifts" from the beyond. If spiritualists took these materializations as definitive proof that people they had cared about in life had not simply ceased to exist in death, they did so only after a context for personal belief had been established by nonmaterial means earlier in the séance. And if they then espoused their firm belief in a Christian afterlife, they did so not on the basis of revelation or the Bible, but that of their own experiences at Rothe's séances. This was a form of liberal theology par excellence, and, as will soon become clear, it posed a significant threat not just to religious authorities but also scientific ones.[12]

If the materialization of solid objects during Rothe's séances sealed the case for the spiritualist interpretation to some, the same phenomena caused others to cry fraud. Materialization mediums like Rothe, indeed, had faced organized opposition for years. Leipzig, for instance, as one of the original centers of modern German occult activity, had also been home to the antispiritualist circle Abila since 1885.[13] And in Berlin, the populace had recently witnessed a series of public exposures and court cases involving prominent materialization mediums. These included Karl Wolter, found guilty of fraud in a court in Resau (a small town near Berlin) in 1889, Valeska Töpfer, found guilty of fraud in a Berlin court in 1892, and a Mr. Pinkert, exposed publicly as a fake by the prominent Berlin occultist Egbert Müller in 1896.[14] As had been true in these earlier cases, those who now accused Rothe of fraud came almost exclusively from the ranks of German psychical research, a movement closely linked to spiritualism and in frequent conflict with it. Whereas spiritualists used the phenomena of mediumism to underpin their belief in the afterlife, psychical researchers sought to use these same phenomena to open the human psyche to experimental probing and scientific theorizing. Rothe's popularity, just as much as her suspicious materialization phenomena, threatened to thwart psychical researchers in this quest for scientific legitimation, and they mounted frontal attacks on the medium and her followers to defend their interests.

Critics from psychical research circles complained that spiritualists were too easy to trick, that they cast their eyes upward to catch a glimpse of the flowers as they materialized from the heavens instead of downward to catch Rothe in the act of pulling the flowers out from underneath her skirt. With surprising care and venom, given the alleged crudeness of the beliefs and tricks in question, these critics staged public exposures and published scathing reports on their investigations with the famous flower medium. One of the first came from the Hamburg occult circle Loge zum Licht in 1894, when two members— a local dentist and a manufacturer—caught Rothe cheating during a séance. Later that year they published evidence of her fraudulence in *Psychische Studien*, Germany's foremost journal of psychical research.[15] Soon after, a Berlin Freemason and seasoned investigator of mediumism named Max Rahn printed corroboratory evidence, gathered during his own sittings with Rothe, in the occult newspaper *Die übersinnliche Welt*. More exposures followed: in 1895 in Dresden, in Zwickau in 1897, and in Chemnitz in 1900.[16]

In 1900 and 1901, two experienced psychical researchers took the mounting evidence of Rothe's fraudulence to the general German public. Although they aimed at different aspects of spiritualism, both framed their attacks using the classical rhetoric of liberalism. They invoked, in other words, familiar tropes featuring themselves as the defenders of a secular and scientific modernity, now threatened by the resurgence of backward-looking superstition. The first, a Breslau lawyer named Erich Bohn, declared himself a servant of truth and blew the whistle on Rothe in a grand "J'Accuse" published initially in 1900 in *Nord und Süd* and then a year later in book form. Admonishing readers that "we are slaves to facts and submit to them," Bohn presented the evidence that he and others had gathered to prove Rothe's fraudulence.[17] His extended discussion of Rothe was justified, he believed, because Rothe posed a serious public threat. Bohn put it thus: "As long as mediums commit fraud in a laboratory, they are not dangerous. But when they go before the public, their activities must be stopped 'ne quid detrimenti res publica capiat.' "[18] Rothe's séances, he reported, took place under conditions totally unsuitable for making the exact scientific observations required to determine whether or not she was an authentic medium.[19] Noting that "church and laboratory exclude each other like prayer and science," he condemned Rothe's séances as purely religious events and bemoaned the fact that mediumism had been claimed as an object of study by spiritualists, when it belonged more appropriately to psychology.[20]

Bohn was soon joined in this public attack on Rothe by a Hamburg doctor, Ferdinand Maack, who took a somewhat different approach to the problem of Anna Rothe. Instead of concentrating on establishing Rothe's fraudulence, in 1901 Maack produced a satirical pamphlet that attacked the scientific credibility of Rothe's followers and ridiculed their despotic arrogance. Whereas Bohn's writings had had a measured, serious tone, Maack's pamphlet—advertised on its front cover as "Sensational. With Illustrations. Interesting!"—was a scathing polemic. Despite the differences in focus and tone, Maack's pamphlet echoed Bohn's principal message: that the occult phenomena of mediumism belonged to science and not to religion, to serious "researchers" and not to ardent spiritualists, in the laboratory and not in the private spiritualist circle. Maack documented the gullibility of spiritualists in embarrassing detail in order to rescue the public image of serious investigators like himself who wanted to use mediumism to explore the human psyche scientifically. Like Bohn, moreover, he also warned his readers about the public threat posed by spiritualism. Spiritualism fostered superstition and weakened the critical faculties. It also encouraged pathological psychic states, not just in the mediums but in séance participants as well. Not least, it distracted individuals from their civic duties and encouraged them to fritter away their time on speculations about their fate in the beyond. Spiritualism was thus a multifaceted menace to liberal society, a sign of just how far the uneducated masses still had to go before achieving the grand goal of full enlightenment. "Spiritualism belongs not in the family," Maack declared in a close echo of Bohn, "but in the laboratory."[21]

Both Bohn and Maack endeavored to show that although the occult phenomena of mediumism deserved serious scientific investigation, the studies conducted by spiritualists were a threat to Germany's social order. Was occultism to become an object of laboratory investigation, a scientific gateway to the "new America" of the human psyche?[22] Or was it to remain in the hands of unenlightened spiritualists whose domestic séances only helped spread outdated religious beliefs and crass superstitions to the masses? What was at stake for Rothe's critics in the German psychical research movement was not whether occultism per se should be allowed in modern Germany, but which kind.

Such aggressive attacks on Rothe's authenticity and her followers' credibility prompted an organized defense from the German spiritualist community that betrayed how much the two sides had in common. Several aspects of this commonality are particularly striking. First, Rothe's defenders and accusers were all actively engaged in the investigation of spiritualist mediums. Their controversy, in other words, was a controversy within Germany's growing modern occult movement. Second, Rothe's defenders and accusers shared a common social background in Germany's propertied and educated middle class *(Besitz-und Bildungsbürgertum)*. It was no accident that when the Commission für Medienschutz (Commission for the protection of mediums) was established in February 1900 in Chemnitz to defend Rothe, it consisted of fifty members whose ranks included six merchants, four magnetists and a medical doctor, five manufacturers and factory owners, two engineers, and an architect, all led by a bookseller.[23] Rothe's accusers had a similar background: Bohn was a lawyer, Maack a doctor, her exposers in Hamburg a dentist and a manufacturer. Yet a third point of commonality in the debate over Rothe was that both sides shared a liberal rhetorical strategy. The Commission für Medienschutz espoused the common spiritualist view that bringing mediums before the public was a necessary element in the general enlightenment and welfare of humanity. Rothe's critics, similarly, sought to expose Rothe's fraudulence so as to protect the German public from this newest threat to its welfare; at the same time, they continued to view their own investigations of mediums as necessary to the promotion of scientific progress in a new realm of experimental research.[24] Public progress, welfare, and enlightenment—all terms drawn from liberal discourse—structured both sides of the debate.

Was Rothe a boon to the progress of German civilization? Or was she an obstacle? The acrimony of the Rothe controversy around 1900 reflected the conviction shared by both sides that it was indeed German civilization that was at stake. Attached to this conviction was a shared scientific ethos that only made the controversy more contentious. Rothe's defenders and critics alike assembled in research groups, published their séance experiences in the form of scientific articles, testified about the evidence of their senses, and understood themselves to be "investigators." The difference between the two sides, of course, was that whereas Rothe's defenders knew themselves to be investigators of the world of the spirit, her critics saw themselves as investigators of a human psyche not capable of producing material objects. The controversy over the German Eusapia, therefore, turned on the question of which group was competent to interpret this "experiential evidence." Men like Bohn and Maack asserted their scientific credentials, but they were answered by spiritualists who claimed the same authority for themselves. Did the "evidence" consist of fact or the fantastic imaginings of the faithful? Spiritualists, it turned out, saw no conflict between their scientific commitments, their common sense, and their personal knowledge of the beyond. As one spiritualist writer commented in 1901 after criticizing Bohn for his excessively harsh attacks on Rothe: "Thank God that there are still people who, despite their common sense, can still feel rapture, and so let us hope that these phenomena continue to be studied in a serious and scientific manner."[25]

Occultism and Spiritualism in "the Metropolis of Intelligence"

When Anna Rothe arrived in Berlin with her family and impresario in the fall of 1901, the city already had a thriving mass occult movement whose members engaged in beliefs and practices as diverse as spiritualism, Theosophy, astrology, neomesmerism, and psychical research. While some observers viewed popular occultism as an expression of Berlin's experimental culture,[26] others considered it to be a blight on the modern city, a typical expression of what one observer sarcastically called "the metropolis of intelligence."[27] Two groups in particular found the local occult movement alarming enough to voice their concerns publicly: the scientific-academic elites, on the one hand,

and Protestant church leaders, on the other. The first group extolled Berlin as an international center of education, science, and political progress; the second berated Berlin as politically dangerous and spiritually bankrupt; but both groups agreed that occultism constituted a public menace. This section tackles the question of why two groups with such diametrically opposed evaluations of Berlin nonetheless achieved a rapid consensus on the threat posed to their city by popular occultism and provides the context crucial to explaining why the trial of Anna Rothe in 1903 took the form it did.

In terms of size, organization, and spread, the popular occult movement in Berlin was indeed significant by the time of Rothe's arrest in 1902. There were at least nine Theosophical lodges, as many registered circles dedicated to spiritualism and psychical research, and many more private ones.[28] Berlin also had a flourishing occult business sector. The city was home to several occult presses and book stores like the ones run by Karl Siegismund, Paul Zillmann, and Max Rahn, as well as several occult periodicals, including *Spiritistische Rundschau* (f. 1892), *Die übersinnliche Welt* (f. 1893), and *[Neue] Metaphysische Rundschau* (f. 1896).

Berlin occultism also enjoyed popularity across the class spectrum. From the working classes came a variety of self-made mediums and occult entrepreneurs; for instance, Berlin was home to many spiritualist circles whose mediums and members worked in the local garment industry.[29] It also housed men like the tanner August Machner, who had recently made himself over as a psychic painter. Able to produce art while in a state of trance despite his lack of artistic training, Machner made works of sufficient artistic merit to be shown at locations around Berlin, including a gallery on Berlin's fashionable Potsdamerstraße.[30] There were also, finally, local occultists like Paul Zillmann, who began his business life as a magnetist and then expanded his skills to become a character analyst and editor of the occult journal *Metaphysische Rundschau.* Dedicated to "metaphysical research," this journal aimed to establish a worldview that would sit on exact scientific foundations while still pursuing the spiritual goals more commonly associated with the churches.[31]

This pairing of scientific and spiritual goals was an even more dominant pattern among Berlin occultists from the educated middle classes. Typical were men like the spiritualist Egbert Müller and the Theosophist Rudolf Steiner, both of whom constantly stressed their dual commitments to science, on the one hand, and the life of the spirit, on the other. A lawyer by training and a lay researcher of occult phenomena by vocation, Müller had been a leader in Berlin spiritualist circles since the early 1890s.[32] He viewed his spiritualist investigations as a service to science and his tireless organizing on behalf of spiritualism as a service to the public. Berating those who dismissed the observed "facts" of mediumism as chimeras, he blamed the dominance of Berlin's "thinking society"—its ethos of dogmatic materialism and narrow-minded rationalism, its "superstitious fear of superstition"—for stopping the march of spiritual and scientific progress.[33] Steiner, a self-made mystic of petty-bourgeois Austrian background, had earned a doctorate in philosophy and edited Goethe's papers before arriving in Berlin in the 1890s. He quickly built a reputation for himself in Berlin Theosophical circles as the proponent of a "spiritual science" that would investigate the world of the soul according to exact scientific methods.[34]

The occult also enjoyed a significant presence among Berlin aristocrats. In Charlottenburg, Cay and Sophie von Brockdorff presided over a Theosophical lodge in which Steiner first began to propound his spiritual science. Helmuth von Moltke, a general in the German army, and his wife Eliza, well-known spiritualists who eventually became followers of Steiner, were devotees of Anna Rothe. Eliza von Moltke, in fact, expended a great deal of energy trying to convince Albert Moll, one of the city's leading psychiatrists, to give his scientific legitimation to Rothe's abilities.[35] Such exalted circles even produced a famous medium, known simply as *"la femme masqué,"* who regularly attracted hundreds of people to her séances and was supposedly married to another German general.[36] At the very highest levels were three members of Wilhelm II's inner circle of friends, including his best friend Philipp zu Eulenburg, who had patronized magnetists and spiritualist mediums for years.[37] Thus, in terms of sheer size, organization, and diffusion across the class spectrum, Berlin occultism certainly warranted notice from local observers keen on discerning new movements afoot in their metropolis. Why, however, did members of the city's intellectual elites and Protestant clergy take an active oppositional stance against popular Berlin occultism? What menace did they discern in this loosely organized, apolitical, and—by their own account—scientifically naive movement?

Echoing concerns already voiced by psychical researchers like Bohn and Maack, members of the city's intellectual elites claimed that popular occultism was a public menace. Typical in this regard were the warnings aired in 1901 by the psychiatrist Richard Henneberg, who later appeared as an expert witness for the prosecution in the Rothe trial. In an article published in the prestigious *Archiv für Psychiatrie* in the spring of 1901, he warned readers that spiritualism and mental illness shared an intimate connection. Drawing on the case histories of several patients seen in the psychiatric wing of Berlin's Charité hospital, Henneberg argued that engaging in spiritualist practices as a medium could actually cause illnesses like hysteria in individuals with no previous history of mental disease. Careful not to dismiss mediumism itself, he nevertheless condemned the "vulgar spiritualism" practiced in lay circles and warned that it endangered public health.[38]

Henneberg's attempt to pathologize spiritualist practices by framing them as a menace to public health obscured the professional interests at stake in his position and that of the professional colleagues who shared it.[39] The issue turned on the question of which group—lay occultists or psychological experts—would control the right to study, develop, interpret, and apply the novel psychical phenomena displayed by mediums. Behind the liberal rhetoric of spiritualism as a "public menace" lurked the self-interest of the emerging profession of modern psychiatry and psychology. Psychiatrists like Henneberg perceived the popular occult movement as a significant threat to their effort to secure expert scientific status, not least because popular occultists also purported to study, develop, and cure the human psyche. By warning the public about the medical dangers of spiritualist practices, Henneberg drew a sharp line differentiating his own therapeutically motivated investigation of mental phenomena from the disease-causing efforts of lay investigators. At the same time, he reinforced his profession's authority to speak on such matters by framing his own mentally ill patients at Berlin's psychiatric hospital as the victims of the popular occult movement.

In their effort to claim the phenomena of mediumism for themselves by medicalizing and thus seeking to control the "vulgar spiritualism" of the masses, the intellectual elites received helped from an unexpected quarter: the Protestant church. A Protestant minister in Berlin-Charlottenburg named Otto Riemann, for instance, became sufficiently concerned about the spiritualist menace to attend one of Rothe's séances at the Berlin spiritualist lodge Psyche on 20 May 1900. In a pamphlet directed to the general public, he sought to "enlighten" his readers about Rothe's fraudulence by explaining the tricks she used to perform her materializations.[40] Riemann also took his message to the Berlin lecture circuit. In the fall of 1900, he informed an audience of two thousand that Christianity had no need of spiritualism to provide evidence for the reality of the afterlife. His dismissal of spiritualism, however, was not a dismissal of the phenomena of mediumism, for Riemann did not hesitate to inform his audience that spiritualist phenomena might be of some use to the new psychology.[41]

Other prominent clergymen repeated the message that although spiritualism menaced Christianity, its phenomena might properly belong to science. Adolf Stoecker, former court chaplain to the Kaiser and leader of the notoriously demagogic Christian-Social Worker's Party, made the dangers of spiritualism central to his address at a Berlin pastoral conference in June 1900. After describing his own séance experiences, he warned the assembled clergymen that spiritualism was widespread, both in the general population and in Christian circles. Estimating that Berlin contained approximately four hundred mediums and ten thousand spiritualists, he urged pastors to inform their parishioners that dabbling in spiritualism was incompatible with a Christian life.[42] Significantly, he also cautioned that although much of spiritualism was fraudulent, not all of it could be dismissed as a swindle, and what there was of value in spiritualism should be investigated by scientific authorities.[43]

What were the deeper motivations for this attack on spiritualism by Berlin's Protestant clergy? One factor was undoubtedly that church attendance among Berliners had been very low, and dropping, for decades. Barely 3 percent of the Berlin populace attended church in 1869; by 1913, only 1 percent did.[44] In this context, a popular movement such as spiritualism that seemed to arouse more enthusiasm for core Christian beliefs than traditional Protestant teachings was sure to stimulate anxiety, not just about loss of clerical control but also about the proliferation of Christian sects. Another factor was the embarrassing reality that there were Protestant clerics who unashamedly publicized their own spiritualist affiliations. Max Gubalke, for instance, was a Berlin minister who chaired the 1898 congress of the Verband Deutscher Okkultisten (Association of German occultists), a national spiritualist association, and discussed the connections between spiritualism and Christianity at length in his opening comments.[45] Regarding the Christian aspects of Berlin spiritualism, the clergy therefore had cause for anxiety.

What is more puzzling and, for the case of Anna Rothe, more significant, is the question of why church representatives had no qualms about shunting the phenomenological aspects of spiritualism into the hands of the scientific community. Scientists were, after all, the representatives of the materialistic-mechanistic worldview that had done so much to erode Christian faith. Moreover, the ideology of science enjoyed a marked popularity among Berlin's liberal political leaders, headed by the medical researcher and politician Rudolf

Virchow, whose hostility to organized religion was well known. Why, then, did Berlin's Protestant leadership throw its support behind the claims of the scientific community on the question of popular occultism? The answer reflects the reorientation of late-nineteenth-century German Protestant theology with respect to the natural sciences. Following the lead of theologians like Wilhelm Herrmann, clerics had begun to insist that science and religion belonged to wholly separate realms: science to nature and religion to morality.[46] Riemann's and Stoecker's support for scientists' claim to mediumism was tantamount to declaring mediumism a natural phenomenon of no interest to Christian faith. It was also a way of attempting to use scientific authority to control the terrifying challenge posed by "vulgar spiritualism" to the authority of the Protestant hierarchy. Although the church no longer attracted the masses, the popularity of spiritualism demonstrated that religious impulses had not disappeared among the people. If anything, the liberal theology of the spiritualists—their insistence that their Christian faith was empirically and rationally grounded in their own experiences and not in the teachings of the church—demonstrated that religiosity was alive and well, even in the decidedly un-Christian metropolis of Berlin. The problem, of course, was that this was not a form of religious feeling calculated to conserve an epistemological order founded on the strict separation of scientific and religious realms of authority.

Lay occultists, for their part, viewed occult phenomena as the property of the public and tended to see their occult researches as an occasion for the reintroduction of a scientifically grounded ethical perspective to modern life. This group counted many spiritualists, magnetists, and Theosophists in its ranks.[47] Theirs was a viewpoint guaranteed to arouse hostility among both traditional religious authorities and scientific leaders, who saw their own realms of power being infringed. While the scientific-academic community had a professional stake in pulling occult phenomena away from questions of value and placing them instead within the confines of controlled investigative settings (ideally, a modern research laboratory), church representatives reasserted the authority of the church to speak on matters of religious and ethical import. By adhering to a picture of nature without moral import, the late-nineteenth-century scientific community had left the church free to speak at least on matters of the spirit with cultural authority; in return, the church had buttressed the cultural authority of science to determine the nature of the physical universe. Lay occultism threatened both groups, not just because its practitioners claimed scientific and spiritual authority for themselves but because their activities threatened to erase the lines according to which scientific and religious authorities had reached their truce.

When Rothe arrived in Berlin to practice her trade as a medium in the fall of 1901, she therefore entered a minefield. There were ardent spiritualists eager to experience one of her séances. There were more skeptical psychical researchers hoping to test her powers and, if necessary, expose their fraudulence. There were doctors, psychologists, and psychiatrists with a professional stake in claiming the phenomena of mediumism for their own use. And there were church officials appalled at the spread of a new form of unbelief among their traditional constituency. By the fall of 1901, the latter three groups had succeeded in building a case against Rothe as a "public menace," and the state lost little time in acting. Soon, policemen had infiltrated several of Rothe's Berlin séances, and by the spring of 1902 Rothe was "safely" under arrest.

German Spiritualism on Trial in Berlin and Beyond

Instead of assuaging the general anxiety over popular occultism in Berlin, Rothe's imprisonment merely focused the antispiritualist animus on a specific person. Her capture became an occasion for critics to push forward with their campaign to obliterate spiritualists' faith at what they must have thought was one of its main sources: a working-class woman with a thick Saxon accent and a diminutive physical presence who had never aspired to scientific legitimation. How they accomplished their aim—and how spiritualists attempted to thwart them—is the topic of this section.

The antispiritualist campaign proceeded in two venues: the national press and the Berlin courtroom. While Rothe sat in prison awaiting trial, critics used the German press to turn the two main arguments raised about popular occultism in Berlin—that it was a public menace and that its phenomena belonged to professional scientists—against Rothe herself. These arguments then entered the courtroom in March 1903 when the state tapped the cultural authority of expert witnesses to convict Rothe of fraud, despite the fervent testimony of her followers to the contrary. Antispiritualists "won" the legal case against Rothe by pulling epistemological rank; whether or not they won the case on the popular front turned out to be a completely different matter.

While Rothe languished in jail through 1902, her opponents continued to sharpen the case against her. Although motivated by different reasons, these critics established a united front dedicated to the public development of two main claims: that Rothe was a fraud and a significant public menace and that the investigation of mediums was a dangerous pastime unless conducted by properly trained scientific authorities. These claims were developed both in religious periodicals and in more secular ones. Riemann, the Berlin cleric who had already weighed in against popular occultism before Rothe's arrest, published an article elaborating on the social menace posed by Rothe and her followers in the very first issue of the new Protestant journal *Reformation* in 1902. Claiming that he had seen for himself how spiritualists damaged their health, family, wealth, social standing, and mental state because of their erroneous faith, he called on the state to protect society from this newest danger. He then advised spiritualists to leave the investigation of mediumism to scientists, who had the requisite training to investigate and explain it through natural terms like hypnosis, the play of the psyche and the unconscious, thought-transference, and animal magnetism. To those who objected that spiritualists counted among their ranks many experienced investigators like the astrophysicist Karl Friedrich Zöllner, of Leipzig, the former *Gymnasium* teacher C. W. Sellin of Hamburg, and the lawyer Egbert Müller, of Berlin, Riemann—following Maack—took care to cast doubt on their qualifications.[48]

While men like Riemann propounded the case against Rothe in religious periodicals like *Reformation,* others made the same case in more secular venues. The Swiss writer, liberal, and prominent Freemason Otto Henne am Rhyn, for example, in 1902 attacked Rothe in the pages of the German bourgeois family journal *Die Gartenlaube.* He called her a swindler who could hoodwink anyone but the most discerning scientist and insisted that there was a world of difference between spiritualists, who trafficked with the dead, and serious investigators like Bohn and Maack, who sought to explain somnambulism, clairvoyance, and related phenomena in natural terms. Urging readers to leave occultism to the experts, he added a warning about the moral, intellectual, and hygienic dangers posed by Rothe. Her séances, he explained, spread diseases of the brain and nervous system; indeed, they were dangerous not just to those who attended her séances, but even to the unborn, for many of Rothe's followers were women who could then pass on their mental diseases to their children.[49]

When Rothe finally went on trial in March 1903, the case against her had already been made several times over in the German press. The trial recycled old arguments in a particularly dramatic way since it offered spiritualists an opportunity to respond to the case against their beloved medium and to reassert their commitment to popular occultism, all before an appreciative public. It also gave critics an opportunity to pull the entire weight of the state behind their opposition to Rothe and her followers' brand of popular occultism. The trial was not just about Rothe but about the status of the popular occult movement in Berlin and in Germany more broadly.

Rothe's case had several strengths. First, of the one hundred plus witnesses who appeared during the week-long trial, the overwhelming majority testified for the defense, and they did so on the basis of their personal experiences at Rothe's séances. The general character of these witnesses can be discerned in the notes of a court journalist present at the trial, who recorded the testimony of sixteen witnesses who testified on Rothe's behalf. All sixteen—five women and eleven men—had been convinced of Rothe's authenticity. Seven had communicated with dead friends and relatives through Rothe's mediumship; seven had witnessed the materialization of flowers and other objects; several had heard Rothe deliver sermons; and three noted that they themselves had clairvoyant abilities.[50]

A second strength in Rothe's case was the power of conviction she inspired among her followers, a fact that came across with great clarity during witnesses' testimony about the spiritual impact that Rothe had had on them. A female witness testified that during her séances, Rothe delivered sermons more magnificent than any pastor could deliver. A male witness, an actor by profession, testified that he had received flowers from his dead grandmother at Rothe's séances and that Rothe had helped transform him from a freethinker into a religious man. Other witnesses testified that they had contacted their dead relatives through Rothe's mediumship and thereby gathered compelling personal evidence for the reality of life after death.[51] These witnesses' testimony revealed that religious authorities had had good reason to fear the liberal theology of spiritualism: because it was not an ordained cleric but an uneducated woman who delivered these marvelous sermons and converted freethinkers, because these religious events occurred in private circles and not in a church setting, and because it was the evidence of direct personal experience rather than the revealed faith of the church that accomplished these conversions.

Yet another strength of Rothe's case was witnesses' certainty about the truth of what they had experienced with the medium, a truth they framed within a rhetoric of conviction and a language of personal knowledge in which they themselves—and not scientific experts—were the authoritative interpreters of their own spiritualist experiences. Witnesses spoke of being convinced *(über-zeugt)*, of having the identity of séance spirits confirmed *(bestätigt)*, of the materialized flowers being without a doubt true *(ganz gewiß wahr)*, of the certainty of their own knowledge *(ich weiß bestimmt)*. One witness, the lawyer who had defended Rothe in Zwickau a few years before, noted that he took Rothe's productions to be perfectly authentic and confessed his inability to understand how science could deny the reality of supernatural forces in the face of such evidence.[52] Not a single one of these witnesses conceded that Rothe could have committed fraud.

Finally, Rothe's defense was strengthened by having several culturally authoritative figures associated with it. For instance, Rothe was represented at her trial by two of Berlin's most prominent defense attorneys, a detail that pointed perhaps as much to the contemporary significance of the trial as to Rothe's popularity with Berliners of high social rank who were willing to use their connections to help the spiritualist cause.[53] It became clear during the course of the trial, moreover, that people of high social rank like Eliza von Moltke and her daughter were regular attendees at Rothe's séances and treated the medium with a loving intimacy.[54]

Where cultural authority helped Rothe most, however, was in the testimony offered by the two star witnesses for the defense: the president of the Swiss Supreme Court, Georg Sulzer, and the physician and medical reformer Georg von Langsdorff. Sulzer testified that he had attended séances with Rothe from 1899 onward and that he was perfectly convinced of the authenticity of the séance phenomena, including the flower materializations. He confessed that he had first been impressed when a spirit spoke through Rothe about his recent turn to Christianity after years of irreligion and unbelief; later in the séance, he recalled, the spirit of his dead wife had materialized. Upon questioning, Sulzer admitted that he had discovered once that flowers materialized for him at a séance had been purchased by Rothe at a Zurich flower shop. But he quickly waved away this apparently damning discovery. "I can only suppose," he observed to the court, "that Mrs. Rothe brought the flowers while in a state of double consciousness *(Doppelbewußtsein)*, then dematerialized them and re-materialized them [during the séance]." Langsdorff recounted similar evidence. Rothe had provided a channel of communication between his wife and a dead relative's spirit. After recounting how this spirit had cured his wife's rheumatism and then sent her a small gift from the beyond, Langsdorff gazed around the courtroom and concluded his testimony by challenging the public audience: "Now I ask everyone in this hall, when something like this happens to one, should it not be believed?"[55]

Against the defense, remarkable both for the number of its witnesses, the depth of their personal convictions about Rothe, and the details about spiritualism they thus narrated to the public, the prosecution offered a very different kind of case. It had two prongs. One consisted of testimony from the police. The policemen who had arrested Rothe narrated the story of her capture; the female police agent who had actually performed the physical examination on Rothe recounted that she had found many flowers and fruits concealed under Rothe's skirt.

Instead of allowing this evidence of fraud to stand on its own, the prosecution then developed its other line of attack. It brought out three expert witnesses *(Sachverständingen)*. The first was the forensic doctor Georg Puppe, who recounted that when he hypnotized Rothe, she had treated him to an ungrammatical and incoherent sermon delivered in Saxon dialect. It was perfectly clear, Puppe stated, that Rothe was a hysteric and that the sermon came not from higher spirits but from her own self. Next came the psychiatrist Richard Henneberg, already well known in antispiritualist circles for his 1901 article on the sanitary danger posed by spiritualism. Henneberg, concurring with Puppe that Rothe was a hysteric, added his opinion that clairvoyance, whether by Rothe or anyone else, was merely a form of hallucination.[56]

Perhaps the most interesting testimony was given by the third and final expert witness, Max Dessoir, a professor of philosophy and psychology in Berlin. Having belonged to psychical research groups and published in Germany's major occult journals from the 1880s onward, Dessoir had garnered decades of experience with modern German occultism and the phenomena of mediumism. However it was not this first-hand experience, much more extensive than that of either Puppe or Henneberg, that Dessoir invoked in his comments from the witness stand; instead, he relied on a more general train of logic. Rothe must be a fraud, he reasoned, because to assert otherwise would be to override thousands of years of scientific experience *(wissenschaftliche Erfahrung)* and to throw overboard everything that had been scientifically established about the nature of matter.[57]

When the attorneys convened on the last day of the trial to summarize the case for and against Rothe, the prosecution attempted to refocus attention on the question of whether or not Rothe had indeed committed the crime of fraud; the defense, in contrast, hammered away on Rothe's good faith, on her followers' belief in Rothe's authenticity—on the claim, in short, that Rothe's flower materializations did not constitute fraud in the legal sense of the term. In the end, neither good faith on Rothe's part nor the personal knowledge espoused by her followers was sufficient to acquit the medium. When the court returned a guilty verdict, it noted: "What today is the public property *(Gemeingut)* of science, what the majority of educated individuals *(Gebildeten)* recognize as true science must take precedence in this case."[58] And then, in response to Rothe's ardent followers, the court stated: "We hold that the people who went to the defendant's meetings did not receive what they supposed they were paying for. Had the defendant said that she possessed inexplicable natural powers she never would have been convicted, but when she claims to possess supernatural powers she has said something that she cannot maintain."[59] Thus was the spiritualists' testimony handily elided and the testimony of the three expert witnesses allowed to carry the day.

As the trial made clear, at issue between those who considered spiritualism a "public menace" and those who considered it integral to the "public welfare" were two different visions of the character and function of knowledge in a modern culture. There were those, defenders of Rothe, who extolled the value of their direct, experiential knowledge acquired in the séance room and insisted on their own authority to discern what was authentic and true from what was not; and then there were those who privileged the indirect but culturally authoritative knowledge of German experts who declared that Rothe could not have done what her followers said she did. Rothe's followers challenged a point of consensus: that the authority to "discover" knowledge about nature belonged to the scientific community. At least in the Berlin courtroom in 1903, they lost the battle for epistemological authority.

Liberals and the Swamps of Superstition

The eighteen-month prison term meted out to Anna Rothe pleased hardly anyone who had followed the trial. This fact registered as far away as the United States, where the *New York Times* reported: "The question . . . is asked by the whole Berlin public, even by those who consider the manifestations of Frau Rothe deceptive, whether the showing of these alleged wonders was deserving of such a long sentence as has been imposed on the medium."[60] In the airing of public displeasure that followed the trial, indeed, it was not just the verdict itself but Rothe's entire history that came under fire. Her medium-ship, her success, her arrest, her trial, and her sentence—all were subjected to careful analyses and passionate critiques in the days, months, and even years following the announcement of the verdict. Sprinkling their comments with such culturally loaded terms as enlightenment, reason, rationality, superstition, and public opinion, most commentators turned the case of the spiritualist medium into a trial of German liberalism, which was found—on all fronts—to be severely wanting.

Many commentators concentrated their polemic on the illiberalism of the German state, an illiberalism that had been revealed with painful clarity during the trial. One man who insisted on this point was Maximilian Harden, editor of the gadfly journal *Zukunft.* For him, the state's handling of Rothe's case had revealed that civil servants had too much authority to regulate the daily life of ordinary German citizens. Harden offered the hypothetical analogy of a meat vendor who—despite his customers' evident satisfaction with his wares—was accused by a state health official of selling tainted meat and found guilty in court on the basis of testimony offered by court experts. Finding the meat vendor guilty of having harmed his customers was as ludicrous, Harden suggested, as the court's ruling that Rothe had defrauded her followers. The vast majority of witnesses who were her customers had testified, after all, that Rothe had not harmed them, and in most cases had actually helped them to solve serious physical and spiritual problems. Ignoring this evidence, however, the court had judged these witnesses' testimony objectively false. Then, on the basis of expert testimony, it ruled that these witnesses had in fact suffered harm at Rothe's hands.[61] Harden concluded that the agents of the state—the policemen, expert witnesses, and judges—had denied Rothe's followers the truth of their own judgments, put Rothe behind bars unfairly, and made the entire problem of German spiritualism much worse.

Liberal opinion also condemned as barbaric the fact that although Rothe was a hysteric, the state had sent her to prison rather than to a mental hospital for treatment. One writer striving to assess the case "rationally" in the periodical *Die Gegenwart* asserted that Rothe was a hysteric who belonged in a psychiatric ward rather than prison. Although she had staged spectacles, she was not really guilty of having swindled.[62] The lawyer and journalist Ernst Grüttefien echoed this assessment in the city's liberal daily *Berliner Tageblatt,* where he voiced his dismay that although the court doctors had found Rothe to be mentally ill, she had been jailed rather than institutionalized and treated. This was a symptom, he warned, of the antiquated laws still in force in Germany.[63]

Such concerns over the barbarity of the sentence continued to hold sway in later years. In a book-length chronicle of the Kaiserreich published in 1922, the writer Fedor von Zobeltitz took the time to record his discomfort with the sentence, not because he doubted Rothe's fraudulence but because he believed that prison was no place for a hysteric.[64]

Turning their critique from the state's response to Rothe and the socio-cultural forces that had given rise to her in the first place, liberal commentators expressed their disgust with the groups and individuals who had helped the medium become a success. They did not have accomplices like Rothe's impresario Jentsch in mind when they made such accusations; their focus, instead, was on representatives of two culturally authoritative groups who should have "known better" than to embrace such a fraud: Germany's aristocrats and educated classes. Max Dessoir aired this view in the popular Berlin periodical *Die Woche,* where he made no bones about his disgust with the aristocrats and men of education who had encouraged the hysteric Rothe in her delusion. They had treated her with such familiarity and respect, he lamented, that she herself came to believe that she possessed supernatural powers.[65] The responsibility for her fraud, thus, was not her own but a social product of precisely those groups who should be leading Germany forward to a more enlightened future.

If the Rothe story revealed the deficiencies of those who should have been Germany's cultural leaders, it also proved—so far as liberal commentators were concerned—that the only social group truly qualified to investigate mediums was not the general public but the public of experts. As Max Dessoir noted further on in his *Die Woche* article, one of the important lessons to be drawn from the Rothe case was that "common sense" was as powerless to detect a medium's fraud as it was to identify artistic forgery. Dessoir lamented the fact, moreover, that much of the Berlin public continued to believe that there had to be something to the testimony of Rothe's followers, and thus to Rothe herself, because of the strength of belief displayed by witnesses on the stand. Here again, it was a misplaced faith in "common sense" that led the public astray. Against this faith, Dessoir reiterated one of his main points during the trial: that only those trained in techniques of exact observation and magicians' tricks *(Taschenspielerei)* were in fact qualified to evaluate mediums. Inexact reports by uncritical enthusiasts, even in large numbers, he concluded, were not proof of Rothe's authenticity, particularly when the claims made in these reports defied the best scientific knowledge about matter and its workings.[66]

Dessoir's comments hinted, finally, at the dominant theme running through all liberal commentary on the Rothe story: that outside the enlightened confines of expert culture lay a swamp *(Sumpf)* of unenlightened public opinion, a swamp where antiquated, unscientific, mystical, and religious beliefs flourished. In his article attacking the excessive power of the German state, for instance, Harden also speculated that the contemporary craze for occultism "oozed" from religious sources. He insisted that these origins rendered the state's attempt to regulate spiritualism by legal means ludicrous. As Harden saw it, the state had created a martyr of Rothe and in this way had given spiritualists, adherents of a species of faith married to modern knowledge, an occasion to build a church around their medium.[67] Not just Rothe's supporters but the court itself, in other words, had helped spread the swamps of superstition. As one writer declared, it was ominous that the court had ruled on questions that had not yet been settled scientifically. By leaving the solid ground of science and civilization, it had turned Rothe into a martyr whose existence could only fuel the religious currents in spiritualism.[68] The prominent Berlin lawyer and liberal Erich Sello continued this line of reasoning in an opinion piece published in *Zukunft,* where, after criticizing the guilty verdict as unjust, he drew conclusions about the "real" lesson of the trial. The case, he argued, showed how thin the veneer of civilization really was—how there bubbled just under the surface of modern civilization an ancient swamp of moral and intellectual barbarism.[69]

If the problem was the festering swamp of barbarism, the solution proposed was the classical liberal panacea: public education. *Berliner Tageblatt,* one of the city's major dailies, had hit on this theme immediately in its 1 April 1903 front-page story headlined "The Fight against Stupidity." Refusing to see the verdict as a triumph of enlightenment, the paper painted it instead as a symptom of the dangerous deficiencies of German public education. A well-educated public, the article implied, would never have succumbed to the allure of spiritualism. Displaying the classic hostility of Berlin liberals to organized Christianity, the article blamed the church and its dominance within the national school system for the fact that German students never learned to think for themselves: German schools produced unenlightened Germans who lacked the tools to shun stupidity and obscurantism—most recently in the form of spiritualism. This pointed to an even more serious lacuna: the schools were failing to provide Germans with the tools to free themselves from their political servitude and become instead full citizens of a liberal Germany.[70]

Of course, none of this was new. In bemoaning the harsh prison sentence as a sign of the state's unenlightened policies and Rothe's popularity as a sign of the people's unenlightened sensibility, commentators raised the usual complaints leveled by German liberals against both the state and the unruly masses, neither of which could be trusted to conduct the march of progress properly.[71] Nor was there anything particularly novel in the talk about civilization and spiritualism. Bohn had already made the connection in 1901, when he noted in the preface to his exposé of Rothe that the case concerned not just criminal acts but civilization itself.[72] Even earlier than Bohn had been Henne am Rhyn, whose 1902 article on the Rothe case in *Die Gartenlaube* had been preceded almost a decade before by his book *Eine Reise durch das Reich des Aberglaubens* (A trip through the empire of superstition). There, he had condemned spiritualism as a species of "elegant superstition" popular among the modern educated classes. Although its adherents claimed that spiritualism furthered the cause of general human enlightenment, Henne am Rhyn had blasted this assertion as a piece of self-deluded arrogance. These spiritualists, he stated confidently, were culturally atavistic, their superstitions a barrier to their development into good, modern citizens *(Staatsbürger)*.[73]

It is ironic, but highly significant for the main argument of this chapter, that Henne am Rhyn's study of spiritualism and other kinds of modern superstitions was published at the press of Max Spohr. Spohr's publishing firm was devoted to popularizing medicine and science. It had also published many of the major texts of the modern German occult movement: both scholarly texts on the history of occultism by authors like Karl Kiesewetter and more popular ones like the pamphlet *Wie errichtet und leitet man spiritistischer Zirkel in der Familie* (How to establish and lead a spiritualist circle in the family) (published in the same year as Henne am Rhyn's book).[74] That Henne am Rhyn's attack on superstition was published at a press that also published works of "vulgar spiritualism" suggests that it was indeed civilization and enlightenment that was at issue for all sides in the contentious public debates over spiritualism and Anna Rothe.

The Culture of Knowledge in the Metropolis of Science

Ultimately, the story of Anna Rothe demonstrated that despite a widespread consensus that science was integral to the march of progress, the question of who was to control this march, and who was to control science, remained open. This state of affairs prevailed, moreover, in spite of the city's scientific, intellectual, and clerical elites, who clearly would have preferred to bar the very broaching of the question in the first place. It was instead lay participants in the city's popular occult movement who, consciously or not, forced the underlying issue of knowledge and its control into the open and thus threatened to redraw the boundary between science and the Berlin public. What does the contestation of this boundary tell us about the larger culture of knowledge in fin-de-siècle Berlin? This final section uses the Rothe drama to offer a few answers.

Rothe's story suggests in the first place that the culture of knowledge extended beyond the strict boundaries of Berlin's world-class universities and research institutes. Whether the city's intellectual elites liked it or not, participants in the city's popular occult movement had clearly absorbed the view that they could and should determine the truth of the world for themselves. Moreover, they had imbibed the basic principle of the scientific worldview that knowledge should be empirical, acquired through careful investigation and reasoned cogitation. The city's occult movement—as much as its centers of intellectual excellence—belonged to a culture of knowledge in which experience, reason, science, and progress were all joined to the liberal vision of a society slowly evolving toward a more enlightened future.[75]

The drama of Anna Rothe exposes, moreover, some of the fault lines running through this larger culture of knowledge. If her popularity was a testimony to the presence of scientific mentalities among the masses, it was also this triumph of popular enlightenment that gave rise to the whole Rothe scandal in the first place. When spiritualists asserted their right to discover knowledge of scientific and religious import for themselves, they were merely putting their own reason and experience to work. But in so doing they challenged two groups—scientists and clerics—with a joint stake in maintaining a less-populist epistemological order. This was an order in which ethical knowledge ostensibly fell under the control of the church and natural knowledge under the control of the scientific elites. Rothe and her followers threatened not only to erase the very boundary sustaining these elites in their distinct realms of authority but to seize the mantle of epistemological authority for themselves.

Finally, the story of Rothe and her followers affords historians a well-placed window on the complexities of fin-de-siècle German liberalism and the place of science within it. We may take the severity of the court's response to Rothe as a sign of the state's illiberal tendencies, but we must acknowledge that even in this illiberal state Rothe received an open trial and that scathing criticism about the trial and the state's handling of it was publicly aired. The state destroyed Rothe—a fact not to be passed over lightly—but it did so with the collusion of Berlin's scientific elites, supposedly an enlightening force of progress and social emancipation. Moreover, having destroyed Rothe, the state went no further. It neither imprisoned her followers nor forbade them from continuing to pursue their beliefs; indeed, in the years following the trial, spiritualism continued to grow in popularity. It also remained, at least in the eyes of its critics, not only an upstart religion but also an upstart science. In the end, of course, spiritualism's vagrancy rested on a fundamental conflict over not just who was to control what kind of knowledge became science, but how science was to serve the larger social good. As will become clear in the next two chapters, these issues concerning science, knowledge, and power continued to fuel the cultural response to occultism right through the middle of the twentieth century.

CHAPTER EIGHT

Between Church and State

The occultist Balthasar Wehdanner did not hesitate to laud himself in his promotional literature as a modern-day Jesus Christ. A brochure from the early 1930s gushed over his skills as a psychoanalyst, magnetic healer, and expert wielder of the sidereal pendulum and announced that Wehdanner commanded the same magnetic forces Christ had used to wake the dead.[1] For a "reasonable" fee of between 1 mark and 8 marks, another pamphlet announced, Wehdanner would use his paranormal talents to proffer advice about such topics as marriage and career choice; he could also bend his occult skills to the diagnosis and treatment of ailments, whether physical or spiritual. All of these services, his advertisements promised, rested on careful experiments, whose validity "official science" could no longer deny. Prospective customers could consult Wehdanner in his Munich office or by phone and attend a public lecture to learn more about the rigorous research that underpinned his occult talents.[2]

As was true of the Anna Rothe scandal at century's turn, extravagant claims such as these attracted negative attention from authorities both secular and sacred. Occultists' pretensions to scientific status made professional scientists angry, the police worried that occultists might be profiting from fraud, and blithe assurances such as Wehdanner's that he and Christ controlled the same life-giving force set off warning bells among church officials concerned that Christian territory was being infringed upon. But if the threats were old, the responses in the interwar period were new. For one thing, the churches and the state now took a much more systematic approach to the occult menace. The state began soliciting expert opinion from scientists, whose pronouncements about the (de)merits of astrology, mesmeric healing, and the like became a yardstick by which police workers in the field could measure the criminality of various occult acts. Similarly, the churches designated individuals and groups as watchdogs over the occult movement and even practiced what one Roman Catholic called "spiritual hygiene," or prophylactic work designed to immunize the laity against the occult appeal.[3]

While the churches and the state grew more proactive in their response to the occult menace, however, they also found it increasingly difficult to take a consistent stand against it. This was because—in marked contrast to the environment in which the Rothe case had unfolded—professional scientists, doctors, philosophers, and theologians had finally begun to take a real interest in such occult sciences as parapsychology, graphology, and dowsing. As the respected philosopher and University of Tübingen professor Traugott Konstantin Oesterreich noted in his popular 1921 book *Der Okkultismus im modernen Weltbild* (Occultism and modern science), given that the occult sciences were now working in tandem with psychology and biology to bring a new worldview into being, educated Germans from all scholarly fields needed to join the effort.[4] And by the mid-1920s, they had. Indeed, as the paranormal became part of the era's increasingly scientific orientation to social problems, one that permeated the church as much as the state, both secular and spiritual authorities found it increasingly difficult to reject the occult sciences wholesale. In other words, the modernist outlook of church and state significantly complicated their own efforts to police the occult menace into oblivion.

The Churches Keep Watch

Occultists had long given the Christian churches reason to worry. Carl du Prel, for example, had announced in 1892 that the occult sciences belonged to the worldview of the future, one that would finally bring traditional religious beliefs in line with modern scientific findings. Contemporary occultists, he

promised, would accomplish the much-needed synthesis that scientific and religious authorities had long neglected.[5] Already alluring in the prewar years,
this message proved increasingly compelling in the aftermath of World War I,
when Germany's defeat and difficult transition to democracy helped call traditional sources of authority into question. Did Germans' enthusiasm for the occult constitute a menace to Christianity? Or did it offer a way—as du Prel had
suggested—to modernize faith for the postwar era? Against the backdrop of
the Weimar Republic's political, economic, and spiritual turmoil, the churches
found it increasingly difficult to offer a clear response to these important
questions. Officially, they viewed those who tried to extract a scientific religion
or religious science from the occult with deep suspicion and insisted that true
science and true religion should inhabit separate spheres. Unofficially, however, there were multiple signs of rapprochement as committed Christians
discovered just how useful the occult sciences could be in negotiating the
volatile interface between faith and knowledge that the Rothe case had first
brought to national public attention.

In the first place, interwar Protestant intellectuals tended to downplay the
spiritual significance of the occult craze. Presided over by theologians like Paul
Tillich, they articulated a neo-orthodox theology that stressed the incommen-
surability of science and religion and refused to grant any religious status to
the occult.[6] As Tillich observed in his widely read 1926 treatise *The Religious
Situation:*

> Occultism is the epitome of all those ideas and actions which refer to a reality
> which is hidden to the natural consciousness. . . . [W]hat is important for our
> evaluation of the religious situation [of today] is the question what the relation-
> ship of such an occult world-between-the-worlds would be to the religious
> sphere. On this point it may be said that what religion means—that is the
> divine—is the absolutely hidden, that which transcends all experience, including
> occult experience. In the presence of the eternal even the occult is temporal, this-
> worldly, finite. In and of itself the occult sphere has no religious meaning.

Spiritualism, astrology, Theosophy, and Anthroposophy—none of these, he
asserted, offered a religious view of the world. Thus, he quickly dismissed the
relevance of occult beliefs to the contemporary landscape of faith.[7]

But if the "occult world-between-the-worlds" offered no theological menace to Protestant intellectuals, it did nonetheless in the eyes of many church
workers still offer a practical one. In a series of position papers published for

the church in the 1920s, for instance, M. Krawielitzki lambasted the Gottesbund Tanatra, a spiritualist group founded in 1923, as a "blasphemous sect" whose belief in reincarnation, positive regard for homosexuality, and perverted Christianity exposed the faithful to dangerous demonic influences. Like the Jehovah's Witnesses and the Salvation Army, he warned, the Gottesbund Tanatra threatened to lure upstanding Protestants into the sect-filled swamps of vulgar superstition.[8] Echoing and amplifying on Krawielitzki's analysis in a handbook for clerics published in 1928, Walther Buntzel portrayed Theosophy, spiritualism, and other such beliefs as a danger to the integrity of Protestantism. In what must have been a confusing aside to readers, however, he noted that when understood as the science of novel mental and physical phenomena, the occult might in fact be of interest to Protestants engaged in the scholarly study of religious psychology.[9]

Tolerance for the occult as science but intolerance for the occult as sect informed the activities of the Apologetische Centrale (Center for apologetics), an organization founded in 1926 that finally gave Protestant observers an institutional base from which to coordinate their watch on the dangerous strains of German occult practice.[10] Among its many activities, the center kept extensive files on various aspects of the occult movement, published booklets and articles to educate lay people and church workers about occult activities, and staged public events in which church workers and occultists debated common questions before lay audiences.[11] The Apologetische Centrale also shared its information freely with church employees, lay people, and state civil servants. To this end, it wrote to police departments describing sect activities in various parts of Germany. Similarly, when the physician Otto Neustätter began to organize an exhibit on the theme "superstition and health" at the 1930 International Exhibition on Hygiene in Dresden, a representative of the Apologetische Centrale wrote to Neustätter offering the collection for his use.[12]

As the files of the Apologetische Centrale demonstrate, what Protestant church officials feared from the occult was less a theological threat than a demographic menace. The success that many occult "sects" were beginning to have with a Protestant constituency gave particular cause for concern. The Horpena (also known as the Bund der Kämpfer für Glaube und Wahrheit), for instance, did well in the traditionally Protestant province of Saxony and attracted the critical wrath of local clerics. In a piece written around 1927, a minister Kircher in Coswig took an explicit public stance against Max Däbritz, the main promoter of this Christian-spiritualist association. Having spoken several times with Däbritz and seen his effect on former followers, the minister labeled the Horpena as dangerous and soul-damaging and called on the church hierarchy to protect the community from the group's false teachings. Theologically at issue, Kircher explained, were the Horpena claims concerning reincarnation, the divinity of humanity, and magic. He reserved his harshest tones, however, for Däbritz' magnetic power and its encroachment on Protestant territory.[13]

Similarly, the Theosophical artist and guru Bô Yin Râ featured in the files as a "false prophet" whose teachings had caused a veritable exodus from the church. In an internal document written for the Apologetische Centrale, Dora Hasselblatt deplored his teachings as perverted Christianity but argued that only by understanding his appeal could the church hope to stem the hemorrhage of former Protestants to his train. By preaching that Christ was but one of the Theosophical masters, Bô Yin Râ had convinced his followers that he himself was one of Christ's modern messengers. He rejected the concept of sin, she continued, and thus grossly misrepresented the truths of salvation and resurrection. All in all, she concluded, the teachings of Bô Yin Râ appealed because they spoke to the deep need of modern men and women for a hazy, mystical, and undogmatic Christianity that required no formal religious education.[14]

While most of the published and unpublished documents of the Apologetische Centrale criticized occult sects strongly, some of the material suggested the possibility of a more sympathetic stance toward religiously tinged occultism. As a correspondent identified only as "an educated woman" wrote to the center's director Karl Schweitzer in 1924, the writings of Bô Yin Râ had completely changed her understanding of the Bible and of God. Noting the difficulties she had had feeling her faith as a student of Protestantism, she explained that Bô Yin Râ's teachings had helped her to experience God directly.[15] The center also received sympathetic testimony from church representatives. Writing from the rectory in Leipzig in 1928, Johannes Berger described his own experiences with the Horpena in a favorable light and admitted that he thought it a mistake for the church to battle the sect. In his opinion, the church would eventually have to reckon with new sciences like astrology and spiritualism and perhaps even accept the possibility of personal reincarnation. None of this, he assured his correspondent, was cause for alarm, as even the occult could lead a person to revealed religion.[16]

Ambivalence about just what kind of threat or opportunity the occult posed for Protestant faith emerged most clearly in the extensive publications of the Apologetische Centrale. In a fly sheet clearly directed to lay people, terse paragraphs warned the faithful that consulting clairvoyants, card readers, or astrologers and dabbling in occultism, spiritualism, or Christian Science were all superstitious activities and, as such, constituted an offense against God.[17] Other fly sheets went further, calling spiritualism, Theosophy, and astrology instruments of the devil.[18] But other pamphlets muddied the waters. When *Die Bereitschaft* (The alert), a pamphlet published serially, devoted its August 1928 issue to astrology, for instance, its author bemoaned the superstitious astrology practiced daily on Germany's public streets and markets, but noted with approval the emergence of a scientific astrology movement. The pamphlet provided titles and prices of brochures and fly sheets written for the church, detailed information on various astrological groups and periodicals in Germany, and included an excellent annotated bibliography, listing books both sympathetic and hostile to astrology, and a short advice column. Written in the spirit of open enlightenment, the pamphlet provided all the information needed to dive into Germany's astrological subculture, whether in its scientific or superstitious variants.[19] In other words, even prophylactic pamphlets like *Die Bereitschaft* communicated to readers the dualistic stance of organized Protestantism toward the occult.

While Protestant representatives debated, opposed, engaged, and struggled to come to terms with the new occult beliefs and practices, their Roman Catholic counterparts found themselves in a similar situation, but they resolved it somewhat differently. Officially, the Roman Catholic Church opposed the occult unequivocally. Decrees issued during the course of the nineteenth and early twentieth centuries discouraged and even forbade Catholics from taking part in occult events. In the midst of the table-turning craze that swept Europe and the United States in the 1850s, for instance, Catholic priests were notified that table-turning and spirit conjuring represented a new menace to the faith. They were instructed to shield their parishioners from this danger and were themselves forbidden from taking part in spiritualist experiments.[20] In 1917 and 1919, the Holy Office in Rome issued decrees extending these prohibitions to séances (27 April 1917) and Theosophy (18 July 1919).[21]

While at the official level the Catholic church thus sought to curb the curiosity of the faithful, not all segments of the Catholic community shared this hostility. When, for instance, Carl du Prel died in 1899, the Catholic periodical *Die Stadt Gottes* eulogized the philosopher of mysticism as a "powerful ally of Christian philosophy" and recommended his works to educated Catholics interested in attempts to explain biblical miracles naturally.[22] Du Prel, it should be remembered, had first hatched his interest in occult phenomena by delving into various instances of religious ecstasy in Christian history, events toward which the Roman Catholic Church has always maintained an open attitude.[23] Moreover, his project of bringing religious experience in line with the findings of modern scholarship, particularly the new science of psychology, resonated with modernist reformers within the Roman Catholic Church who had embarked on a similar project of their own in the 1890s. Dedicated to modernizing the church's traditional views for twentieth-century purposes, these reformers quickly incurred the wrath of the Catholic hierarchy, which feared the perversion of basic Christian tenets and the undermining of its own spiritual authority. By 1907, Pope Pius X had issued an encyclical condemning Catholic modernism as heretical, and he soon took vigorous action against the movement's leaders.[24] Modernism within the Catholic community, however, by no means disappeared, and it left a noticeable mark on the Catholic response to the occult sciences.

Catholic traditionalists identified two main areas of concern vis-à-vis the new occult beliefs and practices. They feared, in the first place, that the occult in its more vulgar form might lead to pantheism. Pantheism, which postulates the unity of God and the world, had been consistently condemned as an error by the Roman Catholic Church. Did occultists' focus on the transcendent (*übersinnlich*) realm threaten to collapse the all-important distinction between the supernatural (*übernatürlich*) and natural worlds on which Catholic religious authority rested? The Catholic commentator Josef Dörfler, for one, conceded that as long as occult researchers limited themselves to the study of mediumism from an animist (or natural) perspective, they need have no fear of trespassing on Christian territory. However, he proclaimed the alliance of modern science and the church in denying spiritualism, not least because spiritualism espoused the pantheistic error.[25] Other Catholic writers condemned Theosophy and astrology for the same reason. The Jesuit Julius Beßmer criticized Theosophy in 1922 as a pantheistic philosophy that denied the reality of the supernatural sphere and thus conflicted directly with revealed religion. Like Dörfler, however, he allowed for the possibility that occult phenomena might be psychological, and he urged readers to leave their study to the new psychological experts.[26] A priest writing in a journal for the clergy in 1935 reiterated the church's long-standing opposition to astrology on the grounds that its pantheism effectively removed all responsibility, guilt, and sin from the individual.[27]

As distressing as the apparent pantheism of occult belief was, perhaps of even greater concern to Catholic traditionalists was the implicit challenge the occult movement posed to the church's religious authority. Dörfler, for instance, called spiritualism blasphemous because it professed a new revelation that superseded Christ's.[28] Similarly, the Catholic philosopher Alois Mager, who wrote extensively about modern experimental psychology and the phenomena of mysticism in the mid-1920s, blasted spiritualism as an attempt to bypass both scientific thought and Christian faith in an effort to bring people into immediate contact with the spiritual beyond.[29] And Beßmer had raised a related criticism concerning the dangerous syncretism so characteristic of the occult movement, especially in its Theosophical variants. Theosophy's claim to tap the original sources of all religions and to bring them all—pagan and Christian—into harmony with each other especially bothered him.[30] All in all, this strand of Catholic opposition to occult activity tended to reinforce the status quo of separate spheres. The occult belonged to science, the soul to the church, and any group threatening to remove this distinction by investing paranormal phenomena with spiritual significance threatened the integrity of both regimes of belief.

But if the intent behind shunting occult phenomena into the hands of scientific experts had been to remove the paranormal from the realm of Christian faith, the ploy by the mid-1920s had begun to backfire as the Catholic sympathy expressed for du Prel in 1899 less than three decades later blossomed among some quarters into a full-fledged embrace of parapsychology. One modern-minded priest named Gregor von Holtum, for example, informed readers in 1926 that the occult had become part of the modern sciences, was contiguous with revealed religion, and should thus be of interest to all concerned with modern intellectual trends.[31] The philosopher Anton Seitz developed this line of thinking at length in *Okkultismus, Wissenschaft, und Religion* (Occultism, science, and religion), a three-volume work published in 1926–27. Here, Seitz differentiated between two species of occultism. Vulgar occultism, which included spiritualism and Theosophy, was the mortal enemy of true knowledge and true faith, a superstition with mass appeal among both the ignorant and the educated tantamount to a "contemporary sickness." But as vulgar as such strains of occultism could be, occult phenomena themselves clearly held scientific interest for serious researchers in both religion and psychology. Taking his cue from Max Dessoir, the philosopher, experienced occult researcher, and new psychologist, Seitz identified their source with the unconscious, which he defined as the "waste basket of mental trash" deposited there by consciousness, an underworld ruled by a veritable second self. Betraying his debt to the psychologists' analysis of the phenomena but also his allegiance to the Roman Catholic worldview, he concluded that the occult sciences, properly understood, merely investigated abnormal phenomena stemming from the "unconscious depths" of the soul and related them to the supernatural sphere.[32]

Catholic commentators such as these, who explicitly recognized the occult as a bridge between the realms of faith and knowledge, between the supernatural and natural worlds, eventually established a toehold for themselves within the church. Their leading representatives in the interwar period were Johannes Maria Verweyen, a philosopher at the University of Bonn since 1918, and Gerda Walther, a collaborator of Schrenck-Notzing's and a member of Munich phenomenological circles. Both had found their way to an updated Catholic faith married to parapsychology after sampling the many other *isms*—among them atheism, monism, materialism, Marxism, and Theosophically tinged Buddhism—that had proliferated in the wide experimental field of fin-de-siècle Germany.[33] This pattern of rapprochement between occultism and Catholicism eventually blossomed in the 1950s, when representatives of the Roman Catholic Church emerged to take on parapsychology in a positive, Catholic light. They established a journal, *Erkenntnis und Glaube* (Knowledge and faith), and dedicated it to the study of a very wide range of paranormal phenomena, including astrology, telepathy, clairvoyance, prophecy, ghosts, dreams, Marian apparitions, spiritualism, coincidence, and fate. Acknowledging their roots in the interwar period, the editors noted their debt to Verweyen and Walther, researchers whom they praised as having pioneered the scholarly study of parapsychology's religious implications.[34] At least for Catholic intellectuals with a modernist temper, therefore, what had begun as a tense relationship in the nineteenth century had by the twentieth become a much more comfortable one.

The State Intervenes

While the churches kept careful watch, the state used its legal powers to keep occult activities under surveillance and, when necessary, took action against what it deemed to be dangerous occult currents. To separate the menacing from the benign, the state turned increasingly to scientists, doctors, and other technically trained professionals for advice, thereby helping to put control over occult phenomena into the hands of qualified experts. Professional pronouncements, however, did not necessarily end up supporting state repression. Indeed, whereas expert opinion in the Rothe case had helped solidify the guilty verdict in 1903, experts' changing relation to the occult sciences in the 1920s at times helped establish occultists' innocence. Expert opinion, it turned out, shaped the means by which occult services were proffered and utilized in the interwar period, but could not underpin the quashing of occult activity wholesale. Expert opinion, in short, increasingly complicated the state's relation to occult activities.

This complexity in the stance of the state toward the occult movement in the 1920s can best be followed in Bavaria, where a special provision in the criminal police code *(Polizeistrafgesetz)* known as article 54 made it possible to prosecute dangerous occult activities more thoroughly and energetically than was possible elsewhere in Germany. Article 54 made the for-profit practice of magic, spirit conjuring, prophecy, fortune-telling with cards, divination, or dream interpretation punishable by fine or imprisonment. It referred to these crimes collectively as *Gaukelei,* a term that translates into English as a form of fraud or trickery and carries connotations of acts by jugglers, buffoons, tumblers, charlatans, and impostors.[35] At the end of World War I, the Bavarian military authorities extended this provision under the rubric of the Bavarian wartime legal code and forbade the unauthorized staging of lectures and demonstrations on spiritualism, occultism, and related topics. Written permission to do so was granted only to those with scientific qualifications; offenses were punishable with prison terms of up to one year or with large fines.[36]

In the 1920s, Bavaria continued to lead the country in the successful prosecution of criminal occult activity, again thanks to article 54. When the jurist Albert Hellwig reviewed recent trends in the legal prosecution of German astrologers in 1927, for instance, he worried that because the national penal code contained no provision against prophesying for profit, the state's only recourse in recent years had been to prosecute astrologers for fraud *(Betrug),* a strategy that had yielded only poor results. Among the numerous recent cases prosecuted in Berlin, Dresden, Bremen, Munich, and other large cities, he complained, only a handful had resulted in a conviction. The Bavarian law against Gaukelei, in contrast, had yielded a high rate of conviction and Hellwig reviewed its results enthusiastically, detailing nine cases from the 1920s that had resulted in guilty verdicts.[37]

Because article 54 gave the Bavarian state such broad powers to observe and curb occult activity, its criminal archives are particularly rich in documentation from which to reconstruct the state's changing relation to the occult movement. And because occultists faced a more hostile legal front here than elsewhere in Germany, Bavaria provides a good test case in the outer limits of possible police action against the occult menace in the pre-Nazi years. What the state's criminal archives suggest is that even though article 54 made Bavaria the most hostile legal territory for profiting from occult practice, occultists still found ways to flourish. It also shows that because expert opinion did not remain fixed, the scope of article 54 did not remain constant. As more of the occult practices crossed the line into the realm of professional scientific activity, so, too, did more practitioners find their way to a legal living by occult means. This situation, then, only helped fee-charging occultists thrive all the more.

To gauge this change and the role of expert opinion in causing it, it is helpful to compare the interwar with the prewar situation, when hostility between state officials and occult advocates was high. In Munich in the 1890s, for instance, expert testimony by Carl du Prel and Albert von Schrenck-Notzing did not save the clairvoyant medium Regina Narr from being found guilty of fraud (Gaukelei) and fined 100 marks under article 54. Incensed by what he saw as the fallacious logic of article 54, its old-fashioned Enlightenment prejudices, and outdated respect for the materialist worldview, du Prel demanded that it be revised so as to convey a modernized understanding. The Bavarian criminal police code, he insisted, must be rewritten in light of recent scientific work proving that clairvoyance could not simply be dismissed as a logical impossibility. When practiced by a person who did not possess the requisite faculties, du Prel allowed, prophecy should of course be punishable as fraud, but to punish all prophetic acts as swindles was to commit an injustice rooted in scientific error. To correct the situation, he boldly urged all members of the German legal system to inform themselves about hypnotism and the latest results of his own research in "transcendent psychology."[38] Nor did du Prel's complaints against the state and its treatment of the occult movement end here. In an 1894 issue of *Zukunft*, he blasted the Munich police for hounding him and his psychical research circle. The police, he wrote, mistakenly feared that his group incubated anarchist tendencies; rather than persecuting those interested in the occult, he observed confidently, the state should embrace such researchers and even establish university chairs for them since occult investigations constituted a powerful antidote to the materialist worldview informing anarchism.[39]

If du Prel's experiences demonstrated that the Bavarian state had kept a tight lid on all varieties of occult activity before the war, events during and after World War I showed the state beginning to take a more nuanced approach to occult acts, doing so—ironically—along the lines du Prel had originally suggested. "Vulgar" occultism practiced by those without scholarly credentials, particularly for profit, was an occasion for police action, while more "scientific" forms of occultism grew unimpeded.[40] Two cases that unfolded during the war show just how far the state was willing to go in its battle against the popularity of "vulgar" occult activity. The first case concerns a former postal worker, Adolbert Haugg, who made himself over as a spiritualist leader and popular hypnotist just before the outbreak of hostilities. As head of the spiritualist group Freibund, Haugg had been under police surveillance since at least 1914, and by May 1917 he had received an unfavorable surveillance report from a policeman named Franz Heigl, who had attended a series of Haugg's lecture-demonstrations. Heigl found Haugg's attacks on "academic knowledge" (*Kathederweisheit*) repugnant and called his occult musings "trash," opining that Haugg was someone who would use any loophole available to evade official control.[41] A few weeks later, the policeman was dismayed to hear Haugg call the war ministry impudent for forbidding him to use the term *experiment* in the placards advertising his meetings. Even more disturbing, Heigl reported, had been Haugg's disparaging speeches. The spiritualist had blasted the churches, the state, and the medical establishment for their suppression of hypnosis, then fulminated against the local police as agents of the military dictatorship; finally he had observed sarcastically that all that remained for the state to take was his right to hold his evening sessions—something, Haugg concluded, that must not be allowed to happen since hypnotism deserved the widest possible public. When Haugg began hypnotic experiments with female members of his audience, the policeman's dismay was complete. "I am convinced," he wrote, "that this kind of mischief produces very unhealthy effects."[42] On 31 May, the military authorities forbade Haugg from staging any further events involving hypnotism or mediumism, and mention of him no longer appeared in the police files.[43]

Haugg's antiauthoritarian blasts against the state and the scientific-medical establishment proved to be a recurrent theme among other local occultists during the war, as the second case shows. Like Haugg, Hanna Vogt-Vilseck and her spiritualist club Die Sucher (The seekers) practiced a form of "vulgar" occultism that fell under police observation and action. Shortly after founding the club in the spring of 1918, Vogt-Vilseck received a notice from the military authorities forbidding her from staging any more events dealing with spiritualism, demonology, occultism, and the like.[44] In October, Vogt-Vilseck wrote back contesting the order, denying the charge that her lectures caused public harm and stating that she had continued to give her lectures and that her audiences came happily and went home suitably edified. She informed the state tartly that she would no longer give notice of her activities and observed how much she looked forward to the establishment of a new government that would increase freedom of speech. Insisting that her lectures did not endanger public security, she advised the state to bend its attention to the activities of the ultranationalist Vaterlandspartei (Fatherland party), which did pose such a threat and whose speeches should be banned.[45]

Case files such as these are as revealing for what they omit as for what they include. Absent is material indicating that Theosophical and psychical research groups faced the kind of intense police scrutiny and intervention that spiritualists like Vogt-Vilseck and Haugg endured. Theosophical groups, in fact, seem to have had little contact with state authorities beyond receiving official permission to form as clubs. For its part, the police department kept files with information and news clippings on Theosophical groups, but it seems not to have put the groups under surveillance or any other pressure.[46] Even the negative comments submitted by an informant in 1923 about Neuland, a group in Munich that mixed Theosophy with aristocratic communism (*Edelkommunismus*), apparently caused no reaction.[47] Members of psychical research groups, after du Prel's complaints in 1894, also seem to have been left alone, except when the state went to them looking for expert testimony on its cases involving fee-charging occultists.[48]

With the restoration of freedom of speech and assembly under the republic, the state again found its hands tied. Unless occult enthusiasts sought to turn a profit on their paranormal activities, the state could do little against them, no matter how "vulgar" their occultism. Even this apparently clear standard, however, could become blurred whenever expert opinion shifted and effectively redefined what counted (or did not count) as prophecy.

Take, for instance, the case of astrology, whose practitioners did not have much luck in pleading the scientific merits of their field. Caught during a 1921 police dragnet against the local astrological community, A. M. Grimm, one of Munich's leading astrologers, received a sentence on the basis of article 54. In 1922, at the Bavarian Supreme Court in Munich, he appealed the verdict of fraud (Gaukelei) on the grounds that because recent scientific studies had demonstrated the efficacy of astrological predictions, his astrological activities had been performed in good faith and did not constitute Gaukelei. Ignoring the scientific claims, the court rejected the appeal on the grounds that the issue was not whether Grimm had prophesied in good faith, but whether he had prophesied for money.[49]

Faced with this hostile environment, the astrological community in Munich soon learned to evade both the police and article 54. A list kept by the Munich police department detailing *Gauklertricks* testified to the creative lengths that astrologers went in order to make a living. Policemen were warned to be on the watch for people selling astrological textbooks with "free" horoscopes tucked inside (this constituted hidden payment for horoscopes) and to keep alert for fortune-tellers trying to evade observation by advertising anonymously for customers in local papers.[50] But despite such systematic attention on the part of the local police, astrologers still found plenty of room to turn a profit, if not to evade state surveillance altogether. Ludwig Stenger, for instance, earned an income in an elaborate scheme not by casting horoscopes but by supplying the astrological tables necessary for casting horoscopes. Two women would buy these tables and put them to use in a two-part scheme. One taught fee-based astrology classes, where she collected students' birth information; the other used this information and Stenger's tables to cast horoscopes that were then returned to the students at no charge under the rubric of the course.[51] The police found themselves unable to take action against this operation because both offering occult courses and trafficking in astrological publications were entirely allowable according to article 54, a standard that police files from the 1920s frequently invoked. When, for instance, Margarethe Schicl, the widow of a chauffeur, was caught selling printed astrological material at a fair in Altöt-ting in 1927, she claimed that she had a permit to sell such astrological publications. Upon inquiry to the Munich branch, the police department in Altötting learned that Schicl did have a permit that authorized her to sell such material and that this did not count as Gaukelei under article 54.[52]

If astrologers thus learned to take evasive action to earn a living despite article 54, when they tried to broaden their scope of action by forcing the state to recognize their field as scientific, they were sorely disappointed. When the

Astrologische Gesellschaft (Astrological society) of Munich applied to become a club in 1923, a police representative wrote to the local court recommending that the group's formation be blocked for two reasons: first, the group's plan to set up a lending library would increase access to astrological texts, which were otherwise prohibitively expensive; second, expert opinion had recently established that astrology was not a science.[53] A few days later, a representative of the Astrologische Gesellschaft sent a letter to the Bavarian interior ministry protesting this second assertion: Munich had no scientific commission for establishing whether or not astrology was a science, the astrologer wrote indignantly, and were it to convene one with such serious scientists as Carl du Prel (an impossibility since du Prel had died in 1899) or the astronomer H. H. Kritzinger, astrology would emerge as nothing more than psychological astronomy and scientific divination. The letter writer urged that the club be admitted to the official rosters, but the appeal was rejected in September on the basis of an expert opinion solicited two years earlier from Hugo von Seeliger, a professor at the University of Munich and one of the leading astronomers of his day.[54] In 1921, Seeliger had written an official brief dismissing astrology as sheer delusion and lamented that neither the Enlightenment nor education had managed to stamp out the practice. Admitting that not all astrologers were swindlers and that some truly believed in the efficacy of their practice, Seeliger nevertheless deplored the appeal that their mathematical machinations held for the superstitious public. Intelligent people found astrology both laughable and distressing, Seeliger noted; those with more restricted mental faculties found it of immense worth.[55] In a short follow-up to this brief, Seeliger noted that, no matter whether practiced in good faith or not, astrology and cure mongering were on the same level and thus gave the state an excellent legal reason to treat them similarly.[56]

While Bavarian astrologers thus had to content themselves with earning their living by evasive maneuvering because they could not secure scientific status for their practice, other kinds of character analysts found themselves facing a progressively less hostile environment that pointed up the state's changing relation to some forms of occult activity. Palm readers and graphologists, for instance, had begun the decade faring little better than astrologers. In 1922, accordingly, when an informant submitted a report to the Munich police department concerning the profitable activities of the palmist Karl Höcker, punitive action followed almost immediately. Within the month, charges had been pressed against Höcker and, convicted of Gaukelei, he was given the option of paying a 1,000-mark fine or spending twenty days in jail.[57]

But by the mid-1920s, the legal system had begun to modify its response to such forms of character analysis, a change that occult service providers were quick to sense and exploit. When a female customer curious about her marriage prospects consulted the character analyst Rosa Amann in 1926, for instance, she paid a small fee in exchange for detailed information about her two suitors. Caught by a policeman on her way out of the door, the customer reluctantly testified against Amann, who was found guilty of Gaukelei and sentenced to a 20-mark fine or a two-day jail term. Although article 54 had thus far worked as it had for decades, Amann soon mounted a successful challenge to the guilty verdict by arguing in a higher court that she had not foretold the future but merely analyzed character, that she had not made a profit on prophecy but merely received a fee for simple psychological services. The court concurred, noting that Amann's comments about her customers' two suitors did not really constitute prophecy.[58]

Amann's insistence that she had analyzed character but not prophesied the future proved to be a useful ploy for other providers of occult services, who soon discovered that the state would allow them to earn a fee for certain occult acts but prosecute them under article 54 for profiting from others. The trick then became to charge for the legal services and perform the others, if at all, for free. In one typical case that unfolded in 1924, the occultist Karl Henkes (an employee at the Munich graphological institute Auer Dult) exploited this loophole masterfully. Henkes read palms without charge, but earned about 30 marks for each graphological analysis he performed. Customers typically wanted both forms of analysis done, but since Henkes charged nothing for the suspect practice of palm reading and contemporary expert opinion had discovered scientific merits in graphology, he evaded prosecution, much to the frustration of the Munich police, who complained that the fight against fortune-telling became progressively more difficult whenever the courts refused to punish such infractions.[59]

In large part, these legal shifts could be attributed to the change in expert opinion, which had gradually begun to recognize certain previously occult arts as "scientific." An expert opinion solicited by the Munich police department in 1930 from Professor Specht of the University of Munich crystallized this new orientation. In his report on physiognomy and Gaukelei, Specht divided physiognomy into two branches. The first, movement physiognomy, investigated the connections between character and movement (including the movement of the writing hand) and counted among its proponents such authorities as the philosopher Ludwig Klages and the psychiatrist Emil Kraepelin. Movement physiognomy, Specht declared, was a genuine branch of study. The second branch, form physiognomy, took the traditional approach of trying to read character from body type. Specht admitted that there was some scientific evidence to support this view, but argued that the issue had yet to be settled satisfactorily. He advised the police to decide on a case-by-case basis whether physiognomic activities constituted Gaukelei. In closing, he noted that physiognomy, both old and new, contained as much art as science and that serious thinkers would perhaps never be able to close the books on it since the phenomena belonged to that realm of life into which rational scientific methods had trouble penetrating. He recommended that article 54 be amended to take note of these facts.[60]

The courts certainly had begun to take note, amending article 54 to bring it in line with the latest "scientific" opinion in much the way du Prel had recommended three decades earlier. When, for instance, the renowned clairvoyant Erik Jan Hanussen appeared in Brückenau in 1931, the police found their path of action blocked. As they soon discovered, Hanussen met privately with paying customers and performed personalized graphological analyses for them. When the Brückenau police wrote to their Munich colleagues asking for advice on how to handle this, the Munich department replied that character analysis performed according to graphological techniques was allowed "since the possibility of discerning specific character traits of the writer from [his] handwriting is recognized on the part of serious science."[61] Caught between the experts it consulted, the changing profession of psychology, and the occultists it sought to control, the state now found itself recognizing some forms of character analysis—notably, graphology—as legal. Henkes, Hanussen, and other fee-charging occultists quickly learned to exploit the loophole thus created.

Church and state alike found it very difficult, if not impossible, to battle the occult menace effectively in the interwar years. Relying uneasily on the position that religious faith and scientific knowledge adjudicated over two separate spheres of reality, the churches were willing to grant legitimacy to the scientific study of occult phenomena, but not to tolerate occultists' efforts to integrate these phenomena into religious practice. Similarly, through the early 1930s, the state proved permissive toward those who absorbed occult phenomena into the sphere of scientific investigation, but relentless toward others who—so the state claimed—sought to profit by selling their occult prophecies. In their effort to curb popular occult activity, however, officials working for church and state found themselves hampered by a growing sympathy that experts themselves extended to some realms of occult practice. When the National Socialists took power in 1933, they inherited this evolving pattern of ambivalence. They broke it only when they finally redefined the issue of occultism, not in epistemological but in ideological terms. The next chapter considers this development in detail.

CHAPTER NINE

The Spectrum of Nazi Responses

In 1947, the British historian Hugh Trevor-Roper published a book that has lured generations of readers with its promise to reveal just what top Nazis thought and did as the Third Reich fell in ruins around them. Currently in its seventh edition, *The Last Days of Hitler* was an attempt to preempt the construction of a "Hitler Myth": the myth that Hitler and his closest colleagues had *not* died in 1945, that they had in fact eluded capture and might be "out there" plotting a return to power. Trevor-Roper documented the fate of Hitler and his closest associates, recreating their death and physical destruction by fire, gun, and poison in graphic detail. When, finally, Heinrich Himmler had committed suicide in front of British soldiers by biting into the cyanide capsule concealed in his mouth, Trevor-Roper brought the curtains crashing down on his well-plotted "history . . . of a savage tribe and a primitive superstition."[1]

As this last line of the drama suggests, Trevor-Roper was not above engaging in his own brand of myth making. *The Last Days of Hitler* cast the Allied forces as the torchbearers of civilization, Hitler and his colleagues as the brutal barbarians who had sought to plunge Europe into a new dark age. The plot invoked the now-familiar theme that the Nazis were the enemies of progress and reason, a theme that Trevor-Roper played for all it was worth. In this, the German occult movement provided valuable material. Trevor-Roper recounted the story of Himmler and his personal astrologer Wilhelm Wulff, the rumors concerning Hitler and his fascination with magic, and the episode in which Joseph Goebbels tried to cheer up his Führer in 1945 with a horoscope that predicted an improvement in Germany's fortunes. The cumulative effect of such scenes was to leave readers with two distinct impressions: first, that Hitler and his colleagues inhabited nothing less than a "fool's paradise" in the last days of the war; and second, that the occult provided a fair measure of the foolishness in those critical final days.[2] As I have discovered in countless conversations with those who first learned about the connection between National Socialism and the occult by reading Trevor-Roper's engaging drama, these have been the impressions that stuck.

The understanding of the occult as a sign of a "fool's paradise"—or, as the German cultural historian Walter Laqueur put it, "lunacy in the higher ranks of the SS"—is a vision that I want to challenge.[3] The many historians who have joined Trevor-Roper and Laqueur in casting the German occult movement as a pathetic prop to the Third Reich, I believe, have missed a darker, richer, and more complex story of that relationship. Whatever else they were, Hitler, Himmler, and their colleagues were neither fools nor mystics, though they may at times have been both foolish and mystical. Nor was their relationship to the occult movement nearly as one-sided as Trevor-Roper's drama suggested. Himmler, for instance, certainly consulted occult seers, but in his capacity as police chief and SS head in the Third Reich he also presided over a twelve-year attempt to eradicate the occult movement from Germany. In other words, although there were certain cultural affinities between occultism and Nazism, these affinities never translated into a sociopolitical alliance of occultists with the state. Indeed, as a careful examination of printed and archival sources shows, the larger story of the Nazi regime and the occult movement is one of escalating hostility. Like so many before them, state officials after 1933 tended to see the occult movement as a dangerous force of antiquated superstition whose charismatic proponents threatened to lead the public astray. Unlike their predecessors, however, they also saw the occult movement as an ideological menace, one that promoted a corrosive individualism and dangerous internationalism antithetical to the Nazi worldview. Unfettered by the rule of law that had always bound officials in pre-1933 Germany, moreover, they did not hesitate to suppress the occult movement brutally, even on occasion taking hostility to a murderous conclusion.[4] To note this institutionalized persecution is in no way to equate what occultists endured with the better-known sufferings of the regime's ethnic victims. Occultists, it is crucial to realize, could always avoid punitive action by ceasing their paranormal activities. In contrast, Jews, Gypsies, and other ethnic groups could not—in the eyes of the regime—opt out of their racial heritage or their status as targets of systematic extermination. With this important caveat in mind, this chapter takes a closer look at the fate of the German occult movement under the Third Reich.

Ideological Tensions

Although the relationship between the Nazi state and the German occult movement was predominantly one of hostility, there were important affinities that underlay and complicated this hostility. These affinities showed up with particular clarity in the constellation of health practices and programs endorsed by many officials in the regime, some of which tapped the same currents of Lebensreform as the occult movement. In the 1920s, a deep antagonism toward conventional medicine and the strong conviction that modern life had damaged their souls and bodies led many Germans of all political persuasions, including fascism, to embrace nature cures, folk remedies, vegetarianism, fresh-air exercise, occult medicine, and other, similar practices. Germans committed to both National Socialism and Lebensreform, indeed, dedicated themselves to recreating a life in harmony with the laws of nature and biology and made their organicism an important element in their movement's worldview.

Such attitudes, of course, were not the exclusive property of Nazi party members; rather, they tapped a deep current of ambivalence that Germans held about the recent triumph of biomedicine and the construction of the modern health bureaucracy. The "natural" or "organic" strain in Nazism, in other words, was neither discontinuous with the German past nor tangential to the regime's ideology. Already in the latter years of the Weimar Republic, Germans had become increasingly unhappy with conventional medicine and had turned with greater frequency to unlicensed lay healers, most of them practicing some form of naturopathy. By 1935, there were fourteen thousand such practitioners registered in Germany—the equivalent of three lay healers for every ten academically trained physicians.[5] Popular interest in natural medicine, moreover, quickly found an echo in the health programs of the regime. As the historian Robert Proctor has recently reminded us, such naturalism was part and parcel of the Nazi quest for a "sanitary utopia" in which pioneering work in public health—an antismoking campaign, a concern with food additives, and a "war on cancer"—was joined to genocide.[6]

In a quest to address the disease-causing aspects of modernity, many Germans turned to various forms of occult medicine, and in some cases this turn went hand in hand with a willingness to sample other services that occult practitioners offered. Among those who turned to occult health practices were top Nazi leaders, whose reasons for dabbling in the occult affords us a well-placed window on the affinities between occultism and Nazism. Adolf Hitler, for instance, had a lifelong fear of getting cancer that in September 1934 induced him to have a dowser examine the Chancellery for evidence of cancer-causing "earth rays" *(Erdstrahlen)*.[7] Although Hitler's willingness to use a dowser did not translate into a wider embrace of occultism—Hitler, indeed, despised occultists' mystical inclinations—two of his most trusted cohorts did cultivate deeper connections to the occult milieu.[8] They were Rudolf Hess and Heinrich Himmler, each of whom will be considered in turn.

Hess, the deputy leader of the Nazi party and the man credited with introducing the concept of Lebensraum to Nazi ideology, was also an enthusiast of naturopathy, and he spent many years working to have it accorded the same status as orthodox medicine. A lifelong follower of homeopathy and a fanatical proponent of organic food, he followed a strict diet. A magnet suspended over his bed, he hoped, would deflect any health-damaging radiation from his body while he slept at night.[9] Astrological horoscopes, magnetic therapies, and consultations with clairvoyants were regular features of his life.

Hess's predilection for such pursuits, in fact, became a tool for casting him as mentally ill in May 1941, when he took it upon himself to parachute into Britain and attempt to end the war on the western front. A public relations disaster for Germany, his "treason" was blamed on the pernicious influence of his occult advisers and rapidly became an excuse for a brutal crackdown on the German occult movement more generally. Hans Frank, who was the leading jurist of the Nazi party and attended the meeting with Hitler following Hess's flight, reported how the Führer had sworn revenge on his former friend and castigated the astrologers who had manipulated him into action. It was high time, Hitler had reportedly insisted, to rid Germany of such superstitious riffraff. Whatever the truth of this private account, it is a matter of public record that the regime's chief propagandist Joseph Goebbels mounted a public campaign to save face for Germany by painting Hess as a lunatic occultist. Immediately after Hess's flight became known, Goebbels issued a communiqué casting Hess as suffering from hallucinations brought on during consultations with astrologers, mesmerists, and other occult seers. The responsible parties, Goebbels assured listeners, were being questioned so that their degree of culpability could be assessed and punished.[10]

Himmler, head of the German police and organizational architect of the "Final Solution," had a more cautious but nonetheless real connection both to fringe medicine and the German occult movement. Like Hess, Himmler had a life-long interest in natural healing and was very critical of modern hospitals and university-trained physicians. His interests in herbalism, homeopathy, mesmerism, and *Biochemie* (holistic medicine), in fact, led him to establish a special garden in the concentration camp of Dachau, where slave laborers cultivated therapeutic herbs for their organically minded masters.[11]

Himmler's predilection for fringe medicine arose at least partially from his own experiences as a patient and was eventually complemented by his willingness to sample the unique services of occult seers. Severe intestinal spasms had plagued him for years and refused to improve under the care of regular doctors. In desperation, Himmler had finally consulted a practitioner of Chinese manual therapy named Felix Kersten at some point in the 1920s. When Kersten's treatment afforded him some relief, Himmler became a convert to alternative medicine. Once war broke out in 1940, Kersten was trapped in Germany and, despite his Finnish citizenship, soon found himself pressed unwillingly into service as Himmler's full-time doctor. Kersten is memorable not only for being Himmler's doctor but also for the account he eventually published about his private wartime chats with Himmler. Among their many topics of conversation were astrology, occultism, and religion. Himmler, Kersten's memoirs revealed, had consulted one or two astrologers during the war, although apparently without much faith in their predictive powers. Moreover, although Himmler had also expressed a deep antipathy toward Catholicism, the religion of his Bavarian youth, this by no means meant that he had no religious inclinations. Kersten's memoirs showed that Himmler in fact believed in some form of reincarnation and was sufficiently enthused about Oriental religions to carry a well-worn personal copy of the Bhagavad Gita with him everywhere he went.[12]

The occult interests that Himmler discussed so knowledgeably with Kersten during the war reflected the six-year relationship he had cultivated with the occult seer Karl Maria Wiligut during the 1930s, a relationship, indeed, that constituted the most dramatic link between the occult and a top Nazi official. Known as Himmler's "Rasputin," Wiligut had served as an Austrian officer during the Great War before discovering around 1920 his special talent for clairvoyantly recovering knowledge about ancient Germanic history, a knowledge he claimed by virtue of his blood relation to a long chain of sages known as the "Uiligotis of the *Asa-Uana-Sippe*." Whatever its source, Wiligut's detailed knowledge covered ancient Germanic military practices, religious beliefs, and political systems whose spirit closely echoed the fantastic imaginings of the Ariosophical leader Guido von List, whose writings Wiligut knew. By the early 1920s, Wiligut had become convinced that Jews, Freemasons, and the Catholic Church—whom he (and other völkisch writers) blamed for Austria's defeat in 1918—were persecuting him; by 1924, he had been committed to a mental asylum in Salzburg, where he was diagnosed as suffering from schizophrenia with paranoid and megalomaniac dimensions and confined until 1927. Despite his confinement, Wiligut corresponded regularly with Ariosophical colleagues and in 1933 one of these, an SS officer, introduced him to Himmler, who eagerly jumped at the chance to harness Wiligut's clairvoyant talents for information about how the ancient Teutons had lived. In September of 1933, Himmler appointed Wiligut, under the pseudonym Karl Maria Weisthor, to head the "Department for Pre- and Early History," a subsidiary of the SS *Rasse-und Siedlungshauptamt* (Race and settlement main office). Two years later, Himmler had put the occult seer on his personal staff and was regularly consulting him for help in setting up the symbolic and ceremonial aspects of the SS. Wiligut, for example, contributed to the design of the infamous *Totenkopfring,* or death's head ring, worn by all SS members; he also persuaded Himmler in 1935 to make the Wewelsburg castle the ceremonial home of the SS and offered many suggestions for imbuing official SS occasions with an aura of ancient Germanic authenticity. But by 1939, in part because embarrassing information about his institutionalization for insanity became public, Wiligut's star had waned and he was forcibly retired from the SS.[13]

Himmler may have lost his occult muse but he did not cease his occult dabblings. His astrological consultations were reported in further detail in 1968 by his personal astrologer Wilhelm Wulff. In an autobiographical account introduced by the historian Walter Laqueur as "altogether reliable," Wulff recounted that he had become Himmler's astrologer in much the same way that Kersten had become Himmler's doctor: by force.[14] A native of Hamburg,

Wulff had become interested in astrology as a young art student before the Great War. After finding himself in financial straights during the 1920s, he had turned his astrological talents to profit. The flight of Rudolf Hess to Scotland in 1941 precipitated a crackdown on German astrology and Wulff, along with many of his colleagues, was arrested and placed in a concentration camp. He was released only on condition that he put his astrological talents to work for Himmler.

What the cases of Hess and Himmler reveal is that occult beliefs and practices had indeed made inroads with Germans at the very top of the regime and that they had done so concomitantly with fringe medical practices. Hess's magnets, horoscopes, and clairvoyants existed on a continuum, just as Himmler's dependence on an alternative healer accompanied his willingness to sample the services of the astrologer Wulff and consult the Bhagavad Gita, a text also central to the Theosophical portion of the occult movement. But in the end these well-documented facts boil down to ambiguous affinities. Hess was clearly interested in fringe medicine and occultism, but there is nothing— beyond the reported angry comments of Hitler and Goebbels, whose hostility to occult mysticism is well documented—to suggest that he undertook his mission to Britain under the influence of nameless occult seers.[15] Similarly, Himmler indubitably consulted occult practitioners, but there is nothing to suggest that the advice he received in this way ever found its way into important political decisions. Wiligut, it is true, had used his clairvoyantly gleaned knowledge to help Himmler create the SS image, but it would be going too far to finger Wiligut's occult visions as the source of the police chief's racist and murderous policies against the Reich's enemies. Furthermore, despite these well-documented forays by Hess and Himmler into the occult milieu, it would be a mistake to conclude that all the regime's officials shared in such occult interests, or that occultism and Nazism had a seamless affinity for each other. Indeed, as the reaction to Hess's flight and Wulff's sojourn in a concentration camp suggest, many leaders—including Hitler himself—could be extremely critical of the occult movement and would not hesitate to turn their criticism into punitive action against occultists themselves.

One of the leaders most hostile to occultism, in fact, was Joseph Goebbels, the regime's main propagandist. In a private diary no doubt doctored for future public scrutiny, Goebbels called Hess's flight to Britain in 1941 "a tragi-comedy . . . [about which] one could simultaneously laugh and cry. . . . The whole thing arose from the atmosphere of his faith healing and grass eating

[*Grasfresserei*]. A thoroughly pathological affair." Whether or not Goebbels actually believed that Hess had acted in an occult frenzy, he clearly relished the opportunity the fiasco had afforded the regime to crack down on occultism. As he wrote in his private diary on 16 May 1941: "The whole obscure swindle is now finally rooted out. The miracle men, Hess's darlings, are going under lock and key."[16] In comments such as these, Goebbels revealed his utter contempt for all things occult. To him, they were nothing more than a superstitious throwback to the Middle Ages and a plague on the Nazi social body.

This was an assessment that other top Nazis echoed. Martin Bormann, chief of the party chancellery, made his own antipathy to occultism perfectly clear in a secret report issued in May 1941 in the wake of the Hess scandal. The report linked superstition, faith in miracles, and astrology together as channels for the distribution of propaganda hostile to the state. Occultists, in his opinion, were using medieval methods to sow discontent among the masses by predicting Germany's imminent defeat.[17] When comments like Goebbels's and Bormann's are viewed within the context of the punitive action that the regime in fact took against the occult movement, one must therefore ask: Where did this antipathy come from? And what were its ideological sources?

The answer, it turns out, has to do with the völkisch milieu in which Nazism evolved. Highly complex, this milieu had been attracting men and women dedicated to creating a new religion appropriate to the German race since the 1880s. By the end of the Great War, it encompassed groups attempting to "Germanize" Christianity and others who rejected Christianity as unsalvageable and instead quested after a Germanic neo-paganism. Activists in the völkisch milieu agreed on the need for German renewal but disagreed, often intensely, on the appropriate means by which to effect it. The occult constituted one such area of contention. Whereas völkisch theorists like the Ariosophist Guido von List saw the occult as a tool for Germanic salvation, other völkisch leaders did not. The criticisms with which this latter group assailed occultists, in fact, eventually found their way into the rationale behind the Nazi regime's persecution of the entire German occult movement.[18]

During the 1920s and early 1930s, the völkisch movement included several important theorists who lumped occultists with Freemasons and maligned both groups as participants in an international conspiracy against German culture. For these theorists, one of the worst crimes of the Freemasons had been to promote a dangerous cosmopolitanism that led to Jewish emancipation in the nineteenth century. Such views became part of official ideology in 1933, when

Hitler came to power. Although at this point Freemasonic circles in Germany counted only seventy-six thousand members, the regime nevertheless moved against the Freemasons as important ideological enemies of the Third Reich.[19] The strong international ties and the hierarchical, hermetic nature of the lodge structure, official ideology held, made Freemasonry inimical to the ideals of the "national community" *(Volksgemeinschaft)* based on the purity of race and blood.[20] In order to understand the official Nazi response to occultism, thus, it is also necessary to understand the völkisch response to Freemasonry, with which occultism was persistently linked in the Nazi worldview.

The chief theorist of Freemasonic criminality was Alfred Rosenberg, who was head of the party's Foreign Affairs Department during the Third Reich and is today remembered as the "philosopher" of National Socialism. In publications like *Die Spur des Juden im Wandel der Zeiten* (The tracks of the Jew through the ages) (1920) and *Das Verbrechen der Freimaurerei* (The crime of Freemasonry) (1921), Rosenberg developed the notion that Germany had been undermined by an international conspiracy of Jews and Freemasons who espoused a universalistic humanity alien to the German soul. Like Jews, he argued repeatedly, Freemasons were natural conspirators and the born enemies of the German people. Not content to limit his views to books and longer essays, Rosenberg also took his message to the popular press. In a piece published in 1921 in *Völkischer Beobachter* (The racial observer), the official newspaper of the Nazi party, for instance, Rosenberg accused Freemasons of viewing Orientals, Negroes, and mulattos as their "brothers." Such attitudes, he believed, made Freemasons and Jews allies against Germandom.[21] He reiterated this message in 1930 when he published his famous tome *The Myth of the Twentieth Century,* which claimed that it was thanks to Freemasons' "preaching of 'humanitarianism' and the doctrine of human equality [that] every Jew, Negro or Mulatto can become a citizen of equal rights in a European State." This humanitarianism, he continued, had also spawned the "pornographic journalist," the new practice of racial intermarriage, and the stock exchange.[22] Here were the standard punching bags of Nazi ideologues—the free market, the liberal press, and cosmopolitanism—but instead of being preceded with the more typical adjective *Jewish* they were instead linked to Freemasonry.

While Rosenberg solidified the ideological link between Jews and Freemasons, he did not make the connection between Freemasons and occultists explicit. Instead, this service was performed by Mathilde Ludendorff, a doctor with first-hand knowledge of Germany's occult movement and a völkisch activist whose vision of Germany's true enemies—Jews, Freemasons, the Roman Catholic Church, and occultists—became particularly influential in the upper echelons of the SS.[23] Helped by her husband Erich Ludendorff, who had been the virtual dictator of Germany at the end of World War I and had since channeled his energies into völkisch organizing, she eventually succeeded in having occultists classified as ideological enemies of the Third Reich.

Mathilde Ludendorff trained as a psychiatrist in Munich with Emil Kraepelin just before the outbreak of World War I and developed her strong antipathy toward the occult movement during her days as a medical student. It was in this period that she first encountered patients whom, she claimed, had been made ill as a result of their occult activities. Munich, of course, had been a hotbed of occultism in the prewar years, and Ludendorff had soon gone on the attack against the movement's most distinguished leader, the psychiatrist Albert von Schrenck-Notzing. Ludendorff's first publication, in fact, was a carefully reasoned and devastating critique of Schrenck-Notzing's experimental conclusions.[24]

Ludendorff's scholarly demolition of Schrenck-Notzing's research results quickly metamorphosed into ideological attacks against the entire occult movement following her conversion to völkisch thinking in the early 1920s. After she cofounded the völkisch Tannenbergbund with her husband in 1926, these attacks increased in vehemence.[25] Appalled by the inroads that occultism, especially astrology, had made in the movement by the early years of the Weimar Republic, she wrote a series of popular essays arguing that astrology was nothing more than a vehicle of foreign powers—Jews and Freemasons, among others—bent on dulling and enslaving the German people. History, she wrote, gave ample testimony to the fact that astrology was nothing more than a Jewish perversion of astronomy. So long as the mixing of the races was allowed to continue, she warned, so, too, would the belief in astrology thrive.[26] By 1933, she had turned her suspicious gaze on spiritualists and Anthroposophists. In an essay entitled "The Miracle of the Marne," she revealed how the Battle of the Marne had been lost by General Helmuth von Moltke after he had fallen under the power of the medium Lisbeth Seidler and her control Rudolf Steiner, the founder of the Anthroposophical Society.[27] In essays like this, occultists joined Jews, Freemasons, and socialists on the list of those who had given Germany the "stab in the back" that had ensured its defeat in World War I.

In addition to what she wrote in her public essays, Mathilde Ludendorff seems to have had at least one more reason for her rabid hatred of German occultism, and in retrospect this must have been the main reason underlying all her diatribes. Quite simply, she viewed the occult as a worldview competing with the völkisch one. As a follower put it in 1937, what Ludendorff had tried to reveal in her public writings was that the German people were in danger of having extricated themselves from Christianity only to fall headlong into the error of occultism instead.[28] In light of Ludendorff's efforts, with the help of her husband, to found a religion appropriate to the German people, this interpretation makes a great deal of sense, particularly when we recall that many German occultists certainly did understand themselves as offering a "new worldview" for Germany's "new man."[29] But whatever the reasons for Ludendorff's venomous attacks on German occultism, she had succeeded in linking occultists and Freemasons. After 1933, these links became institutionalized in the machinery of the Nazi police state.

The Institutionalization of Hostility

The state's hostility to the occult movement achieved its institutional form first in the *Sicherheitsdienst* (SD—the security service) and later under the umbrella of the *Reichssicherheitshauptamt* (RSHA—the Reich security main office). At their most benign, the SD and the RSHA limited themselves to running surveillance on Germans suspected of occult activities; at their most dangerous, however, they functioned as an efficient bureaucratic machine that arrested, interned, and even murdered occultists for ideological crimes against the Third Reich, especially the crime of proving inassimilable to the Volksgemeinschaft. In order to understand this facet of the state's response to occultism after 1933, therefore, it is necessary to examine the inner workings of the SD and RSHA in some detail.

Until the establishment of the RSHA in 1939, the primary responsibility for monitoring and controlling occult activities in Germany fell to the SD. Department II, which focused on domestic matters, organized a special desk under the direction of Helmuth Knochen for the investigation of groups classified as "hostile to the state" *(staatsfeindlich).*[30] Occult groups, along with Christian sects, Freemasons, and other worldview organizations, all fell under its provenance.[31] When the SD was absorbed into the RSHA in 1939, this desk was then integrated into Department VII, where a team conducted "research and evaluation from the perspective of worldview" and an SS officer named Kolrop assumed charge of a special desk dedicated to monitoring sects, including occult ones.[32]

As this bureaucratic arrangement suggests, Germans with ties to the occult movement were institutionally defined as sectarians, a distinction they shared with Mormons, Christian Scientists, Methodists, Baptists, Quakers, Seventh Day Adventists, and Jehovah's Witnesses. Whereas the Christian sects were officially classified as religious ones, however, occultists who adhered to Theosophy, Anthroposophy, Rosicrucianism, Ariosophy, astrology, the teachings of Bô Yin Râ, Mazdaznan, New Thought, and spiritualism were considered—along with Freemasons—to be members of "worldview sects."[33] What connected these very different groups, so far as the SD and RSHA were concerned, was that they espoused an independent belief system and obstinately maintained their separation from the state. In the eyes of Nazi officials, this stubbornness turned sects into a distinct barrier to the creation of a united Volksgemeinschaft.[34]

In the 1930s, the activities taken by the SD and RSHA to guard against the sectarian menace centered mostly on surveillance and harassment, albeit with a few major exceptions. As the war began and suppression on the home front intensified, however, the police bureaucracy helped in coordinating a series of brutal crackdowns on domestic occultism.

The projects pursued by the SD and RSHA were varied. An RSHA program description drawn up circa 1939 listed a representative spectrum of goals for a statistical study of sects on which Kolrop's team was to embark. The team would monitor meetings for any communist and pacifist elements that might be at work and gather information to aid the eventual dissolution of sects altogether. This information, in fact, was to result in the publication of a special reference work to help police outposts coordinate their response to local sectarian activity. Accompanying this reference work would be a series of special reports on individual sects like the Seventh Day Adventists and two spiritualist groups known as the *Gottesbund Tanatra* (Tanatra association of God) and the *Bund der Kämpfer für Glaube und Wahrheit* (Association of fighters for faith and truth).[35]

In this flurry of reports generated by the police bureaucracy, officials often found themselves at pains to specify just what made sects "hostile to the state." In the late 1930s, Kolrop codified these efforts into a list of the top ten dangers that sects posed to the Nazi state. They were:

1. Sect members consider their religious community more important than the Volksgemeinschaft and refuse to carry out the will of the Führer. They promote "egocentrism."
2. Sects like Jehovah's Witnesses have become hotbeds of communist agitation and organization.
3. Many sects form part of an international community headed by Freemasons and Jews.
4. Sect members refuse to give the Heil Hitler salute.
5. Sect members often refuse to do military service.
6. Sect members resist absorption into Nazi umbrella groups.
7. Sect members refuse to work in military industries.
8. Many sects practice faith healing, a treatment that might easily damage the health of the German people.
9. Many sects—especially spiritualist ones—promote stupidity and exploit members' gullibility in order to make money.
10. Most sects deny the racial teachings of Nazism and are, in any case, hotbeds of homosexuality.

Striving to sum up the varied dangers that sects posed to National Socialism, Kolrop finally came out with a simple declaration: sectarian activity threatened the Volksgemeinschaft merely by promoting an alternative worldview; it thus encouraged disunity in the Third Reich. In other words, it was not so much that members of sects were seen as political opponents of Nazism, but that their adherence to an independent worldview—one distinct from National Socialism—necessarily defined them as resisting the will of the state. This resistance, both to giving up their own worldview and accepting the National Socialist one, was at the most basic level what cast them as ideological foes of the Third Reich.[36]

Although the SD and the RSHA lumped all sects together as ideologically suspect, they did not thereby assume that all sects menaced the Volksgemeinschaft in the same way. As it turned out, police observers detected many different ways in which sectarians refused allegiance to the new order. Jehovah's Witnesses, for instance, were persecuted particularly for their refusal to give the German salute, swear the German oath, or perform army service.[37] Members of occult groups may have participated in this type of refusal, but it was probably not these failings that landed them on the Nazi blacklist; the documents suggest that instead it was two specific transgressions that earned occult groups the epithet staatsfeindlich. The first was that, in denying rigid racial hierarchies, they denied a basic tenet of the Nazi worldview. Among the groups that observers had in mind were Theosophical ones, for whom the "brotherhood of humanity" was central, and various spiritualist ones that espoused a similar humanitarian philosophy. The second transgression concerned occultists' alleged ability to mesmerize and manipulate the masses. As one report put it, occultists "hypnotized" the masses with spiritualist mischief (*Unfug*) and poisoned their minds with medieval superstitions. This latter transgression put occultists in the same class as Freemasons since—as one observer noted—both kinds of groups were full of intellectuals who did not hesitate to use their cultural authority to spread ideas in direct conflict with Nazi ideology. Sects like the Jehovah's Witnesses, who attracted older women and simple people from the lowest classes, in contrast, seemed more benign. Occultists thus rated the same danger level as Freemasons because they were perceived as offering a worldview whose popularity among intellectuals gave it a dangerous cultural authority with the masses.[38]

Such inconsistent views on the dangers posed by occult sects revealed tensions in the state's attitudes toward the occult—tensions with which officials in Wilhelmine and Weimar Germany had already struggled. Were occultists powerful mass hypnotists or outdated cranks who preyed on the weak? Just as earlier critics of the spiritualist medium Anna Rothe had not been able to grasp how Rothe's "crass tricks" had inspired a deep Christian faith among her followers, Nazi observers could not grasp what was so compelling about occult leaders like the völkisch spiritualist Joseph Weissenberg. Able to see occultists only as unruly dissidents from the dominant ideology, Nazi observers—like some of Rothe's critics before them—were forced to attribute mysterious powers to the very occultists they sought to expose as charlatans.

Whatever the inconsistencies in their attitudes toward the nature of the occult appeal, the officials of the SD and RSHA were careful to gather numerical evidence to prove just how large this menace in fact was. An internal report issued by the SD in 1937, for instance, provided evidence that sects, including occult ones, were thriving in Nazi Germany. Of the estimated three hundred sects active in the Reich, many supposedly contained several thousand members. Weissenberg's followers numbered 250,000, the report estimated. They thus far outstripped smaller sects like the Baptists, which had between 80,000 and 90,000 members, but did not top the Jehovah's Witnesses, which counted approximately 350,000 members.[39]

Informed by numerical proof such as this, those looking out from the SD and RSHA at the spiritual landscape of Nazi Germany in the late 1930s were alarmed at the rapid sectarian spread following the seizure of power in 1933. Searching for the underlying causes of this growth, the officials of the SD and RSHA were inclined to accuse organized Protestantism for failing to attract believers and thus forcing those with strong religious urges to turn elsewhere for spiritual fulfillment. Indeed, these Protestant failures had precipitated an even worse malady, for once these religiously inclined men and women had set up their "alternative" groups, Marxists, Communists, Freemasons, and other enemies of Nazism had infiltrated and used them as a covert organizing tool.[40]

Whether or not this latter claim was true—and there is no evidence to support it—the files of the SD and the RSHA show that its workers did not stop with this analysis of the occult threat but in fact drew up specific recommendations for combating it. An anonymous report dated January 1937, for instance, lamented the dismal legal tools available to wage the war against occultism. Occult activities, the report's author claimed, escaped state action because of legal loopholes that no one had yet bothered to close. Although such activities stupefied and confused the public and promoted non-Nazi and non-Germanic thinking, the author pointed out, they were neither Marxist nor Jewish and thus remained without penalty. To rectify this dangerous situation, the author recommended that at the very least legal measures be enacted against literature written from an astrological, characterological, or occult perspective.[41]

Eventually, the regime not only censored occult publications but also embarked on a much more sweeping series of operations against occult activities in general. These actions came in two great waves, the first in 1937, the second in 1941. An official decree in July 1937 dissolved Freemasonic lodges, Theosophical circles, and related groups throughout Germany.[42] Occult activities now became illegal. Then, in 1941, in the wake of Hess's flight to Britain, police action against occultists rose to fever pitch.

Reinhard Heydrich, the chief of the SD, revealed the extent of this police response in a June 1941 report on the secret actions pending against the occult movement. The justification for this crackdown, he explained, was simple: "In the current fateful struggle of the German people, it is necessary to maintain the spiritual as well as physical health of both the individual and the entire Volk." Occult teachings were once again declared illegal, as they had been in 1937, and all occultists were declared "parasites" on the Volksgemeinschaft. But this time, the ban was accompanied by a host of further police measures. Police were ordered to confiscate all address lists, cards, correspondence, occult paraphernalia, and related objects immediately, if necessary by house searches of suspects. They were ordered to shut down any presses printing occult materials, to confiscate any publications they found there, and to arrest all astrologers, occultists, spiritualists, prophets, faith healers, Christian Scientists, Anthroposophists, Theosophists, Ariosophists, and adherents of any similar creeds. Detainees were either to be sent to concentration camps or put to work on useful projects. The crackdown, which was to go into effect on 9 June 1941, also required local police stations to submit detailed reports on their actions and the state of occult activities in their districts within a week.[43]

With the crackdown of 1941, the ideological program first developed by Mathilde Ludendorff in the 1920s reached its institutional apex. The ultimate irony embedded in this development was that it occurred under the aegis of police chief Himmler. For if Himmler the public Nazi presided over a brutal suppression of occult activity in Germany, in his more private moments, as we have seen, he was inclined to maintain a somewhat more open attitude toward specific occult practices. This Janus-faced attitude toward German occultism even appeared at times in the files of the RSHA. Presented with a police report on astrological activities in Germany in 1940, for example, Himmler had reputedly expressed the wish that the occult hocus pocus be stopped, but he added that room should nonetheless be left open for legitimate research on astrological questions.[44] Was the occult a social menace or a future science? Like many figures before him, figures of an utterly different political persuasion, Himmler clearly could not resolve the issue consistently.

The Occult Underground

Occult activity certainly took place in Nazi Germany, but with nowhere near the exuberant freedom it had enjoyed previously. As legal measure followed upon legal measure and crackdown upon crackdown, German occultists faced two choices: either to cease their paranormal activities or to take them underground.[45] This section looks at those who opted for the second route.

When Hitler rose to power in 1933, occult life was indeed flourishing in Germany. As the doctor Wolfgang von Weisl observed acerbically in a 1933 essay: "In the year 1910, monism—the science of the half-educated—was modern. Today, occultism—Anthroposophy, Theosophy, spiritualism, parapsychology, astrology, and their accompaniments—has taken the place of monism and become the science of the half-educated as well as the *Ersatz*-church of the uneducated." Weisl saw this not only as a German phenomenon, but more broadly as a European one. The thousands of men and women who followed the spiritualist leader Weissenberg near Berlin were of the same ilk as those others who made the pilgrimage to the Austrian town of Graz, the "Mecca of Spirits," to consult the famous mediums Frieda Weißl and Maria Silbert, or those seekers who took the train to visit yet other occult virtuosos like a certain Mr. Vlcek in Prague or Rudi Schneider in Paris. These were the men and women who consulted astrologers and tarot-card readers, who read the dozens of occult periodicals that appeared in the German press, who attended the hundreds of lectures and demonstrations sponsored by Theosophical, spiritualist, and parapsychological circles throughout Europe.[46]

If Weisl's picture of a broad European stage upon which all manner of occultists performed for cosmopolitan audiences reflected the situation in 1933, it was a portrayal he would have been forced to alter just a few months later since almost immediately following the Nazi seizure of power, a gathering wave of official hostility engulfed the fifty-year-old occult movement. Although initially some groups that had been active before the seizure of power continued their programs and a few new groups sprang up, decrees issued from 1935 onward and the police actions that accompanied them eventually forced most occultists underground.

Berlin's Zentralbibliothek der okkulte Weltliteratur (Central library for occult world literature) was a typical example of an older group that remained viable in the early years of the Third Reich. Continuing its pre-1933 tradition, the library sponsored a biweekly lecture series under the direction of Joseph Stoll. The roster for the fall of 1937 included the medical doctor Walter Kröner speaking on "Magic in Today's World," the trance-painter Heinrich Nüßlein presenting his occult paintings, and the philosopher Johannes Maria Verweyen giving a talk on Christian mystical phenomena in light of parapsychology.[47] While groups like the Zentralbibliothek der okkulte Weltliteratur carried on with such activities after 1933, new groups emerged to join them. Hanns-Maria Clobes, for instance, managed to establish the Archiv für Reinkarnation (Archive for reincarnation) in Leipzig in the mid-1930s. The archive collected books, newspapers, articles, and testimonials pertinent to the achievement of its aim, which was to assemble evidence for the reality of life after death. The lively correspondence that Clobes carried out with occultists as part of this project demonstrated the wide extent of occult activity throughout Germany through 1937.[48] Representatives from Theosophical, spiritualist, astrological, parapsychological, and other occult circles eagerly contributed material for Clobes's archive.[49]

The archive's correspondence also revealed the way in which dedicated occultists understood the significance of the occult worldview for the new Germany. Continuities with the past abounded, as the case of the spiritualist Erwin Schurig made clear. Schurig, the forty-year-old owner of a small press near Dresden, wrote to Clobes in 1937 explaining the rationale behind his allegiance to the occult group Neugeist (New thought). Until 1923, Schurig confessed, he had been a monist who denied the existence of God, but a persistent sense of spiritual emptiness had propelled him to seek a more satisfying philosophy. This he had finally found in Neugeist, which restored his faith in the divine and inspired him to spread the spiritual worldview. His task, as he understood it, was to combat materialism, and he did so not only by furnishing readers with scientific proof of life after death, but also by instilling in them a sense of responsibility for their earthly thoughts and actions. Schurig spread this message through printing and distributing low-priced pamphlets on the theory that the spiritual worldview was something that an individual could come to only in the peace of a private moment of contemplation.

Perhaps more importantly, Schurig's testimonial showed the intellectual and cultural continuities in the occult movement. Before 1933, most occultists had manifested a concern with erecting a scientific system of belief for modern-minded men and women. Schurig testified to the continuing appeal of this program in an eloquent passage he sent to Clobes:

> We . . . can establish that the Bible will satisfy modern man only when he receives a scientific foundation for biblical teachings. How few Christians believe in an afterlife, the belief on which all of Christianity is based!
>
> Modern man requires scientific knowledge to believe. And how much things have changed on the scientific front! I have in mind atomic theory . . . that has single-handedly thrown the materialist worldview overboard.
>
> If it was once science that drew the masses away from God under the slogan "enlightenment," so now will it be science that will fill them with enthusiasm for God.[50]

Here were the highest aspirations of long-dead occultists like Wilhelm Hübbe-Schleiden, the early leader of the Theosophical movement in Germany, and

Georg von Langsdorff, the early leader of the country's spiritualist movement, all echoed virtually without change in the self-understanding of an occultist writing in 1937.

But while groups like the Zentralbibliothek and individuals like Clobes and Schurig continued to sound pre-1933 themes, other parts of the occult movement began to display signs of nazification. The Esoterische Studiengesellschaft (Esoteric study group) in Leipzig, for example, which continued to meet much as it had before the Nazi seizure of power, sponsoring frequent public lectures on characterology, chirology, graphology, and occultism, showed signs that it had made adjustments to the new realities of Nazi Germany. A promotional pamphlet published in 1936 betrayed such pressures on its final page, where it closed by declaring the group's solidarity with Hitler's antimaterialism, on the one hand, and aggressive nationalism, on the other. Antimaterialism, of course, had been a standard feature of Theosophical groups like the Esoterische Studiengesellschaft for decades, but the mention of nationalism was decidedly new. Theosophical groups, both within Germany and out, had generally espoused a robust internationalism and commitment to universal brotherhood. Perhaps, however, this closing declaration of solidarity was little more than window dressing, an opportunistic accommodation to the new regime, since the lecture series itself contained nothing on nationalism, race science, or other such central Nazi concerns.[51]

Although such attempts to nazify were not always cosmetic, even occultists genuinely enthusiastic about the new regime found it difficult to earn official sanction. In 1935, for example, the Ariosophist Ernst Issberner-Haldane published his book *Arisches Weistum* (Aryan wisdom). It included chapters on spiritualism, astrology, clairvoyance, telepathy, and chiromancy, all of which he pitched as forms of ancient Germanic practice. Consistent with his title, Issberner-Haldane took care to voice not only his wish that the occult sciences serve the cause of National Socialism, but also the opinion that Jews belonged to a lower race and that the witch burnings of the Middle Ages had been a crime against the German people.[52] Despite its enthusiastic anti-Semitism and narrow German nationalism, however, *Arisches Weistum* did not fare well among official observers. When the book ended up in police hands in 1935, its reader expressed skepticism about the Nazi merits of the text, which he judged to be much closer to Anthroposophy—well on its way to being labeled officially staatsfeindlich—than National Socialism. The text's primary threat, the policeman concluded, was that it might be spreading false information about the racial history of Germany.[53] Despite its roots in the same völkisch milieu that had nurtured Ariosophy, in other words, the Nazi regime of the mid-1930s remained officially suspicious of occultists' motives and skeptical of their Nazi credentials.

Nor was it only bureaucrats who regarded such nazification efforts by occultists with a suspicious eye. In 1935, Ernst Pistor, editor of the anti-Semitic periodical *Judenkenner* (Jew-connoisseur), published a short piece detailing the recent crackdown in Saxony on the Leipzig branch of the Mazdaznan sect. Pistor noted with satisfaction that despite members' attempts to "nazify" themselves after 1933 by draping their temple with swastikas and filling it with "Heil Hitlers!" the Saxon police had not been fooled; instead, the police had rightly discerned that Mazdaznan was nothing more than a mask for international Jewry. Using anti-Semitic slurs like this, Pistor concluded that the state had been perfectly justified in banning Mazdaznan.[54]

Other occult groups soon found themselves under similar bans, whether or not they had tried to bring their beliefs and practices in line with the new regime. In 1935, the Horpena joined Mazdaznan on a national blacklist, followed a year later by the Gottesbund Tanatra and Gnosis.[55] Occult publishing enterprises were shut down as well. In May 1937 several astrological journals, including *Astrale Warte,* were banned in Berlin.[56] Soon, most occult journals had suffered a similar fate.[57]

Restrictive policies like these, of course, did not necessarily translate into the immediate cessation of occult activities, as the official police files show. A telegram to the main office of the Gestapo in Berlin in 1935 noted that despite the ban the Weissenberg sect was still active around Frankfurt/Oder and even surreptitiously publishing its periodical *Johannes Botschaft* in Forst.[58] When such illegal activities did not stop, the state began to deal more harshly with offenders. Thus, in 1939 in Stettin, the sect member Georg Falk was sentenced to ten months in jail for his activities as a magnetist in the tradition of Weissenberg. Six other members of the sect were fined 150–200 reichsmarks as part of the same proceedings. A similar case in Oppeln that same year resulted in the arrest of four sect members who had been caught with approximately fifty kilograms of illegal written material.[59]

The persistence shown by Weissenberg's followers was mirrored in case after case as occultists simply moved their meetings, trade, and beliefs underground. And police files continued to record their transgressions. A 1939 report to the Gestapo office in Dresden, for instance, noted that a member of the

banned spiritualist group Horpena had been arrested.[60] Similarly, the Gottesbund Tanatra, a spiritualist circle, appeared regularly in the files of the SD as a
group whose members refused to cease their activities.[61] A police raid in 1940
on a villa in Kirschlag Linz revealed a covert Anthroposophical school with
daily lectures, discussions, and exercises. The group, headed by a half-Jewish
woman named Teutschmann, escaped lightly, as the police merely dispersed
the group, declining to arrest anyone.[62] And despite the ban on astrological
publications, a report prepared by the German propaganda ministry in 1939
noted that three astrological newspapers published out of Leipzig, Dresden,
and Erfurt were still in circulation, each with a print run of a few hundred to a
few thousand copies.[63]

Finally, there is evidence to suggest that many freelance occultists—those
who earned their living through occultism—continued to practice their paranormal skills in the face of increasing pressure from the state to desist. Typical in this regard was an exorcist named Gollmann, who had been consulted
by a family suffering from a haunted house in Schleswig-Holstein in 1936.
Gollmann, who had taken the case reluctantly because of the legal dangers
involved, had been discovered, and he soon found himself in court facing
charges of having promoted "criminal superstition." As his trial unfolded, it
transpired that his confiscated library had yielded books on prophecy, yoga,
spiritualism, spell casting, and German flora, as well as incense and a deck
of tarot cards, thus providing a fascinating glimpse of a new underworld
wherein herbalism, exorcism, yoga, folklore, and occultism mixed. His sentence—thirteen months' jail and a three-year suspension of his civil rights—
must have seemed unduly harsh, particularly when compared to the increasing tolerance with which such practitioners had been treated in the Weimar
Republic.[64]

Like Gollmann, others continued their occult activities. Thus, an SD station
in Bielefeld reported on 8 March 1940 that fortune-tellers continued to make
predictions about the outcome of the war. An older woman had consulted the
fortune-teller Karl Grünewald, who had informed her that her money would
soon become worthless through inflation and that peace would come in August, but first German troops would have to suffer heavy losses. Another
fortune-teller, Katharina Breuing, the wife of a Nazi party member, had predicted that thousands of soldiers would probably show their displeasure with
the war by refusing to serve and that this might be a very effective maneuver
since the regime could not shoot that many for mutiny.[65]

In addition to such locally operative, fee-charging prophets, there were also the showier stage performers who traveled around Germany on the occult lecture circuit. One such performer was Rolf Sylvéro, whose case will be discussed in more detail below. Another was the magician Walter Höpfner, who was still doing shows in a Leipzig cabaret in 1941. The propaganda ministry's files also contained a report on a Professor W. A. Christiansen, who was still giving lectures with titles like "A Review of Mysterious Forces" in the summer after Hess's flight to Britain. Christiansen claimed that he had even performed his "anti-occult" show several times for such Nazi groups as Kraft durch Freude (Strength through joy), an association for German workers.[66] Indeed, Christiansen's desperate attempt to save his occult livelihood by proffering whatever Nazi credentials he could muster epitomized the situation in which all German occultists found themselves after 1933. Categorized as ideological enemies of the Reich, for reasons as varied as their internationalism or mystical obscurantism, occultists were forced into a criminal underworld. And when the Nazi state discovered them at work there, occultists had no choice but to try to save themselves in whatever way they could, even if it meant casting themselves as "anti-occult." In any case, as the next section will show, that ploy rarely worked.

Dangerzone Superstition

As the foregoing discussion has established, participants in the German occult movement faced a largely hostile state after 1933. A series of legal measures and police sweeps culminating in the crackdown of 1941, moreover, forced most practitioners into an "occult underground" where they continued their occult activities under constant threat of discovery and punishment. Although a very few figures like the astrologer Wilhelm Wulff were plucked from this underworld and forced to ply their trade for Nazi masters, most had to contend with the more pedestrian realities of belonging to a criminalized group in a brutal police state: they suffered intimidation, coercion, suppression, and—in extreme cases—murder.

Even under the general rubric of hostility, however, the official response to occultism was multivalent, and not all forms of occult activity were treated in the same way. What were the themes underlying this complex dynamic? Why was one occultist executed, another merely ordered to desist? This section considers the case histories of three occultists—Erik Jan Hanussen, Johannes

Maria Verweyen, and Rolf Sylvéro—in order to explore these questions more fully. It then examines a series of popular essays published in 1937 under the title *Gefahrenzone Aberglaube* (Dangerzone superstition) to expose the gap between what the regime told the German public about its occult hostilities and how its police in fact acted toward these "parasites" on the social body.

The first case is that of Erik Jan Hanussen, a self-made man who amassed a small fortune as a result of his occult performances and publications in Weimar Germany. An Austrian Jew by birth, Hanussen claimed to have grown up with a troupe of traveling actors to which his parents belonged. When war broke out in 1914, he joined a regiment on the eastern front and served there until being wounded. While recovering from his injuries, Hanussen discovered that he was a gifted hypnotist and clairvoyant. He used his skills to ease the pain and boredom of his comrades, rapidly adding to his repertoire dowsing, horoscope casting, and other such occult practices. When the war ended in 1918, he then integrated all of these talents into a traveling stage show that often drew hundreds of listeners. Eventually, Hanussen even founded his own newspaper, which he filled with astrological analyses of German social and political life as well as all manner of personalized occult advice.[67]

To many, of course, Hanussen's entrepreneurial spirit seemed to be nothing more than naked opportunism, his astonishing success explainable only as a reprehensible by-product of his willingness to hoodwink the German public. During the Weimar years, in fact, he had repeatedly attracted police attention and had even landed in court on charges of fraud *(Betrug)* (of which he was acquitted) in 1930.[68] By the early 1930s, critics across the political spectrum had begun to discern a deeper danger in Hanussen's accomplishments. In their minds, his fame rested not so much on his occult skills, which were in any case fraudulent, but on the way he used his alleged gifts to sway public opinion. With its visually distinctive red-and-black color scheme, for instance, his periodical *Hanussens B. W. Hellseher Zeitung* (Hanussen's clairvoyant newspaper) was a regular item for sale at newspaper kiosks throughout the country. The tabloid carried political horoscopes for different parties and their leaders; it also used occult predictive techniques to treat more mundane topics like the weather and fashion. In September 1932, it carried a front-page article entitled "Hope for Germany's Rise: Hindenburg-Hitler Union" and two horoscopes (one for Germany, the other for the Reichstag), predicted communism's coming weakness, and National Socialism's coming triumph. Such political forecasts were complemented by advice of a more mundane nature: Mrs. G. of

Aussich was informed that now was not the right time to purchase a hotel; troubled lovers and ailing patients were counseled on the appropriate steps to take to improve their conditions.[69] If the personalized advice struck critics as ludicrous, the more political forecasts struck them as positively terrifying.

Hanussen's political predictions, in fact, earned him the nickname "Hitler's prophet" in the left-wing press. In an article published in *Weltbühne* in 1933, the communist writer Bruno Frei accused "political clairvoyants" of Hanussen's ilk of being little more than economic opportunists who would do anything to sell copy or increase box-office receipts. Displaying a marked contempt for the critical faculties of the masses, Frei accused Hanussen of leading Germany's "little man" astray. Hanussen's astrological predictions about Hitler's rise and communism's demise, he warned, were an attack on European civilization and its rational traditions. "Have we labored to attain the scientific worldview in order to possess it," Frei asked, "or [are we willing] to allow today's masses—a political rabble that makes business out of barbarism—to steal it from us?" In the battle against the Fascist hordes, Frei answered, it was also necessary to fight charismatic cheats like Hanussen who used the occult pulpit to propagandize for the Nazis.[70]

Frei's polemics notwithstanding, Hanussen's relationship to National Socialism remains difficult to judge. Rumors that he and Hitler were on intimate terms certainly abounded by early 1933.[71] Hanussen also seems to have socialized regularly with several storm troopers stationed in Berlin. But his star quickly waned following the Nazi rise to power in January 1933. Information about his Jewish ancestry surfaced, probably leaked by Goebbels, who had been tipped off by Frei. Then, at an occult show staged on 26 February, Hanussen "predicted" the Reichstag fire of February 27, an event Hitler quickly exploited to declare a state of emergency and abolish the last remnants of parliamentary government. For Hanussen, the combination of prophecy and "tainted" racial background proved fatal. A few days after the Reichstag fire, "Hitler's Prophet" was arrested and summarily executed by three storm troopers just outside of Berlin.[72]

Why was Hanussen murdered? Unfortunately, the sources give no definitive answers. They do suggest, however, that by late February Hanussen had become a public-relations liability for the regime, and the various articles published about him in the Nazi press after 1933 support this line of interpretation. In 1937, for example, *Das Schwarze Korps* (the weekly newspaper of the SS) carried an article informing readers that clairvoyants like Hanussen were nothing more than "podium occultists." A portrait accompanied a caption stating that Hanussen had been a full-blood Jew who used "demonic affectations, colossal impudence, and . . . brazen tricks" to earn his fame. Hanussen, the caption continued, had been nothing more than a swindler, a swindler so great that he had amassed a fortune enabling him to purchase a yacht, a luxury apartment, and other such decadent possessions.[73] Opportunistically invoking a typical Nazi trope about the evils of "Jewish" capitalism, such texts, while pointing to the state's continuing concern with fraudulence, also highlighted what had changed since 1933. Concerns about the scientific basis or legality of contemporary occult practice no longer mattered: what dominated instead was an obsession with the control of public opinion and corresponding fear that charismatic individuals beyond the regime's ken could sway it. In a pre-1933 state that still respected the rule of law and allowed alternative viewpoints a certain measure of freedom, Hanussen had garnered state suspicion but largely escaped punitive action. After 1933, in contrast, his charisma and racial background became a liability, and his success rapidly turned him into a public-relations threat. What would have been inconceivable in Wilhelmine or Weimar Germany now happened: Hanussen paid for his occult talents with his life.

If the case of Hanussen suggests that the regime feared occultists' power to manipulate the masses, the case of Verweyen shows that there was still another facet of occultism that the Nazis feared: its psychological modernism and emphasis on the importance of individual self-development. A leading exponent of the liberal wing of *Lebensphilosophie,* Verweyen had embraced the full range of human religious experience and extolled the liberatory potential of novel spiritual practices, including occult ones. Born to a Catholic family in 1883, he finished doctoral work in philosophy in 1905 and then, like so many of his contemporaries, embarked on a period of intense personal exploration. He visited Theosophical circles, attended lectures by a Protestant theologian, immersed himself in the works of Nietzsche and Wagner, dabbled in monism, embraced Lebensreform and vegetarianism, and became a Freemason, poet, composer, and ardent pacifist. In the midst of all this, he also found time to finish his habilitation in philosophy in 1908.[74] Over the next two decades, he made a name for himself as a teacher and writer fascinated by religiosity in its widest sense, including the mystical and the occult. In a popularly oriented book on the "new man" published in 1930, for instance, Verweyen predicted confidently that "the men of the future will gaze into new worlds—still today disparaged by so many as 'occult'—and be at home in them."[75] Active in the Theosophical Liberal-Katholische Kirche (Liberal-Catholic Church), moreover, he also extolled the Theosophical leader Krishnamurti, calling his teaching "a message for all, to the entire world—and yet, oddly enough, a message for none, that is, not a message to be accepted . . . mechanically, slavishly by each person, without thereby hindering [Krishnamurti's] true intention. No authority . . . no discipleship, no pupildom, but rather independence of mind and spirit on the way to liberation and . . . bliss."[76] Although Verweyen reverted to Roman Catholicism in 1934 and formally renounced his Theosophical beliefs, he acknowledged that Theosophy had been his "bridge to Christianity and the church," a spiritual path back to the faith of his youth.[77]

Whatever the byways he had traversed, Verweyen's interests and activities clearly tended to the ecumenical, pacifistic, and even anarchical, interests and activities from which his occult predilections were inextricable. This was also what landed him on a Nazi blacklist in 1934, when the regime forced him to give up his chair in philosophy at the University of Bonn and earned him constant surveillance and harassment from the regime over the next several years. By 1939, Verweyen had joined an anti-Fascist circle in Wiesbaden; by 1941, he was under arrest; and by 1945, he had died in the extermination camp of Bergen-Belsen.[78]

What had Verweyen done to earn the wrath of the regime? His anti-Fascist activities after 1939 may have sealed his fate, but it was his advocacy of the psychotherapeutic implications of the occult under the auspices of the Siemens Studiengesellschaft für psychologische Wissenschaft (Siemens study group for psychological science) that had first earned him negative attention. Otto Siemens, for whom the group was named, was a stage hypnotist who had been active around Cologne in the late 1890s. In 1906 Siemens had founded the Erfolg Hochschule (School for success) and quickly attracted a faithful following among local bourgeois circles. Eventually, the group came to count many lawyers, businessmen, civil servants, doctors, engineers, and university professors among its members. As a promotional pamphlet from the 1930s suggests, the group's focus lay in cultivating a species of psychologically oriented self-liberation. The pamphlet challenged potential members with leading questions: Were readers aware of the unconscious creative forces at work within themselves? Did they feel like average members of the masses? Did they suffer from low self-esteem? Did they feel like failures in their daily lives? For those who answered yes to the last three questions, the Siemens Studiengesellschaft offered by way of solution a rigorous method for achieving self-knowledge—as the pamphlet put it, "becoming a personality"—and parlaying this rejuvenated selfhood into success at living. Success, the group preached, was not determined by external circumstances (birth, environment, and wealth, for instance) but rather by one's own ability to think positively. And this was an ability, of course, that could be learned, nowhere better than at the Siemens Hochschule, a branch of the study group.[79]

As the main expounder of the Siemens philosophy in this group, Verweyen quickly became the "charismatic leader" on whom Nazi observers concentrated their attention. The fact that Verweyen belonged to the Freemasonic group Loge zur Sonne (To the sun), moreover, made him even more a target for suspicion since—as one observer speculated—the Siemens study group might be nothing more than a cover for formerly Freemasonic humanitarian activities. As Nazi spies soon discovered, Verweyen was indeed a popular speaker whose talks on "success" regularly drew audiences of close to one hundred. Attendees—a motley crew that included Jews as well as SA members (two of whom were seen happily handing out pamphlets before a meeting in Cologne)—listened with interest as Verweyen propounded his main messages: "Know thyself" *(Erkenne dich selbst)* and "School the self" *(den inneren Mensch zu schulen)*.[80]

What threat did Verweyen's apparently innocuous message of personal uplift through positive thinking pose to the regime? One observer worried about Verweyen's appeal—about his ability to give extremely engaging lectures that hoodwinked foolish listeners. Another amplified on this theme when he ventured the opinion that what drew the listeners together was failure. "Shipwrecked" by life, this spy speculated, these failed men and women had sought an "anchor" in Verweyen's teachings, which promised to help them achieve a personal triumph in the face of terrible adversity.[81] Comments such as these suggest that there were two points, closely linked, that aroused the antipathies of state observers. First, the fact that Verweyen defined the path to success as building up an autonomous self flew in the face of the requirement that Germans tear down the self and melt into the Volksgemeinschaft. As an anonymous writer had put it on a related matter, not only did occultism promote blind faith and spread fraud, it wreaked havoc by promoting a form of occult individualism.[82] Second, the underlying sense of personal agency, the idea that individuals could triumph over accidents of birth or "blood," must have challenged the biologically determinist elements of Nazi ideology.

Hanussen and Verweyen paid for their transgressions with their lives—a price for their crimes that most astrologers, clairvoyants, hypnotists, and other occult seers in Germany did not have to pay. The case of Rolf Sylvéro (pseudonym for Eduard Neumann-Kolmar), a stage performer in the style of Hanussen, is instructive in this regard, for although Sylvéro lost his livelihood under force from the state, he did not—so far as is known—lose his life. Sylvéro, a stage magician, plied his trade until the summer of 1941, when his lecture-demonstrations finally attracted official attention. In a series of testimonials written to the police in an effort to rescue his livelihood in the summer and fall of 1941, Sylvéro claimed that he had turned to work as a magician out of desperation. Born in Alsace-Lorraine, he had volunteered for the German navy in 1915, but suffered an eye injury that resulted in his discharge. Upon returning home, Sylvéro had found that his fellow Alsatians despised him for his treachery and would not give him work. In desperation—brought on, as he implied, because of his loyal service to the German nation—he had turned to occultism to earn a living.[83]

As Sylvéro explained in a letter written to the propaganda ministry in August 1941, his shows were educational as well as anti-occult. During the first half of his shows, he conducted live experiments in telepathy, clairvoyance, and hypnosis; then in the second half, he would explain to his audience just how the "occult tricks" had been accomplished. Notes taken by an official observer who had witnessed the two-part show himself confirmed the structure of Sylvéro's show, if not the rationale underpinning it. Sylvéro had had audience members stuff an envelope full of slips of paper on which they had written their names, which he then read "clairvoyantly" by putting his finger tips on the envelope. Then he hypnotized audience volunteers, who, upon being told that their knees were cold, began to shiver and cover their knees. Having captivated the audience with such feats, Sylvéro would then launch into a lecture exposing the swindle he had just perpetrated against his audience. As Sylvéro put it, such lecture-demonstrations were the only way to educate a public that was still entirely too willing to believe every occult swindler who appeared before them.[84]

Apparently willing to give him the benefit of the doubt, officials from the propaganda ministry set up a small lecture-demonstration in Munich in September 1941 in order to gauge whether or not Sylvéro's performances needed to be regulated. Unfortunately, Sylvéro failed to make a favorable impression, and his observers produced a list of complaints: he did not greet the Führer; even worse, instead of "enlightening" his mostly female audiences, he left them with the impression that they had just witnessed a great magician; such performances were not only bad for Germany's citizenry, but perverted the anti-occult laws as well; and finally, Sylvéro's shows endangered the Volk by awakening a dangerous belief in the reality of occult forces. In January 1942, Sylvéro was prohibited from staging any more lecture-demonstrations.[85] His attempt to cast his shows as debunking had failed.

As these three cases show, occultists in Nazi Germany had to contend with intrusive surveillance and eventual orders to cease their paranormal activities. If they persisted, especially after the crackdown of 1941, they faced imprisonment or internment in a concentration camp. A few influential public figures like Hanussen, who always played to full audiences, or Verweyen, whose occult beliefs were all of a piece with his pacifism, internationalism, and anti-Fascism, were seen as serious threats to the regime and brutally eliminated.

Given its vigorous fight against the occult menace, the Nazi state was surprisingly reticent to publicize its suppression of occultists to the masses. Instead, it either sent a more gentle message of "enlightenment" or, increasingly, maintained a studious silence. To shape public opinion on the occult question, the regime had many methods at its disposal. A list of approved lecturers, for instance, allowed the RSHA to send speakers who were "experts" on occultism to give lectures designed to "enlighten" the public about outmoded "superstitions" that endangered the Reich.[86] Another approach involved promoting the publication of books that took a critical approach to occultism. A typical one was *Hellsehen und Wahrsagen: Ein uralter Traum der Menschheit* (Clairvoyance and prophecy: An ancient dream of humanity), by Hans Weinert, a professor of anthropology at the University of Kiel. Writing as a race researcher, Weinert first reviewed the various techniques for forecasting the future (clairvoyance, dream analysis, astrology, the sidereal pendulum, and so on) and then explained the tricks behind each of these occult techniques. His goal in writing the book was to help the Volk shed their superstitious beliefs and instead use their reason to determine the truth of the matter—that is, that there were no humans with "natural" gifts for seeing into the future.[87]

Nowhere did the "public enlightenment" approach to occultism come through more clearly than in the pages of general circulation newspapers like *Das Schwarze Korps* (The black corps), the weekly newspaper of the SS. For several months in the fall of 1937, *Das Schwarze Korps* devoted a full page on a bimonthly basis to a column entitled *Gefahrenzone Aberglaube* (Dangerzone superstition). Two photographs of a séance in process published in September, for instance, were accompanied by a caption that read: "Is it really an unknown or even spiritual force that makes the table tip? Not in the least!" Then came a simple physical explanation attributing the table's movement to the séance participants themselves, an explanation much like the one that the bourgeois family journal *Die Gartenlaube* had published nearly eighty years before.[88]

But *Gefahrenzone Aberglaube* was not merely debunking and enlightening: its visually appealing montage of photographs and texts was intended to make the additional point that the occult was not only a species of antiquated superstition but posed a significant social threat as well. In this, the column echoed two concerns that had already been broached in the internal documents of the SD and RSHA. One theme was that occultism was a weapon used by an international conspiracy of Jewish and Catholic forces to mystify and confuse the German people. An early column in the series stressed the need to fight not only church obscurantism but also occult charlatanry. Behind both kinds of mysticism, the column declared, stood Jews and the Roman Catholic Church, who sought to use mystical teachings to make Germans' brains more receptive to suggestive manipulation. These insidious Jewish and Catholic forces, moreover, worked through an army of clairvoyants, mediums, spiritualists, and astrologers who had turned mysticism into a veritable industry.[89] This point concerning the link between occultism and "internationally" oriented religions was also made in the illustrations. Catholic clerics and occultists were lumped together in photographs like the one featuring the priest Carl Lampert (an anti-Fascist) dangling a pendulum in an open clearing to find water. Close by, a photograph displayed a meeting of the spiritualist church of Joseph Weissenberg, accompanied by the caption "Women in increasing hysteria, victims of their blind faith in the occult arts of their 'Master' Weissenberg."[90]

The religious mysticism fueling occultists was complemented, the column implied, by the scientific errors of its more research-oriented branches. Astrology, for instance, was shown to be riddled with obvious problems. What was one to make of the fact that a black child and an Aryan born on the same day shared a horoscope and thus, according to simple-minded astrologers, a similar fate? Astrologers who took no note of racial differences clearly had no business calling themselves scientific. Stopping short of wholesale dismissal, however, the newspaper noted that some astrological claims might one day be scientifically proven.[91] Here again, in other words, the possible scientific aspects of occult phenomena had been acknowledged. The modernism that had tempered official responses to the potential of the occult sciences in the Weimar years still had its echoes in the Third Reich.

This, in any case, was one of the last instances in which the state-controlled press published anything at all on the occult movement for the general reading public. Already, from 1933 to 1937 the number of articles on the occult movement in the general press had dropped dramatically, and after 1937 they disappeared almost altogether, even as state activity against the practice of occultism escalated.[92] The gap between the way in which the Nazi regime acted toward occultists and what it told the German public about its actions requires explanation and a brief exchange between Martin Bormann and Joseph Goebbels in 1941 suggests at least one. Bormann had contacted Goebbels in June 1941 with a report on how the police were stifling occult activities and suggested that this police action might be even more successful were Goebbels to mount a public-education campaign to show the masses why occult teachings were so dangerous and deserving of police attention. Goebbels had declined, noting that enlightenment campaigns sometimes backfired (that is, spread the belief they were intended to combat) and that, in any case, precious media time should rather go to the public campaign against communism.[93] Goebbels's comment indicated both the priority he accorded the occult menace—that it was important, but not as important as the Bolshevik one—and his awareness that the very visibility of state action against occult activities in the pre-1933 years had done more to popularize them than eradicate them. Indeed, unhampered by a free press or any of the other attributes of a liberal state, the Nazi regime moved against the occult movement largely in secret and finally succeeded in doing what no German state had been able to accomplish before: the dismemberment of what had been a highly public movement since its inception in the nineteenth century.

This chapter has sought to expose the full spectrum of Nazi responses to the German occult movement, from the private affinities expressed by some officials to the brutal antipathies manifested by the regime's police. Top Nazis like Hess, Himmler, and even, on occasion, Hitler dabbled in occultism to varying degrees, but their dabblings were essentially private, part of their more general embrace of natural medicine. There is no evidence to suggest that their occult interests ever factored into major policy decisions. Moreover, their selective affinity for occultism was dwarfed by the enormity of their regime's hostility toward the occult movement more generally. Public enlightenment campaigns like the one mounted in *Das Schwarze Korps* in 1937 were accompanied by a series of repressive measures that severely curtailed the scope and size of the German occult movement. Labeled ideological enemies of the Third Reich and hounded by the police to dissolve their groups and cease their activities, German occultists responded by trying to accommodate themselves to the new regime and, failing this, by going underground. And whether they practiced their occultism openly or surreptitiously, it became increasingly clear as the Nazi years wore on that dabbling in occultism could lead to prison, a concentration camp, or even a brutal death.

Since the 1880s, of course, various branches of the German occult movement had had to contend with hostile attention from the state, the churches, and the scientific community. In Wilhelmine and Weimar Germany, the occult had threatened to erase the epistemological boundaries between science and religion, as well as those between scientific experts and the lay public. Critics had mounted campaigns of public enlightenment in the press or lent their expertise to a myriad of court proceedings featuring occultists like the spiritualist medium Anna Rothe. But the courts succeeded in punishing occult activities only when lawyers managed to convince the court that a particular occultist had knowingly committed fraud. The eighteen-month prison term imposed on Rothe in 1903, it is worth recalling, was one of the harshest of the pre-1933 period, and its harshness raised a chorus of protest in the liberal press. Most occultists, if convicted, got off with fines or very short prison terms; others were found innocent of wrongdoing in court and guilty in the press only of having practiced a scientifically suspect art. In short, much as critics in Wilhelmine and Weimar Germany may have wanted to shut down the occult movement, they could not. They were unable to achieve this goal, not only because the occult remained deeply compelling to the lay public but also because the state itself recognized that although occult beliefs and practices might be nonconformist or deviant, they had the right to flourish as alternative worldviews in a modern, liberal nation.

All of this changed after 1933 when Hitler rose to power and his regime moved against occultists as ideological enemies of the Third Reich. Whereas before 1933, occultists had endured the criticism of scientific or religious leaders and flourished nonetheless, after 1933 their alternative culture became criminally deviant. Animosity quickly became institutionalized in the regime, and occultists, like so many others who belonged to suspect groups, faced state terror. Although the occult may have played a minor part in the "fool's paradise" inhabited by top Nazi leaders, the fact remains that escalating hostility was the dominant theme in the regime's response to the occult movement.

A Voice from the Beyond?

In 1928, the parapsychologist Willy Jaschke published a book designed to bring the occult to lay audiences. Titled *Maria: Eine Stimme aus dem Jenseits?* (Maria: A voice from the beyond?) it narrated how an enterprising young man named Frank Werner came to make contact with his dead fiancée Maria in a home research laboratory. Although fictional, the story had been compiled from dozens of true-life experiences and, so Jaschke claimed, was thus an ideal introduction to the highly contested realm of mediumistic phenomena: their nature, setting, research, social context, usefulness, legal and scientific status, and apparently irreducible mysteriousness.[1] Serving for Jaschke as an introduction to the occult, *Maria: Eine Stimme aus dem Jenseits?* serves for me as a useful vehicle for summing up the results of my own study of the occult movement as a facet of German modernism.

Frank Werner first discovered the occult in a small, smoke-filled café in Schwabing, then home to Munich's Bohemian sub-culture. He was immersed in a local newspaper when the somber strains of a Beethoven sonata caught his ear and unleashed a wave of anguished memories. As he recalled that, just a few months before, his fiancée Maria had been killed in a train crash, his gaze settled on an advertisement in the newspaper before him. "Who is interested in serious scientific sittings with mediums?" it asked. Remembering Maria's attraction to spiritualism, Werner noted the contact address and sent a short letter expressing his interest. By return mail, the bereaved young man received a note from an Erich Loertzen inviting him to a preliminary meeting.[2]

This encounter introduced Werner to the scientific underpinnings of modern occultism. When he presented himself at the door, he expected to find a spirit-conjurer ensconced in a suitably mystical setting; instead, he found himself in a simply furnished but comfortable room engaged in easy conversation with Loertzen, a young man of good facial color and radiantly clear eyes. Loertzen explained that séances were primarily scientific experiments, that the Bavarian criminal code imposed certain restrictions on these investigations, and that no one really knew what caused the mysterious phenomena of mediumism. Werner signed a document acknowledging these caveats and then followed his host into an adjoining room, where he received a tour of Loertzen's home research laboratory. It had been outfitted with a medium's cabinet, four cameras, ten chairs for participants, a zither, and a work table equipped with a red light. Loertzen's objectivity and sobriety astounded the young man as much as the laboratory's warmth and coziness reassured him. Werner left a few minutes later, eager to return for his first séance the following Friday night.[3]

Experiments conducted on this and other evenings convinced young Werner of the authenticity of occult phenomena. Typically, eight to ten participants, including men and women drawn from all social classes, were present. The mediums, Karl Schneider, of Braunau (Austria), and Luise Weber, of Munich, were young, slim, and (to Werner's eye, at least) perfectly normal. With Loertzen directing the proceedings, the mediums caused many mysterious events to occur: cold winds blew; a silk screen ripped in half; a hand print appeared in a bowl of flour—all without any mechanical intervention.

Satisfied that no fraud had been committed, Werner echoed Karl Friedrich Zöllner and countless other students of occult phenomena when he wondered aloud why anyone who had actually attended a séance could doubt the truth of the proceedings. A retired general attending the séance that evening replied with an anecdote. When trains had first begun to run through the German countryside, the general recounted, two farmers had watched in amazement as the steaming monster thundered toward them. One had turned to the other and commented knowingly, "There's surely an old horse in there!" Those who rejected the authenticity of occult phenomena, the general concluded, were similarly ignorant of what the phenomena actually entailed.[4]

Recalling the impulse that had propelled him into the séance room in the first place, Werner now begged Loertzen to help him contact his dead fiancée Maria. With some reluctance, the parapsychologist agreed. Several sittings went by without results, until one evening the medium Weber notified the assembled that a certain "intelligence" known to one of the participants had presented herself. A note, received by the medium via automatic dictation, followed: "I must accustom myself to [automatic] writing, I cannot quite succeed, I am too deeply touched, but so happy that you miss me, I am always with you in thought, I come to you from a spiritual world and want to lead you higher. Engagement party—broken vase— . . . a pressed rose. Maria." Convinced that Maria now existed in another form and that she still loved him, Werner left the laboratory in ecstasy. Loertzen and the general remained behind, deep in discussion over these events. Had the "intelligence" really been Maria? Neither the general nor the parapsychologist could say.[5]

Frank Werner's story illustrates, in many respects, the major contention of this book: Germans turned to occult beliefs and practices in the late nineteenth and early twentieth centuries, not just to challenge but also to utilize the forces of modernity shaping their mental universe and very experience of life. Particularly important was the Janus-faced potential of contemporary science, a fundamental component of modernity and one that provoked a consistent pattern of ambivalence among Germans both in and out of the occult movement. Students of occult phenomena objected to the faceless, materialistic, and meaningless universe in which the scientific worldview encased them. At the same time, they sought to reinvigorate their world, their lives, and modern science alike by experimentally researching and developing the occult powers of the human psyche, both in themselves and in others.

In *Maria,* the heterogeneous presence of scientific modernity shows up most clearly in the role assigned to trains and laboratories in mediating Werner's turn to the occult. In Germany as elsewhere, the railroad was an ambiguous symbol of progress. On the one hand, it gave dramatic testimony to the power of human ingenuity to conquer nature, to bend even space and time to human needs. But the railroad also functioned as a source of anxiety, seeming to bring in its wake noise, dirt, crime, and, of course, danger to life and limb.[6] Werner's story casts the train in just this ambiguous role. It is, after all, a train crash that kills the young man's fiancée and gives him cause to contemplate attendance at a séance. On the other hand, a train features as an agent of progress in the anecdote told by the general. The old soldier draws an analogy between the machine and the medium, and to the ignorant it is inconceivable that either vehicle can function except by fraudulent means (an old horse; a sleight of hand). For initiates like Werner and the general, in contrast, trains and mediums are progressive elements, able to take one into an unfamiliar but nonetheless real landscape, whether of the human psyche, the spiritual world, or a larger Germany beyond a provincial farmer's understanding.

If the train is thus simultaneously an agent of tragedy, a symbol of mystery, and a vehicle of progress and hope, the laboratory, too, plays a multivalent role in Werner's story. It provides, in the first place, a venue in which the mystical phenomena of mediumism receive scientific authentication as real, albeit unexplainable, events. The laboratory also convinces Werner of Loertzen's authority as a scientific researcher of occult phenomena. And yet, there are odd and significant details in the story. The young man regards Loertzen as sober and objective—attributes of a good scientist—but he sees the research chamber itself as warm and cozy, qualities more commonly associated with a home than with a venue for rigorous research. This peculiar juxtaposition recurs during the climactic séance, when the laboratory and its sober, objective head become the mediators of what is, for Werner, a profoundly intimate experience: contact with his deceased fiancée.

These jarring details reflect some of the central tensions driving the German occult movement from its inception in the late nineteenth century until its suppression by the Nazi regime after 1937. Modern-minded men and women sought to rectify their suffering under modernity's burdens through an embrace of the new occult sciences. Just as the fictional Werner had lost his fiancée to a quintessentially modern tragedy—a train crash—actual participants in the German occult movement felt that they had lost their bearings in a world disenchanted by an ethic of reason whose most thundering success lay with modern science. And, just as Werner engaged in "serious scientific sittings" to assuage his loss, participants in the movement took up occultism, which promised to restore purpose to their meaningless existence on scientific grounds. Other participants, of course, made even more of their turn to occultism than the bereaved Werner. Whereas he sought merely to contact his beloved, they bent occultism to a wider variety of activities: enlightening the self, solving crimes, finding one's inner artist, healing bodies, researching the unconscious, traveling through time and space, selecting a mate, and discovering true identity. But in the end, like Werner they turned to the occult because occultism held out hope of personal relief in what they experienced as an anonymous, irrational world.

The social aspects of Werner's story are, in many ways, also representative of what the modern occult movement had become by the early twentieth century. Werner's amazement at finding men and women of all social classes attending séances, for example, reflected a fact: that participants in occult events did come from a very wide social spectrum. As had already been true of the séances staged by the fruit-and-flower medium Anna Rothe at century's turn, they included both men and women; doctors, psychologists, engineers, teachers, writers, and housewives; members of the petty bourgeoisie as well as the middle class and the aristocracy; residents of both large cities and small towns; men and women with serious, honorable intentions as well as impostors, opportunists, and actors in quest of fame and fortune.

Similarly, the story hinted at the pronounced therapeutic orientation of the modern German occult movement. Werner had expected that Loertzen and his mediums would be wild-eyed, psychologically unbalanced mystics; instead, he discovered that they were young, clear-eyed, slim, and in every way consistent with modern notions of healthfulness. Their normality, in fact, mirrored a major concern of many participants in the occult movement: to lead healthy lives, cultivate the freshness of youth, and bring mind and body into equilibrium. The clear-eyed, youthful occultists in Werner's story point, ultimately, to the German occult movement's larger context in Lebensreform and Lebensphilosophie.

Just as Jaschke's story exemplifies some of the core tensions and social characteristics of the modern German occult movement, it also captures accurately the importance of the marketplace in putting occult ideas and practices into general circulation. Germans who embraced occultism were propelled by intense feelings of purposelessness, bereavement, and unhappiness, but feelings alone were not enough to get them into the movement. In many cases, cheap and widely available publications—such as Jaschke's *Maria*—bridged the gap. In the story, after all, Werner finds his way to the occult proceedings by way of a well-placed advertisement in one of Munich's general-circulation newspapers. And, in fact, presses were particularly important in disseminating occultism to the masses in the decades before World War I; after 1918, the growing marketplace of occult goods (books; instruments; medicines) and services (clairvoyant character analysis; horoscope casting; graphological advice) quickly and efficiently made occultism available to anyone who could pay the modest fees required.

There are, finally, several clues in Werner's story that point to the ambiguous and contested status that occult phenomena retained both for participants and for those, including the churches and the state, who monitored the movement so closely. One of Werner's first acts is to sign a document acknowledging not just that there are legal restrictions on parapsychological research but also that the final explanation for the mysterious phenomena remains elusive. And the story ends on a similarly open-ended note: whereas Werner plunges into the night convinced that Maria still lives in the beyond, his more sober-minded host and cohort remain behind, unable to resolve the question of what the automatically dictated note written by the medium actually signifies. This indeterminacy, indeed, is reflected in the very title of Jaschke's book: *Maria: Eine Stimme aus dem Jenseits?* invokes the question mark still hanging over occult phenomena in 1928. Here, then, is a last poignant sign that the German occult and the German modern belong together in our historical consciousness. The emotional ambivalence that Germans felt about the new world emerging around them had as its intellectual concomitant the uncomfortable—and thoroughly modernist—recognition of the ultimate uncertainty of all human knowledge.[7] Indeed, neither scientific nor legal experts employed by the state could resolve the uncertainty surrounding the occult sciences completely; nor, for that matter, could the churches. Occultism ceased its highly public presence as part of Germany's reformist milieu of cultural experimentation only after 1937, when the Nazi regime suppressed occultism as one of its many ideological enemies.

Appendixes

Note on Sources

Unless otherwise noted, the information collected in the appendixes has been assembled from the following archival sources and published works:

Archival Sources

ADW CA AC 215
ADW CA AC-S 25; 159; 171; 272; 273
BA Berlin NS18/497; R58 1029; R58 1074
BSB Meyrinkiana I,1; XVIa
Cod WHS 800:1; 800:2; 801; 802:2; 812; 812: 1, 16; 812: 2, 1; 815; 821; 826
EZB 1/A2/465/1; 1/C3/298
GSPK I Rep. 89 (2.2.1) Nr. 15340
Landesarchiv Berlin 42–2147–26390;-26675;-27016;-27303;-27591;-27703
StArMü PDM 576; 674; 678; 682; 683; 3543; 5433; 5439; 5608; 5610; 7103; 7105; 7107; 7109; 7110; 7111; 7113; 7114
SdArMü ZA Astrologie; ZA Okkultismus
USHMM 10, 346, 387, 411, 560

Published Works

Daten zur Geschichte der deutschen Psychologie, I, ed. Ulfried Geuter (Göttingen: Verlag für Psychologie, 1986)

Ludwig Deinhard, *Das Mysterium des Menschen im Lichte der psychischen Forschung* (Berlin: Reichl, c. 1910)

Encyclopedia of Occultism and Parapsychology, 3rd ed., ed. Leslie Shepard (Detroit: Gale Research, 1991)

Hans-Jürgen Glowka, *Deutsche Okkultgruppen 1875–1937* (Munich: Arbeitsgemeinschaft für Religions- und Weltanschauungsfragen, 1981)

Nicholas Goodrick-Clarke, *The Occult Roots of Nazism* (New York: New York University Press, 1985)

Handbuch zur "Völkischen Bewegung," 1871–1918, ed. Uwe Puschner, Walter Schmitz and Justus H. Ulbricht (Munich: K. G. Saur, 1996)

William C. Hartmann, *Who's Who in Occultism, New Thought, Psychism, and Spiritualism* (Jamaica, NY: Occult Press, 1927)

Ekkehard Hieronimus, *Lanz von Liebenfels: Eine Bibliographie* (Toppenstedt: Uwe Berg, 1991)

Ellic Howe, *Astrology and the Third Reich: A Historical Study of Astrological Beliefs in Western Europe since 1700 and in Hitler's Germany, 1933–45* (Wellingborough, Northants.: Aquarian, 1984)

Carl Kiesewetter, *Geschichte des Neueren Occultismus: Geheimwissenschaftliche Systeme von Agrippa von Nettesheym bis zu Carl du Prel* (Schwarzenburg: Ansata, 1977)

Norbert Klatt, *Der Nachlaß von Wilhelm Hübbe-Schleiden in der Niedersächsischen Staats-und Universitätsbibliothek Göttingen* (Göttingen: Klatt, 1996)

———. *Theosophie und Anthroposophie* (Göttingen: Klatt, 1993)

Lexikon der deutschen Verlage. Eine Chronik der deutschen Verlagsfirmen, enthaltend die Geschichte der Zeitungs-, Zeitschriften und Buchverlage, der Kunst-und Musikverlage, sowie der Katalogantiquare (Leipzig: Verlag Curt Müller, 1930)

Ulrich Linse, *Geisterseher und Wunderwirker: Heilssuche im Industriezeitalter* (Frankfurt-am-Main: Fischer, 1996)

———. "Der Spiritismus in Deutschland um 1900," in *Mystique, mysticisme, et modernité en Allemagne autour de 1900*, ed. Moritz Baßler and Hildegard Châttelier (Strasbourg: Presses Universitaires, 1998), pp. 95–113

Horst Miers, *Lexikon des Geheimwissens* (Munich: Wilhelm Goldmann, 1993)

Uwe Puschner, *Die völkische Bewegung im wilhelminischen Kaiserreich: Sprache—Rasse—Religion* (Darmstadt: Wissenschaftliche Buchgesellschaft, 2001)

Diethard Sawicki, *Leben mit den Toten: Geisterglauben und die Entstehung des Spiritismus in Deutschland, 1770–1900* (Paderborn: Ferdinand Schöningh, 2002)

Rudolf Schmidt, *Deutsche Buchhändler, deutsche Buchdrucker* (Berlin: Frank Weber, 1902–8)

Sphinx. Monatsschrift für die geschichtliche, und experimentale Begründung der übersinnlichen Weltanschauung auf monistischer Grundlage 3 (1887)

Spiritistische Rundschau. Monatsschrift für Spiritismus und verwandte Gebiete 8–9 (1900–1902)

Rudolf Tischner, *Geschichte der okkultistischen (metaphysischen) Forschung von der antike bis zur Gegenwart: 2, Von der Mitte des 19. Jahrhunderts bis zum Gegenwart* (Pfullingen in Württemberg: Johannes Baum Verlag, 1924)

Verband Deutscher Okkultisten, *Bericht über die Verhandlungen auf dem Dritten Congress des "Verbandes Deutscher Okkultisten" am 31. Mai und 1. Juni 1898 in München* (Selbstverlag, c. 1898)

Wahrheit-Sucher, unparteiische Monatsschrift vereinter Wahrheitsucher, ed. Leopold Engel (July 1896–June 1897)

James Webb, *The Occult Establishment* (La Salle, IL: Open Court, 1976)

Abbreviations and Symbols Used in the Appendixes

b = banned in
d = defunct in
e = extant in
f = founded in
‡ = *völkisch*

Clubs

Note that the National Socialist regime officially banned occult groups in 1936–37.

Type	Club Name	Location	Active Dates
Anti-occultism	Abila	Leipzig	f. 1885
	Deutsche Gesellschaft zur Bekämpfung von Mißständen im Gesundheitswesen	Munich	Active under the Nazis
	Sternwarte	Munich	e. 1921
Ariosophy[1]	‡Bund der Reinen	Stuttgart	e. 1924–33
	‡Deutsche Arbeitsgemeinschaft für Menschenkenntnis und Menschenschicksal	Düsseldorf-Unterrath	f. 1925
		Oestrich im Rheingau	f. 1925
	‡Deutscher Schafferbund[2]	National (based in Hamburg)	f. 1911
		Freiburg-im-Breisgau	f. 1911
		Hamburg	f. 1911
		Rostock	f. 1911
	‡Edda Gesellschaft	Dinkelsbühl (Franconia)	f. 1925
	‡Gesellschaft Orion	Stuttgart	e. 1924–33
	‡Swastika Circle	Berlin	f. c. 1920
Astrology, dowsing, graphology, palmistry, pendulum	Akademische Gesellschaft für astrologische Forschung	Berlin	f. 1924
	‡Association of Scientific Palmists of Germany	Berlin	e. 1927

Type	Club Name	Location	Active Dates
	Astrologische Gesellschaft in Deutschland	Leipzig	f. 1909
		Berlin-Steglitz	f. 1920
		Munich	f. 1923
	Bund astrologischer Forscher		
	Bund der Sternfreunde		e. 1920s
	Deutsche graphologische Gesellschaft	Munich	f. 1896
	Deutsche Kulturgemeinschaft (Kulturgemeinde) zur Pflege der Astrologie	Berlin	f. 1927
	Deutsche Studiengemeinschaft für wissenschaftliche Astrologie	Freiburg	f. 1927
	Deutscher Astrologenbund	Berlin	e. 1929
	Gesellschaft für astrologische Propaganda		e. 1933
	Gesellschaft für wissen- schaftliche Astrologie	Munich	e. 1910
	Gewa, eine astrologische Gesellschaft zur Erlernung der wissenschaftlichen Astrologie	Munich	f. 1924
	Internationaler Verein der Wünschelrutenforscher, e.V.[3]	Berlin-Steglitz	f. 1921
		Hannover	f. 1921
	Kosmos Gesellschaft deutscher Astrologen	National	f. circa 1907
	Kosmos Verein zur Förderung der wissenschaftlichen Astrologie	Bad Schmiedeberg	e. 1924–26
	Uranische Volksgemeinschaft	Munich	d. 1938
	Uranus Gesellschaft für astrologische Forschung	Munich	e. 1932
	Verein für Pendelforschung	Berlin	f. 1929–b. 1941
Occultism (general)	Adonisten Bund[4]	Dresden	f. 1928–b. 1936
		Pilnitz (Elbe)	f. 1928–b. 1936
	Aranstaat Deutschland	Berlin	e. 1930

Type	Club Name	Location	Active Dates
	Auer Dult	Munich	e. 1924
	Bund der Tatchristen		e. 1929
	‡Christlich-Radikale Volkspartei[5]	Hamburg	f. 1918
	Deutsche okkulte Gesellschaft	Berlin	e. 1923
	Deutsche okkulte Vereinigung	Leipzig	
	Freie Vereinigung zur Förderung der übersinnlichen Weltanschauung	Hamburg	f. 1897
	Freimaurerorden des Goldenen Centuriums (FOGC)	Munich	f. 1840–d. 1933
	Gesellschaft für Okkultismus	Pforzheim	e. 1898
	Internationale Okkulte Reformloge		
	Loge Axmadora	Berlin	e. 1923
	Magische Kunst	Berlin-Tegel	f. 1921–d. 1923
	Magischer Zirkel	Leipzig	e. 1930
	Mazdaznan Bund e.V.[6]	National (based first in Leipzig, then in Freiburg-im-Breisgau)	f. 1907–b. 1936
	Neuland, Gesellschaft für okkulten Wissenschaften	Munich	e. 1923
	Okkultistische Gesellschaft	Munich	f. 1925–d. 1930
		Berlin	e. 1927
	Orden des Okkultisten	Berlin	e. 1923
	Orden Mentalischer Bauherren O.M.B.	Berlin	f. 1922–d. 1929
	Paracelsus	Munich	e. 1931
	Siemens Studiengesellschaft für psychologische Wissenschaft	Bad Homburg	e. 1934
		Cologne	e. 1934
		Düsseldorf	e. 1934
	Verein für okkulte Forschung	Chemnitz	e. 1927
		Leipzig	e. 1927
	Verein für okkultistische Forschung	Gelsenkirchen	e. 1927

Type	Club Name	Location	Active Dates
Occultism (Rosicrucianism)	Westdeutsche okkulte Arbeitsgemeinschaft	Essen	e. 1927
	Xenologische Gesellschaft[7]	Hamburg	e. 1902(?)
	Collegium Pansophicum	Munich	f. 1923
	Esoterische Studien-Gesellschaft[8]	Berlin	e. 1920s–b. 1936
		Leipzig	b. 1936
	Fraternitas Rosicrucian Antiqua		f. 1927
	Fraternitas Saturni[9]	Berlin	f. 1925/8–b. 1936
		Frankfurt	f. 1925/8–b. 1936
		Switzerland	f. 1925–28
	Orden der Rosenkreuzer	Leipzig	f. 1901–b. 1936
		Hamburg	f. 1923–b. 1936
	Pansophische Societät[10]	Berlin	f. after 1918–b. 1936
	Rosenkreuzer Gemeinschaft[11]	Berlin	f. 1909–b. 1936
		Leipzig	f. 1909–b. 1936
		Düsseldorf	f. 1909–b. 1936
	Societas Rosicruciana in Germania	National	f. 1902–d. 1907
Psychical research, parapsychology	Ärztliche Gesellschaft für Parapsychologie[12]	Berlin	e. 1923
	Ärztliche Gesellschaft für parapsychologische Forschung	Berlin	e. 1927
		Munich	e. 1925
	Deutsche Gesellschaft für psychische Forschung	Hamburg	e. 1920s
	Deutsche Gesellschaft für psychologische Forschung	Berlin	e. 1910
		Breslau	e. 1910
		Munich	e. 1910
	Deutsche okkultistische Gesellschaft[13]	Berlin-Charlottenburg	f. 1919
	Gesellschaft für Experimentalpsychologie	Berlin	f. 1888
		Munich[14]	f. 1889
	Gesellschaft für metaphysische Forschung	Munich	e. 1925
	Gesellschaft für psychische Forschung	Breslau	e. 1896

Type	Club Name	Location	Active Dates
		Berlin	e. 1923
		Munich	e. 1927
	Gesellschaft für Psychologie und Charakterologie[15]	Berlin	e. 1928
	Gesellschaft für wissenschaftliche Psychologie	Cologne	e. 1896
	Psychologische Gesellschaft	Dresden	e. 1896
		Düsseldorf	e. 1896
		Munich	f. 1886
		Stuttgart	e. 1896
Spiritualism, magnetism, mesmerism	Bund der Kämpfer für Glaube und Wahrheit (Horpena, Horpenita)	Freital-Zauckerode bei Dresden	e. 1903
		Berlin	e. 1903
	Bund der Wahrheitskämpfer		e. 1930
	Bund für Seelenkultur, Schutzverband deutscher Okkultisten	Hannover	f. 1925
	Bund spiritistischer Vereine	National (based in Berlin)	f. 1900
	Deutscher Spiritualisten Bund	Chemnitz	f. 1901
	Deutscher Spiritisten Verein	Cologne	f. 1904
	‡Christliche Vereinigung[16]	Berlin	f. 1904–7
	Eos	Berlin	f. 1896
		Frankfurt-am-Main	e. 1896
	Freibund	Munich	e. 1915–17
	‡Friedensstadt[17]	Trebbin in der Mark	f. 1920
	Gesellschaft für wissenschaftlichen Spiritismus		
	Gesellschaft "Intelligenz"[18]	Berlin-Charlottenburg	e. 1896
	Gottesbund Tanatra	National (based in Görlitz, with 37 further branches)	f. 1923
		Görlitz	f. 1923

Type	Club Name	Location	Active Dates
	Große Loge von Deutschland des Alten Ordens der Mystiker und Spiritisten[19]	Berlin	e. 1904
		Stettin	e. 1904
	Harmonische Gesellschaft	Hamburg	e. 1896
	Himmelsbotschaft	Seitendorf (Silesia)	e. 1896
	Justinus Kerner zur Eintracht von Deutschland[20]	Berlin	f. 1904
	Leipziger Spiritisten	Leipzig	e. 1896
	Magnetische Gesellschaft	Hamburg-Altona	e. 1896
	Neu-Salems Vereinigung (Lorber Gesellschaft)	Bietigheim (Württemberg)	f. before 1900
	Neue Menschheit	Berlin	e. 1898
	Psyche	Berlin	f. mid-1870s–d. 1881
		National	e. 1896
		Berlin[21]	f. 1884–d. 1896
		Bremen	e. 1896
		Chemnitz	e. 1896
		Düsseldorf[22]	
		Hannover	e. 1896
		Karlsruhe	e. 1896
		Oldenburg	e. 1896
	Psyche zur Wahrheit[23]	Berlin	f. 1897–1904
	Sonnenlicht	Berlin	f. 1890s
	Spiritistischer Zirkel	Hamburg	e. 1896
	Spiritualistischer Bund des rein-geistigen fernwirkenden Verkehrs "Animismus"	Breslau	f. 1893
		Gera	f. 1893
	Spiritualistische Vereinigung	Pforzheim	e. 1896
	Die Sucher, Gemeinschaft für Geistes und Seelenpflege	Munich	f. 1918
	Urania	Berlin	f. 1890s
	Verband Deutscher Okkultisten[24]	National (based in Berlin?)	f. 1896–d. 1900
	Verein für allseitige Erforschung der Geistfrage	Leipzig	f. 1873
	Verein für harmonische Philosophie	Glauchau	e. 1896

Type	Club Name	Location	Active Dates
		Kunzendorf (Silesia)	e. 1896
		Leipzig	f. 1875
		Limbach (Saxony)	e. 1896
		Mülsen St. Niklas (Saxony)	e. 1896
	Verein für okkultistische Forschung 'Durch Nacht zum Licht'	Waldenburg (Silesia)	e. 1896
	Verein für psychische Studien	Hamburg	e. 1880
		Berlin	f. 1890s
	Verein für spirite Studien	Leipzig	f. 1869–d. 1871
	Vereinigung deutscher Magnetopathen	Wiesbaden	f. 1897–b. 1936
		Leipzig	f. 1897–b. 1936
	Vereinigung für zeitgemäße Volksaufklärung	Munich	e. 1918
	Wahrer Weg	National (based in Leipzig)	e. 1927
		Celle	e. 1927
		Hannover	e. 1927
		Magdeburg	e. 1927
	‡Weissenberg Brüder[25]	Trebbin in der Mark (Saxony)	e. 1927–b. 1935
	Wissenschaftliche Vereinigung Sphinx	Berlin	e. 1892
Theosophy (Adyar)[26]	Altgnostische Kirche von Eleusis	Hamborn am Rhein	e. 1921–24
	Bund der Verheißung (Alois Mailänder)	Darmstadt	e. 1890s
		Kempten	e. 1890s
	Deutsche Theosophische Gesellschaft "Adyar"	National (based in Berlin)	f. 1894–b. 1936
		Berlin (Besant-Loge)	e. 1914
		Breslau	e. 1899
		Düsseldorf	f. 1902
		Düsseldorf (Alcyone-Loge)	e. 1914
		Düsseldorf (Blavatsky-Loge)	e. 1914

Type	Club Name	Location	Active Dates
		Essen (Loge Eckehardt)	f. 1922
		Fürstenwald/Spree	e. 1905
		Hamburg	f. 1898
		Hamburg (Hanga Loge)	e. 1922
		Hannover (Brüderschaftsloge)	e. 1922
		Hannover (Dr. Hübbe-Schleiden-Loge)	f. 1898
		Hannover (Loge für Kunst)	e. 1914
		Hannover (Theognostische Loge)	f. 1922
		Kassel	f. 1902
		Leipzig	e. 1896
		Leipzig	f. 1902
		Lohberg (Glückauf)	f. 1922
		Lowenberg, Silesia (Der Pfad)	f. 1922
		Munich	f. 1894–96
		Nuremberg	e. 1899
		Stuttgart	f. 1902
	Esoterischer Kreis der Theosophischen Vereinigung (Wilhelm Hübbe-Schleiden)	Berlin	f. 1893
	Liberal-Katholische Kirche[27]	Berlin	f. 1916–b. 1937
		Bremen	
		Darmstadt	
		Frankfurt	
		Hamburg	
		Hanau	
		Hannover	
		Munich	
		Nuremberg	
	Loge Isis[28]	Hamburg	f. 1879
	Orden des Sterns im Osten (O.S.O.)	National	f. 1912
	Theosophische Gesellschaft (Rudolf Steiner)[29]	National (based in Berlin)	f. 1902–d. 1912–13

Type	Club Name	Location	Active Dates
	Theosophische Loge (Brockdorff)[30]	Berlin-Charlottenburg	f. 1898–99
	Theosophische Societät Germania	National	f. 1884–d. 1887
	Theosophische Vereinigung (Wilhelm Hübbe-Schleiden)	Berlin	f. 1892
Theosophy (ITV)	Allgemeine Geistige Verbrüderung	National	e. 1922
		Berlin	e. 1923
	Lotus Gesellschaft	Munich	f. 1921
	Ordo Templi Orientis (O.T.O.)[31]	National	f. 1895–1904(?)–b. 1936
	Theosophische Gesellschaft (ITV)[32]	National (based first in Munich, then in Leipzig, then in Berlin)	f. 1896–97
		Berlin	f. 1896
		Cottbus	e. 1900
		Dresden	e. 1900
		Essen	e. 1900
		Nuremberg	f. 1896
	Theosophische Vereinigung[33]	Munich	f. 1904
	Wald Loge	Berlin (Gross-Lichterfelde)	f. 1896
Theosophy (affiliation unknown)	A.M.O.		
	Christlich-Theosophische Gesellschaft[34]	Berlin	e. 1900
	Kommunistisch-Theosophische Gesellschaft	Berlin	e. 1923
	Neu-Theosophische Vereinigung	Munich	e. 1897–99
	Oschm-Rahmah-Johjihjah Lodge	Berlin	e. 1904
	Theosophische Loge	Munich	f. 1904–d. 1907
	‡Vril Gesellschaft (Die Loge der Brüder vom Licht)[35]	Berlin	f. 1923(?)
	Wahnfried	Bayreuth	e. 1897

Type	Club Name	Location	Active Dates
Theosophy (Neugeist)[36]	Gralorden[37]	‡Bad Schmiedeberg (Orden vom heiligen Gral, Pension Gralhöhe)	f. 1890–b. 1936
		Dresden (Gralshort Montsalvat)	f. 1923–b. 1936
		Dresden (Gralbrü-derschaft)	f. after 1923–b. 1936
		Dresden (Brüderschaft zum heiligen Gral)	f. after 1923–b. 1936
		Leipzig (Brüderschaft der Alten Riten von Heilgen Graal im großen Orient von Patmos)[38]	f. circa 1921–b. 1936
	Neugeist Bewegung (Neugeist Bund)	National (based in Pfullingen in Württemberg)	f. 1919
		Pfullingen in Württemberg (Bund der Christlichen Mystiker)	e. 1927
		Cannstatt (Ortsgruppe des Neugeistbundes)	e. 1927
		Location unknown (Theosophie Lehrverein für Geisteswissen-schaften)	

Notes to Appendix A

1. This section includes only Ariosophical groups primarily engaged with occult ideas. It does not include groups more properly labeled esoteric such as the Guido von List Gesellschaft (f. 1907–8), Deutscher Orden (f. 1911), Germanenorden (f. 1912), Deutsch-gläubige Gemeinschaft (f. 1911), Germanische Glaubens-Gemeinschaft (f. 1912–13), and Ordo Novi Templi (O.N.T.) (f. 1914). Although many of these groups had occultists as members, none of them made occult beliefs and practices central to their activities or self-understanding. For the complex relationship between Ariosophy and the German occult movement, see chapter 4.

2. P. Erhard Schlund, *Neugermanisches Heidentum im heutigen Deutschland* (Augsburg, 1978), p. 53.

3. Eventually renamed Reichsverband für das Wünschelrutenwesen.

4. A branch of the Adonistische Gesellschaft, founded in 1925 by Dr. Franz Sättler and based in Vienna. Also called Ateschga-Tagonosyn-O.L.Y. and Ateschga Bewegung. See Helmut Möller, "Licht aus dem Osten: Frans Sättlers wundersame Reise nach Nuristân," in *Wege und Abwege: Beiträge zur europäischen Geistesgeschichte der Neuzeit,* ed. A. Götz von Olenhusen (Freiburg: Hochschul Verlag, 1990), pp. 199–230.

5. Also known as the Haeusser Bund. Schlund, *Neugermanisches Heidentum,* pp. 59–61.

6. Founded in 1889 in Chicago by "Dr." Ottoman Hanish. Emphasized breathing exercises, hatha yoga, and vegetarianism, with alchemy, astrology, magic, and other occult sciences. German headquarters initially in Leipzig, then (after 1924) in Freiburg-im-Breisgau. Also called the Zarathustra Gesellschaft and the Mazdaznan-Tempelvereinigung.

7. Name changed (circa 1919) to Deutsche Gesellschaft für wissenschaftliche okkultistische Forschung.

8. This was the profane face of the Fraternitas Saturni (see listing).

9. A successor to the Pansophische Societät (see listing). Note that this group is still in existence.

10. Also known as the Pansophische Gesellschaft and Loge Pansophia. Fraternitas Saturni (see listing) split off from it.

11. Part of the Rosicrucian Fellowship, founded by the German American Max Heindel, in Oceanside, California.

12. Albert Moll, *Der Spiritismus* (Stuttgart: Franckh'sche Verlagshandlung, 1925), pp. 36–49.

13. In 1923, name changed to Deutsche Gesellschaft für wissenschaftlichen Okkultismus; in 1940 changed to Deutsche metaphysische Gesellschaft.

14. Munich branch created through a split from the Psychologische Gesellschaft of Munich in 1889 (see listing). Also known as Gesellschaft für wissenschaftliche Psychologie. Max Dessoir, *Buch der Erinnerung,* 2nd ed. (Stuttgart: Ferdinand Enke, 1947), p. 126.

15. Albert Moll, *Ein Leben als Arzt der Seele: Erinnerungen* (Dresden: Carl Reissner, 1936), p. 136.

16. An early version of what eventually became the Weissenberg Brüder (see listing).

17. A Lebensreform colony run by the Weissenberg Brüder (see listing).

18. Also known as Geistige Erkenntnis.

19. An outgrowth of Psyche in Berlin (see listing).

20. An outgrowth of Psyche in Berlin (see listing). Also known as Justinus Kerner zur Einigkeit.

21. Two groups split off from Psyche: Psyche zur Wahrheit (for middle- and upper-class membership) and Justinus Kerner zur Eintracht (for workers). Eventually, this group also allied itself with the Große Loge von Deutschland des Alten Ordens der Mystiker und Spiritisten. See listings.

22. Also known as the Spiritistischer Verein 'Edewecht.'

23. An outgrowth of the Berlin branch of *Psyche* (see listing). Urlich Linse, *Geisterseher und Wunderwirker: Heilssuche im Industriezeitalter* (Frankfurt-am-Main: Fischer, 1996), p. 101, gives 1897 as its founding date, whereas Hans-Jürgen Glowka, *Deutsche Okkultgruppen, 1875–1937* (Munich: Arbeitsgemeinschaft für Religions-und Weltanschauungsfragen, 1981), pp. 32-33, gives 1904.

24. An umbrella group that included the Spiritualistische Vereinigung, the Gesellschaft für psychische Forschung (Breslau), the Himmelsbotschaft, Spiritistischer Zirkel, the Verein für okkultistische Forschung 'Durch Nacht zum Licht,' the Gesellschaft für wissenschaftliche Psychologie (Munich and Cologne), the Wissenschaftliche Vereinigung Sphinx, the Gesellschaft für Okkultismus, Psyche (Karlsruhe), and the Wissenschaftlicher Verein für Okkultismus (Vienna).

25. Also called the Evangelisch-Johannische Kirche. Associated with Friedensstadt (see listing).

26. Theosophy was an international movement founded in 1875 in New York by Helena Petrovna Blavatasky and Henry Steel Olcott. In 1878, Blavatsky and Olcott moved their headquarters to Adyar, India, and their movement became known as the Theosophical Society (Adyar). Following Blavatsky's death, this branch of the Theosophical movement was led by Annie Besant. In 1895, a split in the Theosophical movement gave rise to the so-called Theosophical Society International, based in California, under the direction of William Quentin Judge and Katherine Tingley. The German Theosophical movement mirrored these splits. The entries above grouped under the heading "Theosophy (Adyar)" adhered to the Theosophical tradition of Blavatsky, Olcott, and Besant. In contrast, those grouped under the heading "Theosophy (I.T.V.)" adhered to the Theosophical tradition of Judge and Tingley; their German leader was Franz Hartmann. Note that an extra complication to the history of the German Theosophical movement came in 1911-12, when Rudolf Steiner (head of the Theosophische Gesellschaft established in Berlin in 1900) broke off to found Anthroposophy. All of these groups, Theosophical as well as Anthroposophical, were banned in 1936–37. For a summary of this complicated history, see Norbert Klatt, *Theosophie und Anthroposophie* (Göttingen: Klatt, 1993), pp. 61–66.

27. An esoteric church founded in England by James Ingall Wedgewood and Charles Leadbeater under the Adyar umbrella. Its goal was to attract churchgoers to Theosophy and it mixed many different religious traditions, especially Buddhism and Roman Catholicism. Its German members included Franz Hartmann and Johannes Maria Verweyen.

28. Refounded and renamed Zum Licht in 1888.

29. Underwent a major split in 1912–13 after Rudolf Steiner left to found the Anthroposophische Gesellschaft, taking many of the German Theosophists with him. The rump group then continued as the Theosophische Gesellschaft.

30. An independent Theosophical circle presided over by Cay and Sophie von Brockdorff, both of whom were also involved in the other Theosophical groups in Berlin. Before founding his own Theosophical branch in Berlin in 1902 (see listing), Rudolf Steiner began his Theosophical career with this circle.

31. An international Theosophical group with European branches in Germany, Austria, Switzerland, Great Britain, the United States, and the Slavic states. Its European headquarters were in Denmark. The German branch was sometimes referred to as the Illuminaten-Orden.

32. Also known as the Theosophische Gesellschaft (Internationale Theosophische Verbrüderung) and the Theosophische Gesellschaft in Deutschland. Its national headquarters were in Munich (1897), Leipzig (1898-1912), and Berlin (after 1912). It had several branch groups, as listed above, and its followers were often referred to as Hartmannianer, after Franz Hartmann, the society's leader.

33. Renamed Theosophische Gesellschaft München ITV in 1905.

34. Renamed Der Gral, Gesellschaft für Theosophie und Spiritismus.

35. Founded by Karl Haushofer, a close confidant of Adolf Hitler and coiner of the term *Lebensraum.* He adapted the racialist ideas of H. P. Blavatsky, went on an important spiritual journey to Tibet, and kept close ties to the infamous Thule Gesellschaft in Munich.

36. In 1889, an American Theosophical faction led by the mesmerist and Christian Scientist Dr. Phineas Quimby began to emphasize practical healing over Theosophical theorizing. In 1894, this faction formally constituted itself as the New Thought Association. Germany had a New Thought group (known as Neugesit) as early as 1890, when the first Gralorden (see listing) were founded. A separate branch of the German New Thought movement began in 1919 with the founding of the Neugeist Bewegung in Pfullingen in Württemberg (see listing). For the American portion of this movement, see Charles Braden, *Spirits in Rebellion: The Rise and Development of New Thought* (Dallas, TX: Southern Methodist University, 1963).

37. Renamed Neuer Gralorden in 1921.

38. Also known as Ermächtigte Bruderschaft der alten Riten and Ebdar. Founded by Bô Yin Râ.

Presses

Type	Press Name	Location	Active Dates[1]
Ariosophy	‡Guido von List[2]	Vienna, Berlin-Lichterfelde	1910–26
	‡Ostara	Rodaun-Mödlinger (1905–13), Mödling-Vienna (1913–17), Vienna (1906–31)	1905–31, f. 1905
	‡Herbert Reichstein	Oestrich i. Rheing. (1925), Düsseldorf-Unterrath (1926), Pforzheim (1927–31)	1925–31, f. 1925
Astrology, dowsing, graphology, palmistry, pendulum	‡Astra	Dresden (1926), Leipzig (1925–41)	1925–41
	‡Deutsche Ehe	Breslau	1933
	‡Deutsche Zukunft	Leipzig (1908–21), Dresden (1932)	1908–32
	‡Ebertin	Erfurt (1928–41), Aalen (1948–78), Freiburg im Breisgau (1979–2002)	1928–2002
	‡A. M. Grimm	Bad Tölz	1923–34
	Max Hübner	Munich	1927
	Jati	Munich	1921–22
	Pyramiden	Berlin	1925–56
	‡Uranus	Bad Oldesloe (1924), Memmingen (1930–36), Hamburg (1930, 1936–37), Saarbrücken (1934)	1924–37
	‡Erich Wiesel	Dresden	1932–35
	Yoga	Dresden	1930–34
Lebensreform	H. Barsdorf	Berlin	1885–1927, f. 1885
	Johannes Baum	Berlin (1912–20), Pfullingen in Württemberg (1921–)	1912–63, f. 1912
	F. E. Baumann[3]	Leipzig (1895–1912), Bad Schmiedeberg (1912?–1926)	1895–1926

Type	Press Name	Location	Active Dates[1]
	Lebensweiser	Gettenbach bei Gelnhausen, Büdingen-Haingründau, Bern	1926–61
	P. Lorenz	Freiburg im Breisgau	1895–1926
	Mazdaznan	Leipzig	1911–34
	Nirwana[4]	Berlin	1922–25
	‡Sonnen-Verlag	Leipzig (1915), Hannover (1933)	1915–33
	Max Spohr	Leipzig	1881–1923, f. 1881
	Wahrheit	Leipzig	1917–25, f. 1917
	Zukunftspost		
Occultism (general)	E. Bartels	Berlin	f. 1880, 1880–1933
	O. W. Barth	Leipzig (1912–26), Munich (1923–82)	1912–82
	Linser	Berlin	1911–38
	Pansophia	Leipzig	1920s
	Karl Rohm	Lorch (Württemberg)	1904–24
	Paul Schmidt	Berlin	1921–32(?), f. 1921
	Talis	Leipzig	1919
	Vorkämpfer	Sorau	1929
	Xenologischer	Hamburg	1901
Spiritualism, mesmerism, magnetism, psychical research, parapsychology	Wilhelm Besser	Leipzig	1881–1917
	I. F. Conrad[5]	Berlin	1892
	Ernst Julius Günther	Leipzig	1864–1903, f. 1864
	Oswald Mutze	Leipzig	1872–1941, f. 1872
	Neu-Salems-Verlag	Bietigheim (Württemberg)	1907–32
	Max Rahn	Berlin	1893
	Karl Siegismund	Berlin	1886–1943, f. 1886
	‡A. Stahn[6]	Forst i. L.	1926–27
Theosophy	Max Altmann	Leipzig	1905–33, f. 1905
	Th. Griebens	Leipzig	1883–1912
	Richard Hummel	Leipzig	1919–39, f. 1919
	Jaeger'sche Buchhandlung	Leipzig	1847–1962
	Kober[7]	Basel, Leipzig	1927–53
	Lotus	Leipzig	1901–27
	Magische Blätter	Leipzig	1920–26
	Ernst Pieper Ring	Düsseldorf	f. 1909

Type	Press Name	Location	Active Dates
	Prana	Pfullingen in Württemberg	1900–25
	Paul Raatz	Berlin	1904–22
	C. A. Schwetschke	Braunschweig/ Brunswick (1851– 97), Berlin (1898–)	1829–1929, f. 1829
	[Rudolf Steiner]	Vienna, Berlin	1903–8
	Theosophische Central-buchhandlung[8]	Leipzig	1903–6
	Theosophische Propaganda Zentrale	Nuremberg	1907–22
	Theosophischer Kultur-Verlag	Leipzig	1909–33
	Theosophisches Verlagshaus	Leipzig	1898–1928
	Verlag des theosophischen Wegweisers	Leipzig	1898–1907
	Wilhelm Friedrich	Leipzig	1878–95, f. 1878
	Paul Zillmann	Berlin-Lichterfelde	1896–1918

Notes to Appendix B

1. The active dates reflect the best available information, which was culled both from printed material and various library catalogs.

2. Guido von List, *Urgrund: Eine Einführung in die Gedankenwelt des Wiener Forschers Guido von List* (Berlin-Lichterfelde: Guido von List Gesellschaft, 1936); available at JFC.

3. Georg Lomer, *Neureligiöse Praxis* (Bad Schmiedeberg: F. E. Baumann, 1926); available at JFC.

4. *Haupt Katalog, 1922* (Berlin: Nirwana-Verlag für Lebensreform, 1922) and *Katalog zur Leihbibliothek* (Berlin: Nirwana-Verlag für Lebensreform, 1925); available at JFC.

5. Egbert Müller, *Stellung des Strafrichters zum Spiritismus und der Proceß Valeska Töpfer* (Berlin: I. F. Conrad's Buchhandlung); available at JFC.

6. Elisabeth Grimm, *Geistige Inspiration durch Gottes Gnade gegeben am 20. Dezember 1926* (Forst i. L.: A. Stahn, 1926–27); available at JFC.

7. Alfred Kober-Staehelin, *Meine Stellung zu Bô Yin Râ* (Leipzig: Kober'sche Verlagsbuchhandlung, 1931).

8. This became part of the *Theosophisches Verlagshaus* in 1912.

Other Institutions

Type of Institution	Name of Organization	Specialty	Location	Active Dates[1]
Bookstores, libraries	Askothebu	Occultism, mysticism	Munich	1920s
	I. F. Conrad	Spiritualism	Berlin	1892
	Inveha	Theosophy	Berlin	1920s
	Nirwana[2]	Occultism, Lebensreform	Berlin	1922–25
	J. Scheible's Antiquariat und Verlagsbuchhandlung	Occultism	Stuttgart	1833–1880s
	Karl Siegismund	Spiritualism, hypnotism, magnetism	Berlin	1889–1940s
	Zentralbibliothek der okkulte Weltliteratur	Occultism	Berlin	1937
Health-related businesses	Bombastus-Werke	Spiritualism (also occultism, Lebensreform)	Freital Zauckerode bei Dresden	1903
	Hallein	Occultism, Lebensreform	Hallein	1890s
	‡Heilinstitut 'Schwester Grete Müller'[3]	Spiritualism	Trebbin in der Mark	1920s
	Jungborn	Theosophy	Harz mountains	
	Prana Haus	Occultism, Lebensreform	Pfullingen in Württemberg	1920s
	Psychomagnetisches suggestives Heilinstitut[4]	Occultism	Munich	1920s(?)
Institutes for advice and information	‡Aeterna Bund, e.V.[5]	Occultism	Munich	1932

Type of Institution	Name of Organization	Specialty	Location	Active Dates[1]
	Archiv für Reinkarnation	Theosophy	Leipzig	1936
	Astrologische Zentralstelle, Statistisches Amt	Astrology	Düsseldorf	f. 1923
	Astrologisches Büro[6]	Astrology	Berlin	1927
	Astrologisches Institut	Astrology	Erfurt	1933
	Beratungs-und Prüfungsstelle für astrologisches und verwandtes Schrifttum	Astrology	Berlin	1935
	Büro für wissenschaftliche Astrologie	Astrology	Berlin	1927
	Forschungsinstitut für Okkultismus	Occultism	Berlin	1931
	Graphologisches Institut	Graphology	Hannover	1901
	Haldame (Haldane) Handdiagnostik	Palmistry	Munich, Berlin	1926
	Institut Alcyone	Astrology	Leipzig	
	Institut für metaphysische Forschung	Psychical research, parapsychology	Berlin	1930
	Institut für wissenschaftliche Astrologie und Graphologie	Astrology, graphology	Kiel	1929
	Institut für Wünschelruten-und Pendelforschung	Dowsing, pendulum	Munich	1933
	Institut für Xenologie	Occultism	Hamburg(?)	f. 1912
	Zentrale für praktischen Okkultismus	Occultism	Leipzig(?)	1920s(?)
	Zentralstelle für Lebenserneuerung	Occultism, Lebensreform	Munich	f. 1929
Lecture halls, schools	Eclaros Saal	Occultism	Munich	1910s(?)
	Freie Hochschule für Geisteswissenschaften	Occultism	Berlin	f. 1924
	Kepler Zirkel[7]	Astrology	Hamburg	f. 1919

Type of Institution	Name of Organization	Specialty	Location	Active Dates[1]
	Mazdaznan Kolleg	Occultism, Lebensreform	Herrliberg bei Zürich	f. 1914
	Pansophische Schule	Occultism, mysticism		b. 1936

Notes to Appendix C

1. The active dates reflect the best available information.

2. *Haupt Katalog, 1922* (Berlin: Nirwana-Verlag für Lebensreform, 1922) and *Katalog zur Leihbibliothek* (Berlin: Nirwana-Verlag für Lebensreform, 1925).

3. Associated with the colony of Friedensstadt, run by Joseph Weissenberg (see listing).

4. *Psychomagnetisches suggestives Heilinstitut München* (Munich, c. 1910).

5. Aeterna Bund, *Okkulte Probleme: Okkultistenbund "Aeterna" e.V. München. Zweck und Ziele. Aeterna Bücher, Band 1* (Munich: Aeterna-Verlag, c. 1932).

6. Arthur Hübscher, "Persönliche Erfahrungen mit Astrologen," *Süddeutsche Monatshefte* 24, no. 9 (1927): 212

7. Founded by Alfred Witte; also known as Hamburger Astrologen-Schule and Astrologische Studiengesellschaft e.V.

Periodicals

ARIOSOPHY AND RUNE OCCULTISM

Deutsche Freiheit. Munich, Dinkelsbühl, 1919–26. Continued as *Arische Freiheit.* Dinkelsbühl, 1927. Continued as *Hag All All Hag.* Dinkelsbühl, Mittenwald, 1929–34. Continued as *Hagal.* Munich, Mittenwald, 1934–39.

Zeitschrift für Menschenkenntnis und Menschenschicksal. Oestrich im Rheingau: Herbert Reichstein, 1925. Continued as *Zeitschrift für Menschenkenntnis und Schicksalsforschung.* Düsseldorf-Unterrath: Herbert Reichstein, 1926–27. Continued as *Zeitschrift für Geistes-und Wissenschaftsreform.* Pforzheim, Vienna, Berlin: Herbert Reichstein, 1928–33.

Der Wehrmann. Pforzheim, 1931–32.

Sig-Run. Pasing, 1932.

Die Neue Flagge. Dresden, 1931–33.

Arische Rundschau. Berlin, 1933–?

ASTROLOGY

Astrale Warte. Bad Oldesloe and Memmingen: Uranus, 1925–36, 1949–51.

ASTRO-Magazin. Berlin: Janiszewski, 1929–30.

Astrologische Blätter. Berlin: Linser, 1914–27. Continued as *Die Astrologie.* Berlin: Linser, 1928–38.

Astrologischer Monatsführer für jedermann. Dresden: Yoga Verlag, 1930–34.

Astrologischer Pionier. Erfurt: Astrologisches Institut, 1933–34.

Astrologischer Ratgeber. Erfurt: Ebertin, 1928–29. Continued as *Neue Sternblätter.* Erfurt: Ebertin, 1929–33. Continued as *Mensch im All.* Erfurt: Ebertin, 1933–41. Continued as *Kosmobiologie.* Aalen: Ebertin, 1948-78. Continued as *Meridian.* Freiburg-im-Breisgau: Ebertin, 1979–2002.

Astrologisches Nachrichtenblatt. Bad Tölz: A. M. Grimm, 1925.

Astrologische Rundschau. Leipzig: Theosophisches Verlagshaus, 1909–38.

Astrologische Studien. Berlin: Pyramiden Verlag, 1925–?

Astropolitische Rundschau. 1933–34. Continued as *Weltpolitische Rundschau.* 1934–35.

Deutsche Astrologen Zeitung. Bad Tölz: A. M. Grimm, 1923–34.

Deutsche Ehe. Breslau: Verlag Deutsche Ehe, 1933.

Die Deutsche Zukunft. Dresden: Verlag die Deutsche Zukunft, 1932.

Kosmisches Tagebuch. 1933.

Kritische Studien zur Astrologie. Munich, 1930–?

Moderne Astrologie. Bad Schmiedeberg: F. E. Baumann, 1924–26.

Quellenschriften zur Astrologie. Leipzig, 1920–21.

Scholle und Stern: Das kommende Deutschland. Hamburg: Uranus Verlag, 1932.

Der Seher: Deutsche astrologische Zeitung. Erfurt: Ebertin Verlag, 1928–35.

Sphinx, okkult-astrologische Wochenblätter. Munich: Max Hübner, 1927.

Sterne und Mensch. Dresden and Leipzig, 1925–41.

Wodania Blätter.

Zenit: Zentralblatt für astrologische Forschung. Düsseldorf: Zenit, 1930–38.

Die Zukunft: Astrologische Zeitbilder. Berlin: Paul Schmidt, 1924–32.

Zukunftskurier. Dresden: Erich Wiesel, 1932. Continued as *Der Germane, die deutsche astrologische Volkszeitung.* 1933–35.

Die Zukunftspost. Verlag die Zukunftspost.

OCCULTISM (GENERAL)

Berichte der deutschen graphologischen Gesellschaft. Munich: Deutsche Graphologische Gesellschaft, 1897–98. Continued as *Graphologische Monatshefte.* Munich: Karl Schüler, 1899–1908.

Der Lebensweiser: Zeitschrift für Aufstieg, Erfolg, und Menschenführung. Büdingen-Gettenbach: Lebensweiser, 1926. Continued as *Mensch und Schicksal.* Büdingen-Gettenbach: Welt und Wissen, 1947–60.

Magikon: Archiv für Beobachtungen aus dem Gebiete der Geisterkunde. Stuttgart: Ebner & Teubert, 1841–53.

Magische Blätter. Leipzig: Verlag Magische Blätter, 1920–26. Continued as *Die Säule: der magischen Blätter.* Leipzig: Richard Hummel Verlag, 1927–41.

Mitteilungen der deutschen graphologischen Studiengesellschaft. Berlin: Leopold Radó, 1928–34.

Natur und Kultur: Monatsschrift für Naturwissenschaft und ihre Grenzgebiete. Munich: Herold Verlag, 1903–29.

Die Okkulte Welt. Berlin and Pfullingen in Würtemberg: Johannes Baum, 1920-30.

Der Okkultismus. Bielefeld, 1925–26.

Pansophia. Leipzig: Pansophia Verlag.

Wahrheits-Sucher. Bitterfeld: F. E. Baumann, 1896–97.

Weisse Fahne. Pfullingen in Württemberg: Johannes Baum, 1920–32, 1950–70. Absorbed *Okkultistische Rundschau, Die Burg,* and *Der 6. Sinn.*

Wissenschaftliche Zeitschrift für Okkultismus. Berlin: Adolf Brand, 1898–99. Continued as *Wissenschaftliche Zeitschrift für Xenologie.* Hamburg: F. Maack, 1899–1902.

Das Wort: Monatsschrift für die allseitige Erkenntnis Gottes. Bitterfeld: F. E. Baumann, 1893–1905. Dresden: Engel, 1906–14.

XELARIA, Internationale Zeitschrift für Seelenkunde und-Forschung. Leipzig and Munich: O. W. Barth, 1921.

Zeitschrift für Metapsychische Forschung. Berlin, 1930–41.

Zentralblatt für Okkultismus. Berlin and Leipzig: Max Altmann, 1907–33.

Zum Licht: Esoterische Nachrichten. Bad Schmiedeberg: F. E. Baumann, 1916.

PSYCHICAL RESEARCH, PARAPSYCHOLOGY, SPIRITUALISM

Internationale Blätter für Spiritismus. Munich and Leipzig: Franz Müller, 1900–1901.

Licht, Mehr Licht: Spiritistische Wochenschrift. Paris and Walthershausen bei Gotha: Egling, 1879–86.

Psyche: Deutsche Zeitschrift für Odwissenschaft und Geisterkunde. Großenhain: Haffner, 1865–66?

Psyche: Monatsschrift für Spiritismus und verwandte Gebiete. Berlin: F. Schlosser, 1893–1900. Continued as *Spiritistische Rundschau.* Berlin: K. Siegismund, 1900–1908. Continued as *Okkultistische Rundschau.* Chemnitz, 1909-29. Merged with *Zeitschrift für Seelenleben und verwandte Gebiete* in 1929.

Psyche: Monatlich erscheinende Zeitschrift für den gesamten Okkultismus und alle Geheimwissenschaften. Berlin: Linser, 1914–27. Merged with *Die übersinnliche Welt* (see below) in 1922.

Psychische Studien. Leipzig, O. Mutze, 1874–1925. Continued as *Zeitschrift für Parapsychologie.* Leipzig: O. Mutze, 1926–34. Continued as *Zeitschrift für Parapsychologie und Grenzgebiete der Psychologie* after 1945.

Schriften der Gesellschaft für Experimental-Psychologie zu Berlin. Leipzig: Ernst Günther, 1888–90.

Spirisophie: Zeitschrift für die Harmonie zwischen Vernunft, Religion und Lebensthätigkeit. Berlin: K. Siegismund, 1889.

Der Spiritist: Zeitschrift für Spiritismus und verwandte Gebiete. Zürich: C. Schmidt, 1892–1902.

Spiritisch-rationalistische Zeitschrift. Leipzig: O. Mutze, 1872–74. Continued as *Psychische Studien* (see above).

Spiritistische Wochenschrift. Rostock and Leipzig: Uhlig, 1885–86.

Spiritualistische Blätter. Leipzig: Noeßler, 1883–84. Continued as *Neue Spiritualistische Blätter.* Leipzig: Noeßler, 1885–87; Berlin: K. Siegismund, 1888–98. Absorbed by *Zeitschrift für Spiritismus und verwandte Gebiete* in 1899.

Der Sprechsaal. Leipzig: Wilhelm Besser, 1881–83.

Die übersinnliche Welt. Berlin: Max Rahn (Linser Verlag?), 1893–1902. Merged with *Psyche: Monatlich erscheinende Zeitschrift* and continued as *Psyche und die übersinnliche Welt* from 1902 to 1922. Continued as supplement to *Psyche.* 1922–26.

Der Vorkämpfer für Geistwissenschaft, Tatchristentum, und Glaubensreform. Sorau: Vorkämpfer-Verlag, 1920–31?

Wahres Leben. Leipzig: Schaarschmidt (R. Besser?), 1899–1932.

Zeitschrift für kritischen Okkultismus und Grenzfragen des Seelenlebens. Stuttgart: F. Enke, 1925–28.

Zeitschrift für Spiritismus und verwandte Gebiete. Leipzig, O. Mutze, 1897-1915. Absorbed *Neue Spiritualistische Blätter* in 1899. Continued as *Zeitschrift für Seelenleben und verwandte Gebiete.* Leipzig: O. Mutze, 1915-41. Absorbed *Okkultistische Rundschau* in 1929.

THEOSOPHY

Blätter für universale Bruderschaft. Nuremberg, 1902–4. Continued as *Universale Bruderschaft.* Nuremberg, 1904–11. Continued as *Der theosophische Pfad.* Nuremberg,

1911–25? Accompanied by the supplement *Die theosophische Warte*. Nuremberg, 1917–21?

Es werde Licht! Leipzig: Theosophische Central-Buchhandlung, 1898–99. Continued as *Theosophischer Wegweiser*. 1899–1907.

Lotusblätter. Leipzig and Munich: O. W. Barth, 1921–25.

Lotusblüthen. Leipzig: W. Friedrich, 1892–1900. Continued as *Neue Lotusblüthen*. Leipzig: Jaeger'sche Buchhandlung, 1908–15.

Luzifer: Zeitschrift für Seelenleben und Geisteskultur. Vienna: R. Steiner, 1903–8. Incorporated *Gnosis* in 1903 and occasionally published under the title *Luzifer-Gnosis*.

Metaphysische Rundschau. Berlin: Paul Zillmann, 1896–97. Continued as *Neue Metaphysische Rundschau*. Berlin: Paul Zillmann, 1898–1917.

Prana. Leipzig: Theosophisches Verlagshaus, 1909–19.

Sphinx. Leipzig: T. Griebens, 1886. Gera: T. Hoffmann, 1887–88. Brunswick: C. A. Schwetschke, 1888–96. Continued as *Metaphysische Rundschau*. 1896 (see above).

Theosophie. Leipzig: Theosophisches Verlagshaus, 1910–37? Contained the supplement *Zeitschrift für astrologische Forschung*.

Theosophische Bausteine zur Förderung der theosophischen Kultur. Leipzig: Theosophischer Kultur-Verlag, 1909–?

Theosophische Botschaft, die. Leipzig: Theosophischer Kultur-Verlag, 1927–33?

Theosophische Forum, Das. Stuttgart, 1930–35, 1948–51.

Theosophische Kultur (I.T.V.). Leipzig: Theosophischer Kultur-Verlag, 1909-37.

Theosophische Kulturbücher für wahre Lebenskunst und Lebensweisheit. Leipzig: Theosophischer Kultur-Verlag, 1916–36?

Theosophische Nachrichten. Berlin: P. Raatz, 1897–98. Continued as *Theosophisches Leben*. Berlin: P. Raatz, 1898–1921. Continued as *Bruderschaft*. Berlin: P. Raatz, 1922–23.

Theosophischer Wegweiser. Leipzig: Theosophische Central-Buchhandlung, 1898-1907? Accompanied by the supplement *Theosophische Rundschau*. Leipzig: Theosophische Central-Buchhandlung, 1905–6.

Theosophisches Streben. Munich: Rösch, 1914–28. Continued as *Theosophische Studien*. Düsseldorf: Ernst Pieper Ring, 1929–32?

Der Vâhan. Berlin, 1899. Leipzig, 1900–1906.

Wahrheit-Sucher. Bitterfeld, 1896–97.

Der Wanderer. Leipzig: Theosophisches Verlagshaus, 1906–8.

NOTE TO APPENDIX D

Most of the periodicals listed in the section "Ariosophy and Rune Occultism" are collected in Nicolas Goodrick-Clarke, *The Occult Roots of Nazism: The Ariosophists of Austria and Germany, 1890–1935* (Northamptonshire: Aquarian, 1985), pp. 282–84. Most of those listed in the section "Astrology" are collected in Glowka, *Deutsche Okkultgruppen*, pp. 50-52. For periodicals on psychical research, parapsychology, and spiritualism, see also *Bibliographie der Zeitschriften des deutschen Sprachgebietes bis 1900*, ed. J. Kirchner, 4 vols. (Stuttgart: Anton Hiersemann, 1977), and Ulrich Linse, "Spiritistische Zeitschriften um 1900: Eine Bibliographie," *Mystique, mysticisme et modernité en Allemagne autour de 1900*, ed. Moritz Baßler and Hildegard Châtellier (Strasbourg: Presses Universitaires, 1998), pp. 111–13.

Notes

Abbreviations

ADW	Archiv des Diakonischen Werk, Evangelische Kirche in Deutschland (Berlin)
CA AC	Central-Ausschuss, Apologetische Centrale
CA AC-S	Central-Ausschuss, Apologetische Centrale-Sammlung
BA	Bundesarchiv (Berlin)
BSB	Bayerische Staatsbibliothek (Munich)
Cod WH-S	Cod Wilhelm Hübbe-Schleiden (Nachlaß), Abteilung für Handschriften und seltene Drucke, Niedersächsische Staats-und Universitätsbibliothek Göttingen
EZB	Evangelisches Zentralarchiv (Berlin)
GSPK	Geheimes Staatsarchiv Preussischer Kulturbesitz (Berlin)
JFC	Janos Frecot Collection, Department of Special Collections, Stanford University Libraries
PDM	Polizeidirektion München
SdArMü	Stadtarchiv München
StArMü	Staatsarchiv München
USHMM	United States Holocaust Memorial Museum (Washington, D. C.)
ZA	Zeitungsausschnitte

CHAPTER ONE: The Lure of the Psyche

1. For useful definitions of occultism, see *On the Margins of the Visible: Sociology, the Esoteric, and the Occult* (New York: John Wiley & Sons, 1974), ed. Edward A. Tiryakian; Mircea Eliade, *Occultism, Witchcraft, and Cultural Fashions: Essays in Comparative Religion* (Chicago, IL: University of Chicago Press, 1976); and Marcello Truzzi, "Definition and Dimensions of the Occult: Towards a Sociological Perspective," *Journal of Popular Culture* (winter 1971): 635–46. For a bibliographical overview, see Robert Galbreath, "The History of Modern Occultism: A Bibliographical Survey," *Journal of Popular Culture* (winter 1971): 726–54.

2. Slade's exposure and trial can be followed in the *Times* (London) from 21 September to 1 November 1876.

3. For samples of such "spirit writing," see the tables reproducing the actual slates used in these experiments at the end of vols. 2 (pt. 1) and 3 of Friedrich Zöllner, *Wissenschaftliche Abhandlungen* (Leipzig: L. Staackamnn, 1878–79).

4. Zöllner, *Wissenschaftliche Abhandlungen* 3:197–98.

5. For reproductions of these "spirit footprints," see tables ibid., vols. 2 (pt. 1) and 3.

6. This day-by-day account of the Leipzig experiments is from ibid., 1:725–29 and 2 (pt. 1): 324–51.

7. J. C. Friedrich Zöllner, "On Space of Four Dimensions," *Quarterly Journal of Science* 8 (April 1878): 234.

8. Zöllner, "On Space," p. 236.

9. Janet Oppenheim, *The Other World: Spiritualism and Psychical Research in England, 1850–1914* (Cambridge: Cambridge University Press, 1985), p. 32. Zöllner's book was translated as *Transcendental Physics: An Account of Experimental Investigations from the Scientific Treatises* (London: W. H. Harrison, 1880) and has been reissued several times.

10. See, for instance, the new edition brought out by Rudolf Tischner under the title *Vierte Dimension und Okkultismus: Auswahl aus den Werken Fr. Zöllners* (Leipzig, 1922).

11. Karl Kiesewetter, *Geschichte des neueren Occultismus* (Schwarzenburg: Ansata, 1977), p. 464; originally published as *Die Geheimwissenschaften: Die Entwicklungsgeschichte des Spiritismus von der Urzeit bis zur Gegenwart* (Leipzig: Wilhelm Friedrich, 1891–95).

12. *Astrophysics and Twentieth-Century Astronomy to 1950*, pt. A, ed. Owen Gingerich (Cambridge: Cambridge University Press, 1984), pp. 14 and 92; Dieter B. Herrmann, *Entdecker des Himmels* (Cologne: Pahl-Rugenstein Verlag, 1979), p. 133.

13. *Dictionary of Scientific Biography* 4 (1971), s.v., "Gustav Theodor Fechner," pp. 556–59; see also the essay by Marilyn Marshall in *The Problematic Science: Psychology in Nineteenth-Century Thought*, ed. William R. Woodward and Mitchell G. Ash (New York: Praeger, 1982).

14. Edwin G. Boring, *A History of Experimental Psychology* (New York: Appleton-Century-Crofts, 1950), p. 323.

15. Linda Dalrymple Henderson, *The Fourth Dimension and Non-Euclidean Geometry in Modern Art* (Princeton, NJ: Princeton University Press, 1983), pp. 12–13.

16. The most pertinent philosophical discussion of these issues can be found in Gary Hatfield, *The Natural and the Normative: Theories of Spatial Perception from Kant to Helmholtz* (Cambridge: MIT Press, 1990). An account by an early historian of modern psychology can be found in Edwin G. Boring, *A History of Experimental Psychology*, pp. 305–7; see also the excellent essays by David E. Leary on Kant and R. Steven Turner on Helmholtz in Woodward and Ash, *Problematic Science*.

17. K. F. Zöllner, *Über die Natur der Cometen* (Leipzig: Engelmann, 1872).

18. Zöllner borrowed the term *transcendental physics* from Fichte: Zöllner, *Wissenschaftliche Abhandlungen* 3, p. xxiv.

19. "Der Spiritismus in Leipzig," *Im Neuen Reich* (1878): 724 and 728–29.

20. Zöllner, *Wissenschaftliche Abhandlungen* 2 (pt. 1), pp. 239–44 and 391–96.

21. G. Stanley Hall, *Founders of Modern Psychology* (New York: Appleton, 1912), p. 267.

22. Dieter B. Herrmann, *Karl Friedrich Zöllner* (Leipzig: Teubner Gesellschaft, 1982), pp. 72 and 77; see also Christoph Meinel, *Karl Friedrich Zöllner und die Wissenschaftskultur der Gründerzeit: Eine Fallstudie zur Genese konservativer Zivilisationskritik* (Berlin: ERS-Verlag, 1991).

23. Herrmann, *Karl Friedrich Zöllner*, p. 77.

24. A few of these went on record with this claim with the rector at the University of Leipzig, Dr. Karl Bücher, in 1903: *Encyclopedia of Occultism and Parapsychology*, 2nd ed. (1984–85), s.v., "Zöllner, Johann C. F.," p. 1012.

25. Dr. K. W. Whistling, "Prof. Friedrich Zöllner," *Leipziger Illustrirte Zeitung* (6 May 1882).

26. In addition to the works discussed above, see also Lazar B. Hellenbach, *Mr. Slades Aufenthalt in Wien* (Vienna: J. C. Fischer, 1878), M. Wirth, *Herrn Professor Zöllners Hypothese intelligenter vierdimensionaler Wesen* (Leipzig: O. Mutze, 1879), and F. Michelis, *Ist die Annahme eines Raumes mit mehr als drei Dimensionen wissenschaftlich berechtigt?* (Freiburg: F. Wagner, 1879).

27. For Zöllner's reply to Wundt, see Zöllner, *Wissenschaftliche Abhandlungen* 3:1–82.

28. Wilhelm Wundt, "Der Spiritismus: Offener Brief an Herrn Prof. Dr. Herm. Ulrici in Halle," *Essays* (Leipzig: Wilhelm Englemann, 1885), pp. 352–53 and 356.

29. Ibid., p. 361.

30. Ibid., p. 365.

31. Ibid., pp. 365–66.

32. *The Encyclopedia of Philosophy* 3 (1967), s.v., "Eduard von Hartmann," pp. 419–21.

33. Eduard von Hartmann, *Der Spiritismus* (Leipzig: Wilhelm Friedrich, 1885), p. 1.

34. Ibid., pp. 14–15 and 21.

35. Ibid., pp. 16 and 19.

36. Ibid., pp. 19–20 and 23.

37. See Harry Houdini, *A Magician among the Spirits* (New York: Harper & Bros., 1924), p. 82.

38. *Preliminary Report of the Commission Appointed by the University of Pennsylvania to Investigate Modern Spiritualism*, 2nd ed. (Philadelphia: J. B. Lippincott, 1920), p. 114. In one of those ironic twists so typical of the shifting terrain of the spiritualist movement, the commission's negative assessment of spiritualist phenomena contravened the wishes of its benefactor, Henry Seybert, who believed that the phenomena merited extensive further study.

39. Later commentators followed Fullerton's lead. For example, according to G. Stanley Hall, an early historian of modern psychology, Fechner always remained skeptical about the spiritualist interpretation of the séances with Slade. On Fechner's recommendation, Hall visited Zöllner, who showed him the two sealed slates on which writing had appeared and other props from the experiments. Zöllner claimed that he had shown these objects to his classes as well, although only a half dozen or so students continued to come to his lectures: G. Stanley Hall, *Founders of Modern Psychology*, pp. 166–68.

40. Wilhelm Hübbe-Schleiden, "Zöllners Zurechnungsfähigkeit und die Seybert-Kommission," *Sphinx* 4, no. 23 (1887): 328.

41. *Kandinsky: Complete Writings on Art*, ed. Kenneth C. Lindsay and Peter Vergo (New York: De Capo Press, 1994), p. 143.

42. For information on the holdings of Kandinsky's library, see Sixten Ringbom, *The Sounding Cosmos: A Study in the Spiritualism of Kandinsky and the Genesis of Abstract Painting* (Abo: Abo Akademi, 1970), chapter 1.

43. David Blackbourn, *The Long Nineteenth Century: A History of Germany, 1780–1918* (New York: Oxford University Press, 1998), pp. 200 and 351.

44. James McFarlane, "Berlin and the Rise of Modernism, 1886–1896," in *Modernism, 1890–1930,* ed. Malcolm Bradbury and James McFarlane (New York: Penguin, 1976), pp. 109–10.

45. On fatigue and its connection to modernism, see Anson Rabinbach, *The Human Motor: Energy, Fatigue, and the Origins of Modernity* (Berkeley: University of California Press, 1990).

46. For Weber and his Janus-faced view of modernity, see Detlev J. K. Peukert, *Max Webers Diagnose der Moderne* (Göttingen: Vandenhoeck & Ruprecht, 1989). For modernism and German culture, some of the most useful sources are as follows: the essay by Bradbury cited above; *The Divided Heritage: Themes and Problems in German Modernism,* ed. Irit Rogoff (Cambridge: Cambridge University Press, 1991); *Imagining Modern German Culture, 1889–1910,* ed. Françoise Forster-Hahn (Hanover, NH: University Press of New England, 1996); and *Kultur und Kulturwissenschaften um 1900: Krise der Moderne und Glaube an die Wissenschaft,* ed. Rüdiger vom Bruch, Friedrich Wilhelm Graf, and Gangolf Hübinger (Stuttgart: Franz Steiner, 1989). Also useful for broader issues of interpretation are Carl Schorske, *Fin-de-Siècle Vienna: Politics and Culture* ([1961] New York: Vintage, 1981), and H. Stuart Hughes, *Consciousness and Society: The Reconstruction of European Social Thought, 1890–1930* ([1958] New York: Vintage, 1961).

47. Herrmann, *Karl Friedrich Zöllner,* p. 65.

48. The economic downturn of 1873 also stimulated organizers to establish the Anti-Semitic League in 1879 and circulate an anti-Semitic petition that garnered 250,000 signatures in 1880–81. The increasingly vocal anti-Semitism of professors like Zöllner and the historian Heinrich von Treitschke lent this organizational wave a certain academic legitimacy. Zöllner was the only professor at the University of Leipzig to sign the anti-Jewish petition of 1880. In addition, he wrote the anti-Semitic tract *Beiträge zur deutschen Judenfrage, mit akademischen Arabesken* (Leipzig: O. Mutze, 1894). The press of Oswald Mutze, it is worth noting, was then the main press devoted to occultism in Germany. For further discussion, see Peter G. Pulzer, *The Rise of Political Anti-Semitism in Austria and Germany* (New York: John Wiley & Sons, 1964).

49. Fritz Ringer, *The Decline of the German Mandarins: The German Academic Community, 1890–1933* (Hanover, NH: University Press of New England, 1990), pp. 102–13.

50. Zöllner, "On Space," p. 232.

51. Friedrich Engels, "Die Naturforschung in der Geisterwelt," in Karl Marx and Friedrich Engels, *Werke,* vol. 20 (Berlin: Dietz, 1986), pp. 345.

52. Woodward and Ash, *Problematic Science,* pp. 148–51. It is indicative of the convoluted history of the "new psychology" that Wundt, its most vocal advocate, still occupied a chair in philosophy. For further discussion on the links between spiritualism and early experimental psychology in Germany, see Klaus Staubermann, "Tying the Knot: Skill, Judgement, and Authority in the 1870s Leipzig Spiritistic Experiments," *British Journal for the History of Science* 34 (2001): 67–79.

53. For the transnational discussion of this possibility, see Henri F. Ellenberger, *The Discovery of the Unconscious: The History and Evolution of Dynamic Psychiatry* (New

York: Basic Books, 1970), pp. 311–14. For the British case, see Oppenheim, *The Other World.*

54. Mitchell G. Ash, epilogue to Woodward and Ash, *Problematic Science,* p. 349.

55. Hermann Schubert, "The Fourth Dimension: Mathematical and Spiritualistic," *Monist* 3, no. 3 (1893): 402.

56. One of the benefits of studying the German occult movement is that it exposes a realm of scientific practice that lies in the neglected territory between two modern disciplines of history: cultural history and history of science. See the suggestive comments by Roger Cooter and Stephen Pumfrey, "Separate Spheres and Public Places: Reflections on the History of Science Popularization and Science in Popular Culture," *History of Science* 32 (September 1994): 248–49.

57. "Psychological modernism" refers to the fin-de-siècle reconceptualization of the human psyche as fragmented into various ill-fitting parts that are driven by arational instincts and desires. Although Freud usually receives the credit for this "discovery," he was but one figure in a trend so large that its limits have yet to be properly established. For useful pointers to this larger history, see the essays in the volume *Modernist Impulses in the Human Sciences, 1870–1930,* ed. Dorothy Ross (Baltimore, MD: Johns Hopkins University Press, 1994), particularly the one by Jan Goldstein on "The Advent of Psychological Modernism in France: An Alternative Narrative," pp. 190–209.

58. William James, also a serious investigator of séance phenomena, made this point about telepathy in 1896; see William James, "The Will to Believe," in *The Will to Believe and Other Essays in Popular Philosophy* (New York: Dover Publications, 1956), p. 10.

59. Although he did not mention occultism, the philosopher Georg Lukács made this point about irrationalism in his famous book *The Destruction of Reason.* Writing in 1952, he identified Germany as the " 'classic' land of irrationalism" in the nineteenth and twentieth centuries and argued that irrationalist philosophies had been crucial in clearing a path for Hitler's rise to power. Historians of German occultism have often followed his line of reasoning: Georg Lukács, *The Destruction of Reason,* trans. Peter Palmer (Atlantic Highlands, NJ: Humanities Press, 1981), pp. 4 and 33.

60. G. L. Mosse, "The Mystical Origins of National Socialism," *Journal of the History of Ideas* 22, no. 1 (1961): 85–88 and 96; for the development of this thesis, see also his *The Crisis of German Ideology: Intellectual Origins of the Third Reich* (New York: Grosset & Dunlap, 1964). Note that although the literature on Nazism and the occult is extensive, most of it is sensationalized and/or unreliable. For two reliable overviews of this literature, see Nicholas Goodrick-Clarke, *The Occult Roots of Nazism: Secret Aryan Cults and their Influence on Nazi Ideology* ([1985] New York: New York University Press, 1992), appendix E; and Stephanie Schnurbein, introduction to *Religion als Kulturkritik: Neugermanisches Heidentum im 20. Jahrhundert* (Heidelberg: Carl Winter Universitätsverlag, 1992).

61. See, for example, Rudolf von Sebottendorf, *Bevor Hitler Kam* (Munich: Grassinger, 1933).

62. This interpretation is developed in the following works as well as in those listed in the notes below: Joachim Besser, "Die Vorgeschichte des Nationalsozialismus in neuem Licht," *Die Pforte: Monatsschrift für Kultur* 2, nos. 21–22 (1950): 763–84; Wilfried

Daim, *Der Mann, der Hitler die Ideen gab: Jörg Lanz von Liebenfels,* 3rd ed. ([1957] Vienna: Ueberreuter, 1994); James Webb, *The Occult Underground* (La Salle, IL: Open Court, 1974) and *The Occult Establishment* (La Salle, IL: Open Court, 1976); Jeffrey A. Goldstein, "On Racism and Anti-Semitism in Occultism and Nazism," *Yad Vashem Studies* 13 (1979): 53–72; and Jackson Spielvogel and David Redles, "Hitler's Racial Ideology: Content and Occult Sources," *Simon Wiesenthal Center Annual* 3 (1986): 227–46. Note that Zöllner appears frequently in the works of this school of interpretation. Searching for the roots of modern anti-Semitism in Germany and Austria, for instance, the historian Peter Pulzer turned his attention in 1964 to contributions made by "the cult of grass roots." Here, anti-Semitism mixed with the return of pagan traditions, resistance to the practices of vaccination and inoculation, and a revival of superstitious beliefs including numerology, spiritualism, and astrology. Pulzer mentioned Zöllner's sittings with Slade and his anti-Semitic outbursts in this connection and also singled out Lanz von Liebenfels as a leader in the project to merge racial and anti-Semitic notions with occult ideas: Pulzer, *The Rise of Political Anti-Semitism,* pp. 65–73.

63. Goodrick-Clarke, *The Occult Roots of Nazism,* p. 1; see also his study of Viennese occultism: Nicholas Goodrick-Clarke, "The Occult Revival in Vienna, 1880–1910," *Durham University Journal* 80–81 (1987): 63–68. Goodrick-Clarke is the former doctoral student of Peter Pulzer.

64. The essays that treat occultism are Ekkehard Hieronimus, "Jörg Lanz von Liebenfels," pp. 131–46; Helmut Zander, "Sozialdarwinistische Rassentheorien aus dem okkulten Untergrund des Kaiserreichs," pp. 224–51; and Justus H. Ulbricht, "Das völk-ischen Verlagswesens im deutschen Kaiserreich," pp. 277–301. All are in the *Handbuch zur "Völkischen Bewegung," 1871–1918,* ed. Uwe Puschner, Walter Schmitz, and Justus H. Ulbricht (Munich: K. G. Saur, 1996). Another reexamination of the connection between the occult and German völkisch circles can be found in Ulrich Linse, *Geisterseher und Wunderwirker: Heilsuche im Industriezeitalter* (Frankfurt am Main: Fischer, 1996).

65. Zander also made a few erroneous claims. First, ignoring the integration of occult phenomena for the first time into academic discourse in the 1920s, he claimed that occultism, especially in the 1920s, was dominated by a decided antiscientific mood that reflected on its isolation from the scientific mainstream. Second, not having defined occultism clearly, he included the *Deutschgläubige Gemeinschaft* in his list of occult groups, without providing any evidence that the group had in fact integrated occult concepts like mediumism, clairvoyance, telepathy, or psychometry into its practice.

66. Although he did not link it directly to Nazism, Theodor Adorno published a scathing study of modern astrology in which he made the pronouncement that "Occultism is the metaphysics of the dopes." He argued that occultism was but one of the many movements of the early twentieth century (along with fascism and psycho-analysis) that helped to undermine the Enlightenment and destroy European civilization; see Theodor Adorno, "Theses against Occultism," *Telos* 19 (spring 1974): 7–12, and "The Stars Down to Earth: The Los Angeles Times Astrology Column," ibid.: 13–90.

67. One line of approach to rethinking the occultism-Nazism connection might be to explore the connections between modern occultism and radical political movements in other European countries.

68. Detlev Peukert, *The Weimar Republic: The Crisis of Classical Modernity,* trans.

Richard Deveson (New York: Hill & Wang, 1989), p. xiii; see also *Zivilisation und Barberei: Die widersprüchlichen Potentiale der Moderne* (Hamburg: Christians, 1991); and the highly influential discussion of the German *Sonderweg* ("special path") interpretation of German history in David Blackbourn and Geoff Eley, *The Peculiarities of German History: Bourgeois Society and Politics in Nineteenth-Century Germany* ([1984] Oxford: Oxford University Press, 1991).

69. This emphasis on the occult as a complex adaptation to modernity also echoes recent work in the non-German context. For the United States, see Ruth Brandon, *The Spiritualists: The Passion for the Occult in the Nineteenth and Twentieth Centuries;* Michael F. Brown, *The Channeling Zone: American Spirituality in an Anxious Age* (Cambridge: Harvard University Press, 1997); *The Occult in America: New Historical Perspectives,* ed. Howard Kerr and Charles L. Crow (Urbana: University of Illinois Press, 1982); and R. Laurence Moore, *In Search of White Crows: Spiritualism, Parapsychology, and American Culture* (New York: Oxford University Press, 1977). For Britain, see Logie Barrow, *Independent Spirits: Spiritualism and English Plebeians, 1850–1910* (London: Routledge & Kegan Paul, 1986); Jenny Hazelgrove, *Spiritualism and British Society between the Wars* (Manchester, Eng.: Manchester University Press, 2000); Janet Oppenheim, *The Other World: Spiritualism and Psychical Research in England, 1850–1914* (Cambridge: Cambridge University Press, 1985); Alex Owen, *The Darkened Room: Women, Power, and Spiritualism in Late Victorian England* (Philadelphia: University of Pennsylvania Press, 1990); and Alison Winter, *Mesmerized: Powers of Mind in Victorian Britain* (Chicago, IL: University of Chicago Press, 1998). For France, see Robert Darnton, *Mesmerism and the End of the Enlightenment in France* (Cambridge: Harvard University Press, 1968); Lynn Sharp, "Spiritual Equality: Spiritism's Challenge to the Second Empire," *Proceedings of the Annual Meeting of the Western Society for French History* (1991): 331–36, and "Women in Spiritism: Using the Beyond to Construct the Here and Now," *Proceedings of the Annual Meeting of the Western Society for French History* (1994): 161–68; and Thomas Kselman, *Death and the Afterlife in Modern France* (Princeton, NJ: Princeton University Press, 1993). For Russia and the Soviet Union, see *The Occult in Russian and Soviet Culture,* ed. Bernice Glatzer Rosenthal (Ithaca, NY: Cornell University Press, 1997). For magic, see Simon During, *Modern Enchantments: The Cultural Power of Secular Magic* (Cambridge: Harvard University Press, 2002).

CHAPTER TWO: A Psychological Point of View

1. Carl Gustav Jung, *Memories, Dreams, Reflections,* ed. Aniela Jaffé, trans. Richard and Clara Winston (New York: Pantheon, 1961), pp. 98–99. Jung's thesis appeared at a spiritualist press under the title *Zur Psychologie und Pathologie sogenannter occulter Phänomene* (Leipzig: O. Mutze, 1902).

2. Ibid., p. 107.

3. Dr. K. Andree, "Geisterklopfen und Tischrücken in den Hansestädten," *Beilage zu Nr. 94 der Allgemeinen Zeitung,* 4 April 1953, pp. 1497–98.

4. Jacques Groll, "Aus der Kinderstube des modernen Spiritismus: Ein Beitrag zur Geschichte des Spiritismus in Deutschland," *Spiritistische Rundschau* 10 (1902–3): 102–6.

5. Karl Kiesewetter, *Geschichte des neueren Occultismus* (Schwarzenburg: Ansata

Verlag, 1977), pp. 460–62; originally published as *Die Geheimwissenschaften: Die Entwicklungsgeschichte des Spiritismus von der Urzeit bis zur Gegenwart* (Leipzig: Wilhelm Friedrich, 1891–95).

6. See, for instance, "Klopfgeister und wandernde Tische," *Beilage zu Nr. 105 der Allgemeinen Zeitung,* 15 April 1853, pp. 1674–75, and "Die Spiritualisten und die Wissenschaft: Tischdrehen. Tischklopfen. Tischschreiben," *Die Gartenlaube: Illustriertes Familienblatt* 2 (1861): 23–25.

7. Rambacher was a *Bußprediger* (preacher of repentance): Annie Francé-Harrar, *So war's um Neunzehnhundert: Mein Fin de Siècle* (Munich: Albert Langen & Georg Müller, 1962), pp. 138–41.

8. Louis Büchner, *Force and Matter: Empirico-Philosophical Studies, Intelligibly Rendered,* ed. J. Frederick Collingwood (London: Trübner, 1864), pp. xviii, 105, and 149; originally published as Ludwig Büchner, *Kraft und Stoff: Empirisch-naturphilosophische Studien in allgemein verständlicher Darstellung* (Frankfurt am Main: Meidinger, 1855).

9. Hannah S. Decker, *Freud in Germany: Revolution and Reaction in Science, 1893–1907* (New York: International University Press, 1977), pp. 54–55.

10. Other proponents had included the doctors Karl Christian Wolfart, Friedrich Hufeland, Eberhard Gmelin, Johann Christian Reil, and C. A. F. Kluge: Henri Ellenberger, *The Discovery of the Unconscious: The History and Evolution of Dynamic Psychiatry* (New York: Basic Books, 1970), pp. 77 and 158–59. For a fuller account, see Wilhelm Erman, *Der tierische Magnetismus in Preussen vor und nach den Freiheitskriegen* (Munich: R. Oldenbourg, 1925). For a useful English summary of the German encounter with mesmerism and animal magnetism, see Ellenberger, *Discovery,* pages cited above, and Alan Gauld, *A History of Hypnotism* (Cambridge: Cambridge University Press, 1992), pp. 78–90, 99–110, and 141–59.

11. Frederick Gregory, *Scientific Materialism in Nineteenth-Century Germany* (Boston, MA: D. Reidel Publishing, 1977), p. 106.

12. Arthur Schopenhauer, "Essay on Spirit Seeing," in *Parerga and Paralipomena: Short Philosophical Essays,* vol. 1, trans. E. F. J. Payne (Oxford, Eng.: Clarendon, 1974), pp. 229 and 268.

13. For a useful study of Schopenhauer and his times, see Rüdiger Safranski, *Schopenhauer and the Wild Years of Philosophy* (Cambridge: Harvard University Press, 1990).

14. For sources on mesmerism and spiritualism in the non-German context, see chapter 1 notes, above.

15. Langsdorff was a follower of the republican Friedrich Hecker. For a biographical sketch, see Gunda Wegner, "Das Leben des Georg von Langsdorff: Turner, Revolutionär und Wissenschaftler," *Zeitschrift des Breisgau-Geschichts Vereins "Schau-ins-Land"* 3 (1992): 79–94.

16. Ulrich Linse, *Geisterseher und Wunderwirker: Heilssuche im Industriezeitalter* (Frankfurt am Main: Fischer Taschenbuch Verlag, 1996), pp. 78–79.

17. Wegner, too, makes this connection between Langsdorff's political, dental, and spiritualist activities: Wegner, "Das Leben des Georg von Langsdorff," pp. 89–92.

18. Nicholas Jardine, "*Naturphilosophie* and the Kingdom of Nature," in *Cultures of Natural History,* ed. Nicholas Jardine, James A. Secord, and Emma C. Spary (Cambridge: Cambridge University Press, 1996), pp. 236–37. Note that Nees von Esenbeck represented Breslau at the Prussian National Assembly in 1848; see Matthew Levinger,

Enlightened Nationalism: The Transformation of Prussian Political Culture, 1806–1848 (New York: Oxford University Press, 2000), pp. 218–19.

19. Kiesewetter, *Geschichte*, pp. 463–64. The club was the *Verein für allseitige Erforschung der Geistfrage*. Wittig also founded another club, the *Verein für harmonische Philosophie*, in 1875. For more on spiritualist activity in Leipzig, see Diethard Sawicki, *Leben mit den Toten: Geisterglauben und die Entstehung des Spiritismus in Deutschland, 1770–1900* (Paderborn: Ferdinand Schöningh, 2002), p. 292.

20. This view received an eloquent proponent in the person of Alexander Aksakow, who published his internationally influential *Animism and Spiritism* in 1890; see Alexander Aksakow, *Animismus und Spiritismus* (Leipzig: O. Mutze, 1890).

21. Kiesewetter, *Geschichte*, pp. 464–66.

22. Dr. Freiherrn v. Schrenck-Notzing, "Albert von Keller als Malerpsychologe und Metapsychiker," *Psychische Studien* 48 (April–May 1921): 194–95; Rudolf Tischner, *Geschichte der okkultistischen (metaphysischen) Forschung, von der Antique bis zur Gegenwart, 2, Von der Mitte des 19. Jahrhunderts bis zur Gegenwart* (Pfullingen in Württemburg: Johannes Baum, 1924), pp. 224–25.

23. Quoted in Büchner, *Force and Matter*, p. 135.

24. "Programm der psychologischen Gesellschaft in München," *Sphinx* 3, 13 (1887): 32–36.

25. For a cultural history of this backlash against materialism, see Christoph Asendorf, *Ströme und Strahlen: Das langsame Verschwinden der Materie um 1900* (Gießen: Anabas, 1989).

26. Carl du Prel, "Übersinnliche Gedankenübertragung," *Sphinx* 5 (1888): 28–31. Albert von Notzing, "Telepathische Experimente," *Sphinx* 4 (1887): 386–88.

27. Siegfried Käss, *Der heimliche Kaiser der Kunst: Adolph Bayersdorfer, seine Freunde und seine Zeit* (Munich: tuduv Verlagsgesellschaft, 1987), pp. 72–74. In addition to du Prel, the group's members included Adolf Bayersdorfer, Heinrich Noë, Robert von Hornstein, and Martin Greif. Later, these men all became prominent in aesthetic circles—Bayersdorfer as an art historian and museum curator, Noë as a writer, Hornstein as a composer, and Greif as a poet.

28. Carl du Prel, *Oneirokritikon, der Traum vom Standpunkt des transzendentalen Idealismus* (Tübingen, 1868); and idem, *Der Kampf ums Dasein am Himmel* (Berlin: Denicke, 1874).

29. Note that du Prel was not alone in raising ethical concerns about materialism. Two others were the science popularizer Wilhelm Bölsche, who also dabbled in occultism, and the neo-Kantian philosopher and socialist Fritz Albert Lange, who did not. For information on Lange, see Thomas E. Willey, *Back to Kant: The Revival of Kantianism in German Social and Historical Thought, 1860–1914* (Detroit, MI: Wayne State University Press, 1978), pp. 87–99.

30. Carl du Prel, *The Philosophy of Mysticism* 1, trans. C. C. Massey (London: George Redway, 1889), pp. 1–7; originally published in German as *Die Philosophie der Mystik* (Leipzig: Ernst Günther, 1885). For du Prel's discussion of Kant, see du Prel, *Philosophie* 1:400. For his usage of terms such as *Bewusstsein,* or *sinnliche Bewusstsein* (waking consciousness) and *Unbewussten,* or *transcendentale Bewusstsein* (the unconscious), see du Prel, *Philosophie* 1:420–21. For his discussion of "Empfindungsschwelle" or barriers of awareness and their relation to Fechner's psychophysics, see du Prel, *Philosophy* 2:136–46. For a useful schematic representation summing up du Prel's views

of human consciousness as Janus faced, see the fold-out page at the back of Carl du Prel, *Das Rätsel der Menschen: Einleitung in das Studium der Geheimwissenschaften* (Leipzig: Philipp Reclam, 1892). Note that "transcendent psychology" comes from du Prel's German term *transcendentale Psychologie.*

31. Du Prel, *Das Rätsel,* pp. 4–5.

32. Ibid., p. 4.

33. Carl Du Prel, "Problem: Medium oder Taschenspieler? Der Stand der Streitfrage," *Sphinx* 1 (1886): 369; see also his popular *Der Spiritismus* (Leipzig: Philipp Reclam, 1893).

34. In Germany, hypnotism had excited some interest in the early 1880s, but mostly among German scientists more involved in academic problems than in psychotherapy. It was not until Schrenck-Notzing, Moll, and Dessoir adapted the work of Charcot and Bernheim in the late 1880s that hypnosis began to attract attention (most of it negative) among German clinicians; see Gauld, *History,* pp. 302–6.

35. Both Moll and Dessoir wrote internationally influential texts on hypnotism. Moll was known for *Der Hypnotismus* (Berlin: Fischer, 1889) while Dessoir became famous for his *Bibliographie des modernen Hypnotismus* (Berlin: C. Dunker, 1888) and *Das Doppel-Ich* (Berlin: K. Siegismund, 1889).

36. Ellenberger, *Discovery,* p. 88. For the larger history of hypnosis, see Ellenberger, *Discovery,* pp. 85–101.

37. G. T. Fechner, *Elemente der Psychophysik* (Leipzig: Breitkopf & Härtl, 1860). For the best overview of the history of this complicated topic, see *The Problematic Science: Psychology in Nineteenth-Century Thought,* ed. W. R. Woodward and M. G. Ash (New York: Prager, 1982). Although they do not discuss occultism explicitly, the following works are useful for situating psychical research in the larger history of German psychology: Mitchell G. Ash, *Gestalt Psychology in German Culture, 1890–1967* (Cambridge: Cambridge University Press, 1995); Joseph Ben-David and Randall Collins, "Social Factors in the Origins of a New Science: The Case of Psychology," *American Sociological Review* 31 (August 1966): 451–65; and Anne Harrington, *Reenchanted Science: Holism in German Culture from Wilhelm II to Hitler* (Princeton, NJ: Princeton University Press, 1996).

38. Albert von Schrenck-Notzing, *Phenomena of Materialization: A Contribution to the Investigation of Mediumistic Teleplastics* (New York: E. P. Dutton, 1920), pp. 2, 12, and 34; originally published as *Materialisationsphaenomene: Ein Beitrag zur Erforschung der mediumistischen Teleplastie* (Munich: E. Reinhardt, 1914).

39. Ellenberger, *Discovery,* pp. 87–88. Schrenck-Notzing's most influential work on this score was *Die Suggestions-Therapie bei krankhaften Erscheinungen des Geschlechtsinnes* (Stuttgart: F. Enke, 1892), in which he discussed sexual impotence (male and female), criticized social mores about extramarital sex, advocated the use of condoms, and displayed for his era a remarkable sensitivity to female sexual experience; Gauld, *History of Hypnotism,* p. 483.

40. Decker, *Freud in Germany,* pp. 124 and 241.

41. An important exception is Ellenberger, *Discovery.* Other preliminary studies include Eberhard Bauer, "Periods of Historical Development of Parapsychology in Germany: An Overview," *Research in Parapsychology, 1991,* ed. E. W. Cook and D. L. Delanoy (Metuchen, NJ: Scarecrow Press, 1994), pp. 123–27; Christian Thiel, "Zur Dynamik von Wissenschaft, Grenzwissenschaften und Pseudowissenschaften in der

Moderne," *Zeitschrift für Parapsychologie und Grenzgebiete der Psychologie* 30 (1988): 152–71; and Barbara Wolf-Braun, " 'The Higher Order of the Natural Laws and the Wrong World of Hysterical Mediums': Medicine and the Occult 'Fringe' at the Turn of the Nineteenth Century in Germany," *Historical Aspects of Unconventional Medicine: Approaches, Concepts, Case Studies,* ed. R. Jütte, M. Eklöf, and M. C. Nelson (Sheffield, Eng.: European Association for the History of Medicine and Health Publications, 2001), pp. 227–45. For the American case, see especially Deborah Coon, "Testing the Limits of Sense and Science: American Experimental Psychologists Combat Spiritualism, 1880–1920," *American Psychologist* 47 (February 1992): 143–51.

42. Ludwig Brunn, "Der Prophet," *Sphinx* 7 (March 1889): 159–66.

43. "Der Fluch der Zeit," *Sphinx* 7 (March 1889): 166–67.

44. Max Dessoir, "Die Parapsychologie," *Sphinx* 8 (June 1889): 341–42; see also Pascal Le Maléfan, "Naissance du parapsychologique chez Max Dessoir, philosophe et médecin, 1867–1947," *Fr'en'esie* 10 (spring 1992), 237–48. Note that Dessoir published extensively on the occult; see especially *Vom Jenseits der Seele: Die Geheimwissenschaften in kritischer Betrachtung* (Stuttgart: Ferdinand Enke, 1917); and the edited volumes *Der Okkultismus in Urkunden* (Berlin: Ullstein, 1925).

45. *Mind* 14, no. 55 (1889): 471. "The Congress of Physiological Psychology at Paris," *Mind* 14 , no. 56 (1889): 614. "Report of the International Congress of Physiological Psychology," *Mind* 16, no. 61 (1891): 157.

46. William Crookes, "Address of the President before the British Association for the Advancement of Science, Bristol, 1898," *Science* 8 (4 November 1898): 610–11.

47. Oppenheim, *The Other World,* p. 245. Gauld, *A History of Hypnotism,* p. 401.

48. Sigmund Freud, *The Interpretation of Dreams,* trans. and ed. James Strachey (New York: Avon, 1965), p. 96. The links between the occult and new trends in the mind/brain sciences were also visible in the path-breaking work of the Swiss psychiatrist Théodore Flournoy. His magisterial *Des Indes à la Planète Mars: Etude sur un cas de somnambulisme avec glossolalie* (From India to the planet Mars: A study of a case of somnambulism, with glossolalia) (1899) recounted his observations of the medium Hélène Smith (Élise-Catherin Müller). Just as Freud insisted on a scientific approach to dreams, Flournoy insisted on such an approach to séance phenomena. Both saw these phenomena as tools for investigating the structure and function of the deep levels of the human psyche. For a recent edition with an excellent introduction, see Théodore Flournoy, *From India to the Planet Mars: A Case of Multiple Personality with Imaginary Languages* (Princeton, NJ : Princeton University Press, 1994).

49. Decker, *Freud in Germany,* p. 68. During this period, Lipps also headed the University of Munich's psychological institute, one of Germany's first such institutes: *Daten zur Geschichte der deutschen Psychologie,* vol. 1, ed. Ulfried Geuter (Göttingen: Verlag für Psychologie, 1986), pp. 71–73.

50. Something similar had happened a few years earlier in England, when the Breuer-Freud studies of hysteria were initially published. They received their first public attention when F. W. H. Myers reviewed them in the *Proceedings of the Society for Psychical Research:* Oppenheim, *The Other World,* p. 245.

51. Decker, *Freud in Germany,* p. 104. Moll was a psychiatrist who specialized in criminology and sexuality. He was also a prominent member of the Bund für Mutterschutz (League for the protection of maternal rights, f. 1905), a sexual-reform group to which Freud, too, belonged. For a biographical sketch of Moll, see Sören Wen-

delborn, "Die Entwicklung der Klinischen Psychologie im Berlin der ausgehenden 19. Jahrhunderts—dargestellt am Beispiel Albert Moll, 1862–1939," *Psychologie und Geschichte* 6 (1994): 303–12.

52. Albert von Schrenck-Notzing, *Die Traumtänzerin Magedeleine G.: Eine psychologische Studie über Hypnose und dramatische Kunst* (Stuttgart: F. Enke, 1904), p. 75.

53. Decker, *Freud in Germany,* pp. 285–86.

54. Ernest Jones, *The Life and Work of Sigmund Freud,* vol. 3 (New York: Basic Books, 1957), pp. 383–85, 389, 397, and 402.

55. Ronald Hayman, *A Life of Jung* (New York: W. W. Norton, 1999), pp. 229 and 258–59.

56. Herbert Spiegelberg, *The Phenomenological Movement: A Historical Introduction,* vol. 2 (The Hague: Martinus Nijhoff, 1960), pp. 169–72 and 193–95; see also Gerda Walther, "A Plea for the Introduction of Edmund Husserl's Phenomenological Method into Parapsychology," *Proceedings of the First International Conference of Parapsychological Studies* (July–August 1953): 114–15.

57. Du Prel, *Das Rätsel,* p. 103.

58. Marshall Bermann, "Why Modernism Still Matters," in *Modernity and Identity,* ed. Scott Lash and Jonathan Friedman (Oxford, Eng.: Blackwell, 1992), p. 33.

59. Gangolf Hübinger, *Kulturprotestantismus und Politik: Zum Verhältnis von Liberalismus und Protestantismus im wilhelminischen Deutschland* (Tübingen: J. C. B. Mohr, 1994), pp. 12–16.

60. Kevin Repp, *Reformers, Critics, and the Paths of German Modernity: Anti-Politics and the Search for Alternatives* (Cambridge: Harvard University Press, 2000), pp. 14, 218–19, and 227.

61. Thomas Rohrkrämer, *Eine andere Moderne? Zivilisationskritik, Natur und Technik in Deutschland, 1880–1933* (Paderborn: Ferdinand Schöningh, 1999), pp. 32–34; see also the critique by Anson Rabinbach in "Eine Andere Moderne? Book Review," *Central European History* 34 (2001): 579–85. For allied varieties of modernism for the Weimar period, see Jeffrey Herf, *Reactionary Modernism: Technology, Culture, and Politics in Weimar and the Third Reich* (Cambridge: Cambridge University Press, 1984).

62. Alex Owen, "Occultism and the 'Modern Self' in Fin-de-siècle Britain," in *Meanings of Modernity: Britain from the Late Victorian Era to World War II,* ed. M. Daunton and B. Rieger (New York: Berg, 2001), p. 88.

63. Alfred Russel Wallace, "Wissenschaftliche und übersinnliche Anschauungen, ein Nachweis ihrer Übereinstimmung," *Sphinx* 1 (1886): 85–94. Adolf Bastian, "Spiritismus und Ethnologie," *Sphinx* 3 (1887): 87–90. Eduard von Hartmann, "Die 'Grenzen der Philosophie': Eine Entgegnung auf Freiherrn Dr. von Goelers Aufsatz," *Sphinx* 5 (1888): 265–66.

64. The original title was *Sphinx: Monatsschrift für die geschichtliche und experimentale Begründung der übersinnlichen Weltanschauung auf monistischer Grundlage.*

65. The title was *Metaphysische Rundschau: Monatsschrift zum Studium der praktischen Metaphysik, Psychologie, orientalischen Philosophie und des gesamten Okkultismus* (1896–97); it then became *Neue Metaphysische Rundschau: Monatsschrift für philosophische, psychologische und okkulte Forschungen in welcher enthalten ist Archiv für animalischen (Heil-)Magnetismus, Astrologische Rundschau; Rundschau für Phrenologie und Theosophie.*

66. *Fünfzehn Jahre Metaphysische Rundschau,* p. 10; available at JFC. For further discussion of Guido von List and Ariosophy, see chapter 4.

67. *Neue Metaphysische Rundschau* 1, nos. 1–2 (1897).

68. *Fünfzehn Jahre Metaphysische Rundschau,* pp. 16–28.

69. *Neue Metaphysische Rundschau* 1 (1897–98).

70. *Fünfzehn Jahre Metaphysische Rundschau* (1912), p. 7.

71. Paul Zillmann, "Briefe über Mystik an einen Freund," *Neue Metaphysische Rundschau* 1, nos. 3–7 (1897–98): 197–99. For the full cycle of letters, see pp. 196–201, 229–31, 328–32, and 397–99.

72. E. Honold, *Memoiren einer Spiritisten: Erlebte Wahrheiten gesammelt in 15jährigen okkultem Studium,* 4th–5th ed. (Berlin: Prana, n.d.), pp. 5, 11, 62–64, 69, 74, 78–84; available at JFC.

CHAPTER THREE: The Occult Public

1. For a discussion of "esoteric culture" and its connections to occultism, see Edward A. Tiryakian, "Toward the Sociology of Esoteric Culture," *American Journal of Sociology* 78, no. 3 (1972): 491–512.

2. Theodor Traub, "Der Spiritismus," in *Kirchen und Sekten der Gegenwart,* ed. Ernst Kalb (Stuttgart: Verlag der Buchhandlung der Evang. Gesellschaft, 1905), p. 414.

3. *Reichsbote* 278 (27 November 1901), Sign. 7/3946, EZB.

4. " 'Wie stehts mit dem Spiritismus?' Glossen zum Skandal Rothe Sellin," *Reichsbote,* 25 March 1902, Sign. 7/3946, EZB.

5. Wilhelm Kaesen, "Spiritismus," *Theol. prakt. Quartalschrift* 1 (1923): 35.

6. Report from Alfred Weiml to the Diakonisches Werk on 12 March 1929, CA AC-S 273, ADW.

7. "Schicksal und Willensfreiheit," *Münchner Neueste Nachrichten* 167, 22 June 1927, ZA Astrologie, SdArMü.

8. "Sensationshoroskope und ihre Erklärung," *Völkischer Beobachter* 242, 20 October 1927, ZA Astrologie, SdArMü.

9. James Webb, *The Occult Establishment* (La Salle, IL: Open Court, 1976), pp. 55–61.

10. Ulrich Linse, *Geisterseher und Wunderwirker: Heilssuche im Industriezeitalter* (Frankfurt am Main: Fischer, 1996), pp. 93, 98, and 119.

11. Klaus-Maria Brandauer and István Szábo, *Hanussen* (Objektív FilmStúdió, 1989). For more on Hanussen, see chapter 9.

12. Carl Zuckmayer, *A Part of Myself,* trans. Richard and Clara Winston (New York: Harcourt Brace Jovanovich, 1966), pp. 164–65.

13. Verein Freibund, PDM 576, StArMü.

14. Franz Heigl, "Überwachung (19 May 1917)," p. 1, and Franz Heigl, "Abschrift (26 Mai 1917)," PDM 576, StArMü.

15. "Therese (Claire) Reichart vor Gericht," *Münchner Neueste Nachrichten* 99, 10 April 1926), p. 7; see also Elisabeth von Zech, *Die Hellseherin Claire Reichert* (Munich: H. Frambold, n.d.). Reichart's background in theater is something she shared with many other men and women who managed to earn a living in the occult revival (among the ones mentioned in this chapter are the clairvoyant Erik Jan Hanussen, who

was the son of actors, Hanna Vogt-Vilseck, and the astrologer Karl Brandler-Pracht). For biographical information on Brandler-Pracht, see Ellic Howe, *Astrology and the Third Reich* (Wellingborough, Northants.: Aquarian Press, 1984), p. 81.

16. "Der Anfang des Wahrsagens: 300 amtsbekannte Wahrsager," *Grossdeutsche Zeitung* 73, 28 April 1924, ZA Aberglaube, SdArMü.

17. Harry Price, *Rudi Schneider: A Scientific Examination of his Mediumship* (London: Methuen, 1930), p. viii.

18. Howe, *Astrology*, p. 98. This trio demonstrates the complexity of occult sociability and the need to be careful in linking occultism to Nazism. Edgar Daqué was one of the writers whose nature mysticism inspired Adolf Hitler; Theodor Lessing was a Jewish philosopher with idealist tendencies; Johannes Maria Verweyen converted from monism to occultism to Roman Catholicism and then joined the anti-Nazi resistance before dying as a political prisoner in a concentration camp (see chapter 9). For Daqué, see George Mosse, *The Crisis of German Ideology: Intellectual Origins of the Third Reich* (New York: Grosset & Dunlap, 1964), p. 306.

19. Howe, *Astrology*, p. 80.

20. "Hartmann, Franz," *Biogr. Jahrbuch u. Deutscher Nekrolog* 18 (1913); reprinted in *Deutscher Biographischer Index*, ed. Willi Gorzny (Munich, 1986).

21. See, for example, "Satzungen der Occultistischen Gesellschaft e.V. München," PDM 5610, StArMü.

22. One of these women was the writer Emilie Mataja: Max Dessoir, *Buch der Erinnerung*, 2nd ed. (Stuttgart: Ferdinand Enke, 1947), pp. 116–37.

23. Agathe Haemmerle, "The German Theosophical Society," Cod WH-S 812: 2,1.

24. PDM 3543, StArMü.

25. Ref. Ia Dst. 20. München, den 7.5.32, PDM 7114, StArMü.

26. "Sensationshoroskope und ihre Erklärung."

27. "Überwachung eines Vortrages über Astrologie im Hotel Senefelder-Hof," PDM 7114, StArMü.

28. These difficulties arise because bourgeois women typically acted as mediums on a private and informal basis and were rarely identified by name in the reports written about them. In addition, because of their class background, they probably did not need or even want to give séances for money. Such women would not have featured as suspects in police files or as defendants in the spectacular court cases involving their lower-class colleagues, the sources from which my sample of mediums has largely been derived.

29. For information on Guipet and Gumppenberg, see chapter 5.

30. "Albert Freiherr von Schrenck-Notzing," *Jahrbuch der Millionäre i. Bayern* (Berlin, 1914) and "Dr. Frhr. v. Schrenck-Notzing," *Münchner Augsburger Abendzeitung* 44 (14 February 1929), ZA Personen Schrenck-Notzing, Albert, SdArMü. Siegle's father was Gustav Siegle, a National Liberal who represented Stuttgart at the Reichstag: Barbara Wolf-Braun, "'The Higher Order of the Natural Laws and the Wrong World of Hysterical Mediums': Medicine and the Occult 'Fringe' at the Turn of the Nineteenth Century in Germany," *Historical Aspects of Unconventional Medicine: Approaches, Concepts, Case Studies*, ed. R. Jütte, M. Eklöf, and M. C. Nelson (Sheffield, Yorks.: European Association for the History of Medicine and Health Publications, 2001), p. 245.

31. Dessoir, *Buch der Erinnerung*, p. 130.

32. Albert Moll, *Ein Leben als Arzt der Seele: Erinnerungen* (Dresden: Carl Reissner,

1936), pp. 99–101. Moltke shared her spiritualist leanings with her husband Helmuth, a German general, who faithfully followed his wife into Theosophy and, eventually, Anthroposophy; see also *Light for the New Millennium: Rudolf Steiner's Association with Helmuth and Eliza von Moltke: Letters, Documents, and After-Death Communications,* ed. T. H. Meyer (London: Rudolf Steiner Press, 1997).

33. Dessoir, *Buch der Erinnerung,* pp. 116–37. The connection between Spreti and Hartmann is noted in Norbert Klatt, *Der Nachlaß von Wilhelm Hübbe-Schleiden* (Göttingen: Klatt, 1996), p. 266. These three women had close family connections to male leaders in the occult movement, a fact suggesting that occultism also spread along family lines: Albertine du Prel and Emma von Max were married to Carl and Gabriel, respectively; Spreti was the sister of Franz Hartmann.

34. Isabel Hull, *The Entourage of Kaiser Wilhelm II, 1888–1918* (Cambridge: Cambridge University Press, 1982), pp. 72–73. John C. G. Röhl, *The Kaiser and His Court: Wilhelm II and the Government of Germany* (Cambridge: Cambridge University Press, 1987), p. 66. Röhl also discusses this material in *Young Wilhelm: The Kaiser's Early Life, 1859–1888,* trans. Jeremy Gaines and Rebecca Wallach (Cambridge: Cambridge University Press, 1998), pp. 714–17.

In the Kaiserreich, charges surfaced repeatedly that Eulenburg used spiritualism to manipulate the Kaiser over political issues. Usually, this came with innuendo about homosexual currents in the Liebenberg Circle. This occurred in the *Kladderadatsch* campaign in 1894 and in the trials pitting the journalist Maximilian Harden against Moltke and Eulenburg in 1907–9, which climaxed with the *Daily Telegraph* affair in 1908 and led to Eulenburg's fall; see Hull, *The Entourage,* pp. 68–73. Historians have differed in their assessment of how seriously to take the influence on Wilhelm II of Eulenburg's spiritualist commitments. Isabel Hull concludes that the charges were overblown, that Eulenburg had never done more than entertain his friend with spiritualist stories, and had ceased to do even this much by 1890. John Röhl, in contrast, presents spiritualism as a significant element in the friendship in the years just before and after Wilhelm's accession to the throne in 1888. Hull has the more convincing case. Spiritualism seems to have been one topic among many in the friendship between the two men, but there is no evidence to suggest that Wilhelm II ever had any serious interest in séances or related occult practices.

35. Röhl, *The Kaiser,* p. 66.

36. *Reichsbote* 198 (23 August 1901), and *Reichsbote* 278 (26 November 1901), Sign. 7/3946, EZB.

37. Annie Francé-Harrar, *So war's um Neunzehnhundert: Mein Fin de Siècle* (Munich-Vienna: Albert Langen-Georg Müller, 1962), pp. 42–47.

38. Nicolas Goodrick-Clarke, *The Occult Roots of Nazism: The Ariosophists of Austria and Germany, 1890–1935* (Wellingborough, Northants.: Aquarian Press, 1985), pp. 135–52.

39. *Zeitschrift für Seelenleben* 31, no. 14 (1927): cover.

40. Max Gubalke, *Bericht über die Verhandlungen auf dem Dritten Congress des "Verbandes Deutscher Okkultisten" am 31. Mai und 1. Juni (Pfingsten) 1898 in München* (Selbstverlag), pp. 3–13.

41. This was "Bis hierher hat mich Gott geführt" in "Bericht über die Tätigkeit des Bundes für Seelenkultur, Schutzverband deutscher Okkultisten, auf die Zeit vom Juli 1925 bis April 1927," *Okkultistische Rundschau* 22, no. 7 (July 1927): 124.

42. Moll, *Ein Leben,* pp. 94–97.

43. In one of the inversions that occultism permitted its adherents, the lower-class background and national origins of these mediums probably helped them to succeed in convincing their higher-class employers and patrons of their occult abilities, which were often seen as vestiges of an earlier stage of human evolution. Mediums also came from northern European countries, but not in such large numbers.

44. Eberhard Buchner, *Sekten und Sektierer in Berlin* (Berlin: Verlag von Hermann Seeman, c. 1904), pp. 78–90.

45. Egbert Falk, *Sonnenkinder: Ist Nacktheit Sünde? Ein Kulturroman aus dem Anfang des zwangzigsten Jahrhunderts,* 2nd ed. (Berlin: Otto Mieth Verlag, 1924), pp. 112–13; available at JFC.

46. Rolf Koerber, "Freikörperkultur," *Handbuch der deutschen Reformbewegungen, 1880–1933,* ed. Diethart Kerbs and Jürgen Reulecke (Wuppertal: Hammer, 1998), p. 106.

47. Gustav Meyrink, *An der Grenze des Jenseits* (Leipzig: Dürr & Weber, 1923); see also E. F. Bleiler's introduction to Gustav Meyrink, *The Golem* (New York: Dover, 1976).

48. Gunda Wegner, "Das Leben des Georg von Langsdorff: Turner, Revolutionär, und Wissenschaftler," *Zeitschrift des Breisgau-Geschichts Vereins "Schau-ins-Land"* 3 (1992): 79–94; see also Linse, *Geisterseher und Wunderwirker,* pp. 78–79.

49. Gottfried Kratt, "Erinnerungen an Dr. Carl Freiherr du Prel," *Zentralblatt für Okkultismus* 5, no. 1 (1911): 31.

50. E. Honold, *Memoiren einer Spiritisten: Erlebte Wahrheiten gesammelt in 15 jährigen okkultem Studium,* 4th–5th ed. (Berlin: Prana Verlag, n.d.); available at JFC.

51. Dr. Egbert Müller, *Stellung des Strafrichters zum Spiritismus und der Proceß Valeska Töpfer* (Berlin: I. F. Conrads Buchhandlung [Paul Ackermann], 1892).

52. *Magische Unterweisungen des edlen und hochgelehrten Philosophi und Medici Philippi Theophrasti Bombasti von Hohenheim Paracelsus genannt* (Leipzig: Im Wolkenwanderer Verlag, 1923).

53. The press flourished under the joint directorship of Oswald Mutze and his brother Victor: *Lexikon der deutschen Verlage: Eine Chronik der deutschen Verlagsfirmen, enthaltend die Geschichte der Zeitungs-, Zeitschriften und Buchverlage, der Kunst- und Musikverlage, sowie der Katalogantiquare* (Leipzig: Verlag Curt Müller, 1930), p. 188; see also Ulrich Linse, " 'Das Buch der Wunder und Geheimwissenschaften': Der spiritistische Verlag Oswald Mutze in Leipzig im Rahmen der spiritistischen Bewegung Sachsens," in *Das bewegte Buch: Buchwesen und soziale, nationale und kulturelle Bewegungen um 1900,* ed. Mark Lehmstedt and Andreas Herzog (Wiesbaden: Harrassowitz, 1999), pp. 219–44.

54. See, for instance, A. Aksakov, *Animismus und Spiritismus* (Leipzig: O. Mutze, 1890); William Crookes, *Der Spiritualismus und die Wissenschaft* (Leipzig: O. Mutze, 1898); A. J. Davis, *Der Zauber-Stab* (Leipzig: O. Mutze, 1874), and Allan Kardec, *Das Buch der Medien* (Leipzig: O. Mutze). For a partial list of the Mutze offerings in the early years of the occult movement, see the back cover of *Sphinx* 2 (1886).

55. Carl Gustav Jung, *Zur Psychologie und Pathologie sogenannter occulter Phänomene* (Leipzig: O. Mutze, 1902); see also Richard Noll, *The Jung Cult: Origins of a Charismatic Movement* (Princeton, NJ: Princeton University Press, 1994), p. 144.

56. Daniel Paul Schreber, *Denkwürdigkeiten eines Nervenkranken* (Leipzig: O. Mutze, 1903). Schreber's memoir also attracted the attention of Elias Canetti, who devoted two chapters of *Crowds and Power* to the case, and Walter Benjamin, who

published an account of it in *Die literarische Welt* (July 1928). See the comments of Samuel M. Weber in his introduction to Daniel Paul Schreber, *Memoirs of My Nervous Illness* (Cambridge: Harvard University Press, 1988), pp. xii–xiii.

57. Manfred Hellge, *Der Verleger Wilhelm Friedrich und das "Magazin für die Literatur des In-und Auslandes": Ein Beitrag zur Literatur-und Verlagsgeschichte des frühen Naturalismus in Deutschland* (Frankfurt: Buchhändler-Vereinigung GmbH, 1976), pp. 826 and 841–47.

58. See Franz Hartmann, *Grundriss der Lehren des Theophrastus Paracelsus von Hohenheim von religionswissenschaftlichen Standpunkt betrachtet* (Leipzig: Wilhelm Friedrich, 1898); Karl Kiesewetter, *Die Geheimwissenschaften: Die Entwicklungsgeschichte des Spiritismus von der Urzeit bis zur Gegenwart* (Leipzig: Wilhelm Friedrich, 1891–95); and Carl du Prel, *Experimentalpsychologie und Experimentalmetaphysik* (Leipzig: Wilhelm Friedrich, 1891).

59. For a general discussion of Lebensreform, see Wolfgang Krabbe, *Gesellschaftsveränderung durch Lebensreform* (Göttingen: Vanderhoeck & Ruprecht, 1974). Also see chapter 6.

60. Note that Ferdinand Spohr, the brother of Max Spohr, also ran a Lebensreform press (Verlag Wahrheit) that published a similar mix of titles: *Lexikon*, pp. 191 and 194.

61. Hirschfeld belonged to an international group of sexologists whose members included Richard von Krafft-Ebing, August Forel, Havelock Ellis, Iwan Bloch, and Albert Moll (also involved in Berlin psychical-research circles): Ulrich Linse, "Sexualreform und Sexualberatung," in *Handbuch der deutschen Reformbewegungen, 1880–1933*, ed. D. Kerbs and J. Reulecke (Wuppertal: Hammer, 1998), pp. 211–26.

62. Hans Arnold, *Wie errichtet und leitet man spiritistische Zirkel in der Familie: Ein Leitfaden für die selbständige Prüfung der mediumistischen Phänomen*, 2nd ed. (Leipzig: M. Spohr, 1894).

63. Hellge, *Der Verleger Wilhelm Friedrich*, p. 855.

64. Among these were Friedrich Graf zu Egloffstein, *Wiedergeburtslehre, Sonnenreligion, und Christentum* (1916), and G. Herman (Max Ferdinand Sebaldt), *Sexual-Magie*, 3 vols. (1905). These works are mentioned in Justus H. Ulbricht, "Das völkische Verlagswesen im deutschen Kaiserreich," *Handbuch zur "Völkischen Bewegung," 1871–1918*, ed. Uwe Puschner, Walter Schmitz, and Justus H. Ulbricht (Munich: K. G. Saur, 1996), p. 280.

65. Ulbricht, "Das völkische Verlagswesen," pp. 291–92.

66. Herbert Reichstein, *Die Mystik der Namen*, 4th ed. (Berlin: Herbert Reichstein, 1935), p. 270; available at JFC.

67. Helmut Zander cautions against this in "Sozialdarwinistische Rassentheorien aus dem okkulten Untergrund des Kaiserreichs," in *Handbuch zur "Völkischen Bewegung,"* pp. 237–40.

68. Stark portrays Diederichs as an antimodernist in the völkisch mode: Gary Stark, *Entrepreneurs of Ideology: Neoconservative Publishers in Germany, 1890–1933* (Chapel Hill: University of North Carolina Press, 1981), pp. 74, 90, and 92. For a useful corrective, see Gangolf Hübinger, "Der Verlag Eugen Diederichs in Jena: Wissenschaftskritik, Lebensreform, und völklische Bewegung," *Geschichte und Gesellschaft* 22 (1996): 31–45.

69. *Fünfzehn Jahre Metaphysische Rundschau* (1912); available at JFC.

70. Stark, *Entrepreneurs of Ideology*, p. 249.

71. *Haupt-Katalog, 1922*, pp. vii, 77, and 161; available at JFC.

72. *Haupt-Katalog, 1922*, pp. v–vi.

73. The mail-order catalog was an excellent example of the new commercial outlets that were then proliferating in Germany. Another was the department store. See Peter Stearns, "Stages of Consumerism: Recent Works on Issues of Periodization," *Journal of Modern History* 69, no. 1 (1997): 109–10.

74. *Katalog zur Leihbibliothek* (Berlin: Nirwana-Verlag für Lebensreform, 1925); available at JFC.

75. Dr. med. Gustav Riedlin, *Der Vegetarismus im Lichte der Theosophie* (Freiburg: Verlag Fr. Paul Lorenz, n.d.); available at JFC.

76. The psychical researcher Rudolf Tischner gave an introduction to occult phenomena; the occultist G. W. Surya and the writer Max Kemmerich spoke on spontaneous occult phenomena; further offerings included a course on experimental occultism, a history of occultism in two parts, and an introduction to philosophy. *Studienkurse für Okkultismus: Semester 1923/4*, PDM 5608, StArMü.

77. Heinz Artur Strauß, "Astrologie: Was sie uns heute bedeuten kann: Zum Kursus in der Münchner Volkshochschule," *Münchner Neueste Nachrichten*, 21 November 1930, ZA Astrologie, SdArMü.

78. "Astrologische Ausstellung in München," *Bayerische Staatszeitung* 240, 16 October 1932, ZA Astrologie, SdArMü.

79. Howe, *Astrology*, pp. 114–15: Bert van Solden, *Das astrologische Examen: Band 1, Die mündliche Prüfung* (Memmingen: Uranus-Verlag, 1937).

80. "Preisverzeichnis (Rudolf Sagittarius, Institut für wissenschaftliche Astrologie und Graphologie, Kiel)," CA AC-S 25, ADW.

81. Police report by Johann Knockl on 10 June 1924, PDM 7106, StArMü. Further examples can be found in PDM 7105 and 7111, StArMü. See chapters 7 through 9 for a fuller discussion of how the occult was policed.

82. Abschrift aus Fischers Zeitschrift für Verwaltungsrecht Bd. 60 s. 109 fl., PDM 7111, StArMü.

83. Howe, *Astrology*, p. 105. Howe takes this from Herbert von Klöckler, *Sterne und Mensch*.

84. Reports on Georg Schwab, PDM 7106, StArMü.

85. Carl Christian Bry, *Verkappte Religionen* (Gotha: Verlag Friedrich Andreas Perthes, 1924), pp. 231–32. In the last stanza, "a Waldorf" is a reference to the Waldorf schools, founded by Rudolf Steiner to provide an alternative educational environment for grade-school children. These schools still exist worldwide.

86. For modern consumerism, which took shape in the late nineteenth and early twentieth centuries, see the excellent discussion by Stearns, "Stages of Consumerism." Modern consumerism entailed a wider breadth of goods (for instance, new reading matter produced by the mass press, commercialized leisure forms typified by multiplication of seaside resorts, and novel objects like the immensely popular bicycle) catered not just to the domestic needs of the family but to the new thirst for information, travel, and leisure. It also entailed a dramatic change in the type of commercial outlets available. Department stores and mail-order businesses proliferated, and advertising shifted its focus from goods as useful or cheap to goods as satisfying, comfortable, stylish, and sensual—in short, personally gratifying. For a suggestive look at the American context, see T. J. Jackson Lears, "From Salvation to Self-Realization: Adver-

tising and the Therapeutic Roots of the Consumer Culture, 1880–1930," in *The Culture of Consumption: Critical Essays in American History, 1880–1980*, ed. R. W. Fox and T. J. Jackson Lears (New York: Pantheon, 1983), pp. 3–37.

C H A P T E R   F O U R : Varieties of Theosophical Experience

1. The scandal was caused by the Hodgson Report of 1885. The report was the result of an investigation carried out by Richard Hodgson on behalf of the British Society for Psychical Research into allegations of fraud at the Theosophical headquarters in Adyar. Among other items, Hodgson reported finding a shrine with a removable back wall through which the so-called Mahatma letters were supposedly delivered: Janet Oppenheim, *The Other World: Spiritualism and Psychical Research in England, 1850–1914* (Cambridge: Cambridge University Press, 1985), pp. 175–78.

2. Cod WH-S 807.

3. Kuhlenbeck was later recruited by Heinrich Class for the Pan-German League. George Mosse, *The Crisis of German Ideology: Intellectual Origins of the Third Reich* (New York: Grosset & Dunlap, 1964), pp. 222–23.

4. Fritz Stern, *The Politics of Cultural Despair: A Study in the Rise of the Germanic Ideology* (Berkeley: University of California Press, 1961), pp. 3–94. Note also that although the early issues of *Sphinx* carried articles by Kuhlenbeck, the editorial board apparently never succeeded in recruiting Tolstoi, Lagarde, or Eisner to write for the journal.

5. A similar point could be made about the repackaging of traditional Christian ideas in this reform context; see Justus H. Ulbricht, "Der 'neue Mensch' auf der Suche nach 'neuer Religiosität': Ästhetisch-religiöse Sinnsuche um 1900," *Deutschunterricht* 51 (1998): 38–49.

6. Joy Dixon makes a similar case for British Theosophy in *Divine Feminine: Theosophy and Feminism in England* (Baltimore, MD: Johns Hopkins University Press, 2001), chapter 5.

7. For a recent review of German liberalism, see Dieter Langewiesche, "The Nature of German Liberalism," in *Modern Germany Reconsidered*, ed. Gordon Martel (London: Routledge, 1992), pp. 96–116; and his *Liberalism in Germany* (Princeton, NJ: Princeton University Press, 2000), originally published as *Liberalismus in Deutschland* (Frankfurt: Suhrkamp, 1988). Also useful is the classic by James Sheehan, *German Liberalism in the Nineteenth Century* (Chicago, IL: University of Chicago Press, 1978). For an in-depth discussion of German liberalism as well as its "failures" and its European context, see David Blackbourn and Geoff Eley, *The Peculiarities of German History: Bourgeois Society and Politics in Nineteenth-Century Germany* (Oxford: Oxford University Press, 1984).

8. Several books have been published on particular aspects of the international Theosophical movement, but none offers a thorough overview. For the most complete narrative history to date, see Bruce F. Campbell, *Ancient Wisdom Revived: A History of the Theosophical Movement* (Berkeley: University of California Press, 1980). For a speculative examination of Blavatsky's sources, see K. Paul Johnson, *The Masters Revealed: Madame Blavatsky and the Myth of the Great White Lodge* (New York: State University of New York Press, 1994). Also useful is Joscelyn Godwin, *The Theosophical Enlightenment* (Albany: State University of New York Press, 1994). For a histori-

cal treatment of the Theosophical movement in Russian culture, see Maria Carlson, *"No Religion Higher Than Truth": A History of the Theosophical Movement in Russia, 1875–1922* (Princeton, NJ: Princeton University Press, 1993). For a historical treatment of the British case, see Dixon, *Divine Feminine.* No history of German Theosophy exists, but useful information can be found in the following books: H. R. Fischer, *100 Jahre "Theosophische Gesellschaft": Ein geschichtlicher Überblick* (Calw/Württemburg: Schatzkammerverlag Hans Fändrich, n.d.); Norbert Klatt, *Theosophie und Anthroposophie: Neue Aspekte zu ihrer Geschichte aus dem Nachlaß von Wilhelm Hübbe-Schleiden (1846–1916) mit einer Auswahl von 81 Briefen* (Göttingen: Klatt, 1993); Norbert Klatt, *Der Nachlaß von Wilhelm Hübbe-Schleiden in der Niedersächsischen Staats-und Universitätsbibliothek Göttingen. Verzeichnis der Materialien und Korrespondenten mit bio-bibliographischen Angaben* (Göttingen: Klatt, 1996); and Helmut Zander, *Geschichte der Seelenwanderung in Europa: Alternative religiöse Traditionen von der Antike bis heute* (Darmstadt: Wissenschaftliche Buchgesellschaft, 1999), chapter 42.

9. Dixon, *Divine Feminine,* p. 149.

10. The strange notion of a "universal brotherhood" composed of individuals accepted without regard to sex has yet to be fully explored by historians; see Robert S. Ellwood and Catherine Wessinger, "The Feminism of 'Universal Brotherhood': Women in the Theosophical Movement," in *Women's Leadership in Marginal Religions: Explorations Outside the Mainstream,* ed. Catherine Wessinger (Urbana: University of Illinois Press, 1993), pp. 68–87. For comments by a contemporary, see Julius Duboc, "Weibliche Philosophie," *Die Zukunft* 34 (2 March 1901): 366–73.

11. For the clearest explanation of Theosophical doctrine to date, see Carlson, *No Religion,* chapter 5.

12. This was Matthias Jakob Schleiden, a botanist whose work on the cell and its nucleus became a major stimulus to microscopal investigation and modern cellular biology.

13. For Hübbe-Schleiden's work for Fabri, see Klaus J. Bade, *Friedrich Fabri und der Imperialismus in der Bismarckzeit: Revolution-Depression-Expansion* (Freiburg im Breisgau: Atlantis Verlag, 1975), p. 14.

14. Klatt, *Theosophie,* pp. 14–25.

15. Hans-Ulrich Wehler, *Bismarck und der Imperialismus* (Cologne: Kiepenheuer & Witsch, 1969), pp. 121 and 144–47.

16. Woodruff Smith, *The Ideological Origins of Nazi Imperialism* (New York: Oxford University Press, 1986), p. 146, and "The Ideology of German Colonialism, 1840–1906," *Journal of Modern History* 46 (December 1974): 651.

17. Klatt, *Theosophie,* pp. 204–5.

18. Wilhelm Hübbe-Schleiden, "Weltpolitik: Neue Weltkultur, Weltreligion, Weltrasse: Das Programm der Theosophischen Bewegung. Vortrag gehalten zum 30. Jahrestage in Deutschland zu Berlin um Pfingsten 1914," pp. 8–14, Cod WH-S 416:1–2.

19. Wilhelm Hübbe-Schleiden, personal journal, pp. 5–7, Cod WH-S 1012:1. Some of this is also reprinted in Klatt, *Theosophie,* p. 17.

20. William James, *The Varieties of Religious Experience* (New York: Penguin, 1958), p. 24.

21. For an account of the founding of this group, see Emil Bock, *Rudolf Steiner: Studien zu seinem Lebensgang und Lebenswerk* (Stuttgart: Verlag Freies Geistesleben, 1961), p. 177.

22. One exception to this was Hübbe-Schleiden's participation in the founding

conference of the colonialist group *Alldeutsche Verband* in Berlin in 1891. *Handbuch zur "Völkischen Bewegung," 1871–1918*, ed. Uwe Puschner, Walter Schmitz, and Justus H. Ulbricht (Munich: K. G. Saur, 1996), p. 303.

23. Wilhelm Hübbe-Schleiden, "Psychometrisches Experimente," *Sphinx* 5, no. 27 (1888): 156–59.

24. Klatt, *Theosophie*, p. 260. Hübbe-Schleiden was not the only colonialist who "converted" to other reformist causes. Ernst von Weber, for instance, had also been a high-profile propagandist for German colonies in the early years of the Kaiserreich and joined the new German Theosophical Society in 1884. He left the group in 1886, but then devoted himself to yet another reformist circle in Bayreuth that had grown up around the composer Richard Wagner. For a list of members, see "Mitglieder Verzeichnis der Theosophischen Societät Germania," Cod WH-S 812: 2, 1.

25. Wilhelm Hübbe-Schleiden, "Address of the German Branch to the President of the Theosophical Society" (November 1884), Cod WH-S 812: 2, 1.

26. Wilhelm Hübbe-Schleiden, "Aufruf und Vorwort," *Sphinx* (1886): iv.

27. His comment may have referred more specifically to the antisocialist laws then in force in Germany.

28. Smith, *Ideological Origins*, p. 33.

29. Hübbe-Schleiden, "Weltpolitik," pp. 33–35.

30. Klatt, *Theosophie*, p. 16.

31. Smith, *Ideological Origins*, p. 52.

32. See especially Geoff Eley's argument that social imperialism was never the exclusive preserve of German conservatism and that it appealed also to liberals aiming not to prevent but to promote social reform: Geoff Eley, "Social Imperialism in Germany: Reformist Synthesis or Reactionary Sleight of Hand?" *From Unification to Nazism: Reinterpreting the German Past* (Boston: Unwin Hyman, 1986), chapter 6. Also valuable on liberalism and Weltpolitik is Langewiesche, *Liberalism in Germany*, pp. 236–39.

33. Hübbe-Schleiden, "Weltpolitik," pp. 8–14.

34. Klatt, *Theosophie*, p. 204.

35. Bock, *Rudolf Steiner*, p. 179.

36. Hübbe-Schleiden, "Weltpolitik," p. 39.

37. Bock, *Rudolf Steiner*, p. 175.

38. For Hübbe-Schleiden on Africans, see Klatt, *Theosophie*, pp. 15–16.

39. Klatt, *Der Nachlaß*, p. 183; see also the letter on Lauweriks's election from L. Fuhrmann and J. Zech, Cod WH-S 801.

40. Letter from Hübbe-Schleiden (November 1914), Cod WH-S 801. Wilhelm Hübbe-Schleiden to Annie Besant on 19 December 1915, in Klatt, *Theosophie*, pp. 262–63. This was not to say, of course, that Hübbe-Schleiden was immune to national pride. In a letter written to the British Theosophical leader Annie Besant in December 1915, he called Emperor Wilhelm II a man of peace and condemned England as an aggressor nation. But in the end, Hübbe-Schleiden's nationalism was lukewarm, a product more of external circumstance than internal conviction—so much so that he could acknowledge the parallels between German Theosophy and that other great movement dedicated to universal brotherhood, Social Democracy. Adherents of both movements, Hübbe-Schleiden noted mournfully in the fall of 1914, had more friends outside than inside Germany and harbored deep misgivings about supporting the start of military hostilities: Hübbe-Schleiden, "Wir Theosophen," Cod WH-S 921.

41. Hermann Keyserling, *The Travel Diary of a Philosopher*, vol. 1, trans. J. Holroyd

Reece (New York: Harcourt, Brace, 1925), p. 158; originally published as *Das Reisetage-buch eines Philosophen* (Darmstadt: O. Reichl, 1919).

42. Franz Hartmann, *Denkwürdige Erinnerungen aus dem Leben des Verfassers der "Lotusblüten": Mit besonderer Berücksichtigung der Geschichte der theosophischen Bewegung* 1 (Calw, Württemberg: Schatzkammerverlag Hans Fändrich, n.d.), p. 9. This is also recorded in Franz Hartmann, "Autobiography of Franz Hartmann," *Occult Review* 7, no. 1 (1908): 8. *Denkwürdige Erinnerungen* was originally published in 1898.

43. Hartmann, "Autobiography," p. 10. Although Hartmann had been a medical student in Munich, he did not finish his studies there and did not have a degree when he set sail. Similarly, although he practiced under the title of physician in the United States, it is not clear whether he ever earned a medical degree there.

44. Hartmann says that this chief was the first to instruct him about the core Theosophical teaching of universal brotherhood: Hartmann, *Denkwürdige Erinnerungen,* p. 12.

45. All information in this paragraph comes from Hartmann, "Autobiography," p. 12.

46. Professor Peebles was probably J. M. Peebles, a former Unitarian minister who became an ardent spiritualist, worked sometimes as a professor at the Eclectic Medical College in Cincinnati, and was a key link between American and British working-class spiritualism: Logie Barrow, *Independent Spirits: Spiritualism and English Plebeians, 1850–1910* (London: Routledge & Kegan Paul, 1986), pp. 4–5.

47. Hartmann, "Autobiography," pp. 12–14.

48. Hartmann, *Denkwürdige Erinnerungen,* p. 34.

49. Except where otherwise noted, all information in this paragraph comes from Hartmann, "Autobiography," pp. 16–17.

50. Hartmann, "Autobiography," p. 20.

51. Hartmann, *Denkwürdige Erinnerungen,* pp. 717–22.

52. Hartmann, "Autobiography," p. 20.

53. Hartmann's autobiographical works include *Denkwürdige Erinnerungen* (1898) and *Unter den Adepten: Vertrauliche Mittheilungen aus den Kreisen der indischen Adepten und christlichen Mystiker* (1901). Among his pieces of fantasy fiction, see Franz Hartmann, *Among the Gnomes: An Occult Tale of Adventure in the Untersberg* (New York: Arno Press, 1978), originally printed as *Among the Gnomes* (London: F. T. Unwin, 1895). T. J. Jackson Lears, a historian of American antimodernism, has noted late-nineteenth-century Americans' fascination with the "medieval folk mind," manifested in renewed popularity of stories featuring fairies, gnomes, and other creatures from medieval fairy tales. He associates this interest with the contemporary passion for Orientalism, mind-cure, occultism, and mysticism. The case of Hartmann suggests that similar claims might be made about Europeans in this period; see T. J. Jackson Lears, *No Place of Grace: Antimodernism and the Transformation of American Culture, 1880–1920* (Chicago: University of Chicago Press, 1994 (1981)), pp. 167–75.

54. Hartmann, *Denkwürdige Erinnerungen,* p. 102.

55. For a discussion of Steiner's roots in the intellectual history of the nineteenth century, see Robert Carroll Galbreath, "Spiritual Science in an Age of Materialism: Rudolf Steiner and Occultism," Ph.D. dissertation, University of Michigan, 1970; see also Robert Sumser, "Rational Occultism in Fin de Siècle Germany: Rudolf Steiner's Modernism," *History of European Ideas* 18, no. 4 (1994): 497–511.

56. Rudolf Steiner, *The Story of My Life* (London: Anthroposophical Publishing, 1928), chapter 1 and p. 38; originally published as Rudolf Steiner, *Mein Lebensgang* (Dornach: Philosophisch-anthroposophischer Verlag, 1925).

57. Steiner, *Story*, pp. 11 and 39.

58. Ibid., pp. 76, 110, and 282, and chapter 24.

59. Ibid., pp. 284–85 and 289.

60. Rudolf Steiner, *Theosophie: Einführung in übersinnliche Welterkenntnis und Menschenbestimmung* (Dornach, Switzerland: Rudolf Steiner Verlag, 1973), p. 14; originally published in Leipzig by M. Altmann in 1908.

61. Letter from Eliza von Moltke to Rudolf Steiner on 20 July 1904: Rudolf Steiner, *Zur Geschichte und aus den Inhalten der ersten Abteilung der Esoterischen Schule, 1904–1914: Briefe, Rundbriefe, Dokumente, und Vorträge* (Dornach, Switzerland: Rudolf Steiner Verlag, 1984), pp. 73–74; see also *Light for the New Millenium: Rudolf Steiner's Association with Helmuth and Eliza von Moltke: Letters, Documents, and After-Death Communications*, ed. T. H. Meyer (London: Rudolf Steiner Press, 1997).

62. For biographical information on Wohlbold, see Steiner, *Zur Geschichte*, p. 463.

63. Steiner, *Zur Geschichte*, p. 157.

64. The term *Anthroposophy* came from Thomas Vaughan, who had coined it in his 1650 *Anthroposophie Theomagica*, a work to which Steiner had been exposed during his Vienna days of attending philosophy lectures by Robert Zimmermann: *Encyclopedia of Occultism and Parapsychology*, 3rd ed. (1991), vol. 1, s.v., "Anthroposophical Society," p. 60. For an overview of the Anthroposophical movement, see Norbert Schwarte, "Anthroposophie," *Handbuch der deutschen Reformbewegungen, 1880–1933*, ed. Diethart Kerbs and Jürgen Reulecke (Wuppertal: Peter Hammer, 1998), pp. 595–609.

65. Wilhelm Hübbe-Schleiden in Göttingen to Gretchen Boggiani (postscript), 10 October 1911: Klatt, *Theosophie*, p. 205.

66. Wilhelm Hübbe-Schleiden in Göttingen to Rudolf Steiner, 9 August 1911: Klatt, *Theosophie*, p. 197.

67. "Mitteilungen für die Mitglieder der 'Internationalen Theosophischen Verbrüderung' (I.T.V.)," 2 June 1912, Cod WH-S 815.

68. *Zentrale für praktischen Okkultismus* (n.p., n.d.), pp. 3, 10, and 56. I have tentatively dated this piece to the 1920s because there are no examples of such institutes in the Wilhelmine period and because the address listed on the pamphlet (Blumengasse 12, Leipzig) is that of the headquarters of the Internationale Theosophische Verbrüderung, which stayed at this address through the 1920s. This pamphlet is available at the Stadtbibliothek München.

69. Very little has been written about Monte Verità in its historical context. The information in this paragraph comes from Martin Green, *Mountain of Truth: The Counterculture Begins. Ascona, 1900–1920* (Hanover, NH: University Press of New England, 1980), which documents the main figures and ideas of the colony. See also the very interesting work *Monte Verità: Berg der Wahrheit: Lokale Anthropologie als Beitrag zur Wiederentdeckung einer neuzeitlichen sakralen Topographie*, ed. Harald Szeemann (Milan: Electa Editrice, 1978). Even with the effective end of the Monte Verità colony in 1920, Ascona and the Ticino region of Switzerland of which it was a part more broadly continued to attract Germans (and others) interested in cultivating alternative lives and free self-expression. Among these were important and influential representatives from the German Theosophical movement such as the artist Bô Yin Râ, who settled in

the area in 1925 (Bô Yin Râ is discussed in chapter 6). Useful information can also be found in Ellic Howe and Helmut Möller, "Theodor Reuss: Irregular Freemasonry in Germany, 1900–23," *Ars Quatuor Coronatorum* 91 (1978): 28–46.

70. Hermann Rudolph, *Die theosophische Verbrüderung die einer Bekenntnisfreie Religion: Der Wegweiser in das neue, lichte Zeitalter, und zur Höherentwicklung der menschlichen Rasse* (Leipzig: Theosophischer Kultur-Verlag, 1925), p. 3; available at JFC.

71. Rudolph, *Die theosophische Verbrüderung*, pp. 20 and 22–23.

72. *Handbuch der Ariosophie*, ed. Karl Kern (Pforzheim: Verlag Herbert Reichstein, 1931–32), p. 17; available at JFC.

73. My reading of the völkisch movement relies on recent path-breaking work by Uwe Puschner: foreword to *Handbuch zur "Völkischen Bewegung,"* pp. xiv and xix; Uwe Puschner, *Die völkische Bewegung im wilhelminischen Kaiserreich: Sprache—Rasse—Religion* (Darmstadt: Wissenschaftliche Buchgesellschaft, 2001), pp. 15–16 and 168.

74. Note that while Ariosophy is listed separately in the appendix, technically it is an offshoot of Theosophy.

75. *Handbuch der Ariosophie*, pp. xviii–xix; Puschner, *Die völkische Bewegung*, pp. 15–16 and 204–87; see also Günter Hartung, "Völkische Ideologie," in *Handbuch zur "Völkischen Bewegung,"* pp. 22–41.

76. For a thought-provoking examination of how these complicated ideas played out in the British context, see Dixon, *Divine Feminine*, pp. 59–60.

77. Helmut Zander, "Sozialdarwinistische Rassentheorien aus dem okkulten Untergrund des Kaiserreichs," in *Handbuch zur "Völkischen Bewegung,"* pp. 239–46.

78. Wilhelm Hübbe-Schleiden to Ludwig Deinhard (6 March 1902), in Klatt, *Theosophie*, p. 135. The person in question was Richard Bresch. See also Hübbe-Schleiden's comments about Bresch on p. 152.

79. Nicolas Goodrick-Clarke, *The Occult Roots of Nazism: Secret Aryan Cults and Their Influence on Nazi Ideology* (New York: New York University Press, 1992), chapters 4–6 and 15.

80. For information on Lanz von Liebenfels, see Goodrick-Clarke, *Occult Roots*, and Ekkehard Hieronimus, "Jörg Lanz von Liebenfels," in *Handbuch zur "Völkischen Bewegung,"* pp. 131–46.

81. *Handbuch der Ariosophie*, p. iii; see also the table of contents on p. 199.

82. See the clipping tucked into Herbert Reichstein, *Die Mystik der Namen: Eine Philosophie der Zahlen: Eine Charakterwissenschaft als deutsche Lebenslehre*, 4th ed. (Berlin: Verlag Herbert Reichstein, 1935); available at JFC. Despite the obvious associations, Reichstein denied that his Kabbalograms had anything to do with the Jewish form of mysticism known as Kabbala; see his comments, ibid., p. 9.

83. Hans-Jürgen Glowka, *Deutsche Okkultgruppen, 1875–1937* (Munich: Arbeitsgemeinschaft für Religions-und Weltanschauungsfragen, 1981), p. 94.

84. Max Seiling, *Was soll ich? Weise Lebensregeln, mit einem Anhang: Gesundheitsregeln* (Bad Schmiedeberg: F. E. Baumann, n.d.); available at JFC.

85. Goodrick-Clarke, *Occult Roots*, p. 55; see also Max Seiling, *Mainländer, [sic] ein neuer Messias: Eine frohe Botschaft inmitten der herrschenden Geistesverwirrung* (Munich: Theodor Ackermann, 1888).

86. Goodrick-Clarke, *Occult Roots*, pp. 53–54.

87. Glowka, *Deutsche Okkultgruppen*, p. 94. Presumably because of his publishing activities on behalf of Ariosophy, Puschner includes Zillmann in a list of key figures in

the early völkisch movement. This may be a somewhat misleading characterization, for the reasons noted above: Puschner, *Die völkische Bewegung,* p. 287.

88. All appeared at Zillmann's *Neue Metaphysische Rundschau.* For an excellent overview of Lanz von Liebenfels's publications, see Ekkehard Hieronimus, *Lanz von Liebenfels: Eine Bibliographie* (Toppenstedt: Uwe Berg, 1991).

89. Hieronimus, *Lanz von Liebenfels,* pp. 113–56. For reproductions of his horoscopes, see pp. 185–92.

90. Ibid., pp. 35–44.

91. Ibid., pp. 44–75.

92. Ibid., pp. 90–106.

93. Richard Ungewitter, *Rettung oder Untergang des deutschen Volkes* (Stuttgart: Verlag Richard Ungewitter, 1921), p. 7; available at JFC. Ungewitter also raged against monists, Freemasons, Jews, and Jehovah's Witnesses—all groups later persecuted systematically by the Nazi regime. See chapter 9.

94. W. von Bülow, *Der Ewigkeitsgehalt der eddischen Runen und Zahlen: Grundriß arischer Weisheit und Jungbrunnen des deutschen Volkstums* (Munich: Verlag Hans Stiegeler, n.d.), p. 5; available at JFC.

95. *Handbuch der Ariosophie,* p. iii. For post-1945 Ariosophical activity, see Nicholas Goodrick-Clarke, *Hitler's Priestess: Savitri Devi, the Hindu-Aryan Myth, and Neo-Nazism* (New York: New York University Press, 1998), and *Black Sun: Aryan Cults, Esoteric Nazism, and the Politics of Identity* (New York: New York University Press, 2001).

96. There are many more studies of German eugenics than can be listed here. Among the best are Loren R. Graham, "Attitudes toward Eugenics in Germany and Soviet Russia in the 1920s: An Examination of Science and Values," in *Morals, Science, and Society,* ed. H. T. Engelhardt and Daniel Callahan (Hastings-on-Hudson, NY: Hastings Center, 1978), pp. 119–49; Robert N. Proctor, *Racial Hygiene: Medicine under the Nazis* (Cambridge: Harvard University Press, 1988); and Sheila Faith Weiss, "Wilhelm Schallmayer and the Logic of German Eugenics," *Isis* 77 (1986): 33–46.

CHAPTER FIVE: The Creative Unconscious

1. Sixten Ringbom, "Art in 'the Epoch of the Great Spiritual': Occult Elements in the Early Theory of Abstract Painting," *Journal of the Warburg and Courtauld Institutes* 29 (1966): 416–17; see also Sixten Ringbom, *The Sounding Cosmos: A Study in the Spiritualism of Kandinsky and the Genesis of Abstract Painting* (Abo: Abo Akademi, 1970).

2. *Kandinsky: Complete Writings on Art,* ed. Kenneth C. Lindsay and Peter Vergo (New York: Da Capo Press, 1994), p. 209.

3. Hans Prinzhorn, *Artistry of the Mentally Ill: A Contribution to the Psychology and Psychopathology of Configuration,* trans. Eric von Brockdorff (New York: Springer, 1972), pp. 271–72.

4. Franziska Gräfin zu Reventlow, *Autobiographisches* (Munich: Albert Langen, 1980), pp. 376–88; Thomas Mann, "Okkulte Erlebnisse," *Gesammelte Werke* 10 (Frankfurt: Fischer, 1974), pp. 135–71. See also the climactic séance near the end of Mann's *The Magic Mountain.* Many other German writers showed an interest in occult phenomena, including the popular science essayist Wilhelm Bölsche, who took spiritualism as a

main theme in his 1889 novel *Die Mittagsgöttin,* and Melchior Lechter, who belonged to the Stefan George circle of writers in Munich: Roy Pascal, *From Naturalism to Expressionism: German Literature and Society, 1880–1918* (New York: Basic Books, 1973), p. 176.

5. Thomas Elsaesser, *Weimar Cinema and After: Germany's Historical Imaginary* (London: Routledge, 2000), p. 226; Lotte Eisner, *Murnau* (Berkeley: University of California Press, 1964), p. 109.

6. Friedrich Wilhelm Fischer, "Geheimlehren und moderne Kunst: Zur hermetischen Kunstauffassung von Baudelaire bis Malewitsch," in *Fin de Siècle: Zu Literatur und Kunst der Jahrhundertwende,* ed. Roger Bauer et al. (Frankfurt am Main: Klostermann, 1977), pp. 344–77; Peter Gay, *Art and Act: On Causes in History: Manet, Gropius, Mondrian* (New York: Harper & Row, 1976); John Golding, *Paths to the Absolute: Mondrian, Malevich, Kandinsky, Pollock, Newman, Rothko, and Still* (Princeton, NJ: Princeton University Press, 2000); M. E. Warlick, *Max Ernst and Alchemy: A Magician in Search of Myth* (Austin: University of Texas Press, 2001); see also the exhibition catalogs *Okkultismus und Avantgarde: Von Munch bis Mondrian, 1900–1915* (Frankfurt: Tertium, 1995), and *The Spiritual in Art: Abstract Painting, 1890–1985* (Los Angeles County Museum of Art, 1986). For the Viennese case, see Astrid Kury, *"Heiligenscheine eines elektrischen Jahrhundertendes sehen anders aus . . .": Okkultismus und die Kunst der Wiener Moderne* (Vienna: Passagen Verlag, 2000).

7. "Programm der psychologischen Gesellschaft in München," *Sphinx* 3, 13 (1887): 32–36.

8. For overviews of new developments in the visual arts, see Shearer West, *The Visual Arts in Germany, 1890–1937: Utopia and Despair* (New Brunswick, NJ: Rutgers University Press, 2001), and Peter Paret, *German Encounters with Modernism, 1840–1945* (Cambridge: Cambridge University Press, 2001).

9. Siegfried Käss, *Der heimliche Kaiser der Kunst: Adolf Bayersdorfer, seine Freunde und seine Zeit* (Munich: tuduv Verlagsgesellschaft, 1987), pp. 103–6.

10. Mary Margaret Richter, *Gabriel Max: The Artist, the Darwinist, and the Spiritualist,* Ph.D. dissertation, New York University, 1998, chapter 1. Richter goes on to argue, convincingly, that Max should be seen as "central to any evaluation of art at the end of the [nineteenth] century" (p. 355). Further information on Max can be found in Friedrich Pecht, *Geschichte der Münchner Kunst im neunzehnten Jahrhundert* (Munich: Verlagsanstalt für Kunst und Wissenschaft, 1888), pp. 324–30, and Hermann Uhde-Bernays, *Die Münchner Malerei im neunzehnten Jahrhundert:* vol. 2., *1850–1900* (Munich: Verlag F. Bruckmann, n.d.), pp. 196–201. Note also that Bayersdorfer had signaled Max out as one of Munich's leading "modern" painters as early as 1874: *Adolf Bayersdorfers Leben und Schriften: Aus seinem Nachlaß,* ed. Hans Mackowsky, August Pauly, and Wilhelm Weigand (Munich: F. Bruckmann, 1908), p. 241. For Max's influence on art today, see Stephan Berg, " 'Klopfe nur, wenn du die Richtige bist': Die Seh(n)suchte des Johannes Muggenthaler," *Kunstforum International* 135 (October 1996–January 1997): 254–59.

11. Oskar A. Müller, *Albert von Keller, 1884 Gais/Schweiz-1920 München* (Munich: Verlag Karl Thiemig, 1981), p. 166. Note that Keller served as president of the Psychologische Gesellschaft from 1889 to 1892 as well: "Keller," *Neue Deutsche Biographie* 11 (Berlin: Duncker & Humboldt), p. 428.

12. Maria Makela, "The Politics of Parody: Some Thoughts on the 'Modern' in Turn-of-the-Century Munich," in *Imagining Modern German Culture, 1889–1910,*

ed. Françoise Forster-Hahn (Hanover, NH: University Press of New England, 1996), pp. 185, 187, and 191–92.

13. Richter, *Gabriel Max*, p. 189; quoted from Percy Adlon, *Im Haus des Affenmalers Gabriel Max*, typescript, October–November 1980.

14. "Mitglieder Verzeichnis der Theosophischen Societät Germania," Cod WH-S 812:2,1; Richter, *Gabriel Max*, pp. 311–13 and 337.

15. Maria Makela, *The Munich Secession: Art and Artists in Turn-of-the-Century Munich* (Princeton, NJ: Princeton University Press, 1990), p. 31; see also "Max," in *Neue Deutsche Biographie* 16, p. 457.

16. Uhde-Bernays, *Münchner Malerei*, p. 200.

17. The painting was *Erweckung von Jairi Töchterlein* (Revival of Jairus's daughter), sometimes referred to as *Christus erweckt eine Tote* (Christ revives a corpse). The story comes from the Gospel of Mark, chapter 5. Jairus was the administrative head of the Capernaum synagogue. When his twelve-year-old daughter became sick, he begged Jesus to come cure her. Informed that she had died, Jairus despaired; upon his arrival, however, Jesus announced that the girl was only sleeping, and then miraculously restored her to life. This story was also the subject of Albert von Keller's 1885 *Auferweckung der Tochter Jairi* (see below).

18. Richter, *Gabriel Max*, pp. 234–35. The painting was titled *Geistesgruss* (Spirit greeting).

19. The painting was *Die ekstatische Jungfrau Katharina Emmerich* and now belongs to the Neue Pinakothek in Munich. Anna Katharina Emmerich entered a convent in 1802. When her convent closed in 1811, Emmerich experienced visions and ecstatic states, including stigmata on her hands. Numerous priests and physicians authenticated her experiences and she drew the attention of such writers as the poet Clemens Brentano and Pope Pius IX. Emmerich was a favorite topic in German occult journals of the 1880s and 1890s.

20. The painting was *Die Seherin von Prevorst in Hochschlaf.* Friederike Hauffe had had visions and prophetic dreams since childhood, and these only increased in frequency and intensity after an early arranged marriage. Mesmeric treatment by the local doctor Justinus Kerner brought her relief from pain and allowed her some measure of control over her visions, during which she spoke High German, diagnosed and prescribed for herself and others, and conveyed philosophical teachings. Kerner published his account of her in *Die Seherin von Prevorst* (Stuttgart: Cotta, 1829). Part of this material was then edited by Hermann Hesse and republished as *Blätter aus Prevorst: Eine Auswahl von Berichten über Magnetismus, Hellsehen, Geistererscheinungen aus dem Kreise Justinus Kerners und seiner Freunde* (Berlin: S. Fischer, 1926). Hauffe was a popular topic in German occult journals; see, for instance, the drawings Max submitted to accompany the article of Carl du Prel, "Justinus Kerner und die Seherin von Prevorst," *Sphinx* 2 (1886): 139–56.

21. Many of these paintings have been lost. Reproductions of those that survive can be found in Richter, *Gabriel Max*.

22. Richter, *Gabriel Max*, pp. 66, 227, 240–41 and 245–46. Max became involved in spiritualism in 1879, when he hosted a series of séances at his home with the medium William Eglinton. Initial sittings went well, but by the spring of the following year Max had become suspicious of Eglinton and eventually exposed him as a fraud, much to the irritation of Zöllner.

23. Müller, *Albert von Keller,* pp. 51 and 75–77.

24. The mediums were Lina Matzinger, Lily, Eusapia Paladino, and Madeleine Guipet: Müller, *Albert von Keller* p. 52. For reproductions, see pp. 75, 97–98, 102–7, 112, 116–7, 251–54, and 256–64.

25. Veit Loers and Pia Witzmann, "Münchens okkultistisches Netzwerk," *Okkultismus und Avantgarde,* p. 238.

26. For reproductions, see Hans Rosenhagen, *Albert von Keller* (Bielefeld: Verlag von Velhagen & Clasing, 1912), p. 62, and Albert von Schrenck-Notzing, "Albert von Keller als Malerpsychologe und Metapsychiker," *Psychische Studien* 48 (April–May 1929): 202–3.

27. For the occult and Viennese modernism, see Kury, *"Heiligenscheine."*

28. Albert von Schrenck-Notzing, *Die Traumtänzerin Magdeleine G. Eine psychologische Studie über Hypnose und dramatische Kunst* (Stuttgart: Verlag von Ferdinand Enke, 1904), pp. 1 and 21–22. Note that Madeleine Guipet was often referred to simply as Madeleine G.

29. Georg Fuchs, *Sturm und Drang in München um die Jahrhundertwende* (Munich: Verlag Georg D. W. Callwey, 1936), p. 241.

30. Schrenck-Notzing, *Traumtänzerin,* pp. 2–4. Seidl, who had also built the villas of Keller and Schrenck-Notzing, was part of the vernacular revival in architecture that created a "Bavarian image," combining regional craftsmanship with academic traditions. He designed the Bavarian National Museum, Deutsches Museum (Munich, 1906–13), and the interior of the Villa Lenbach (Munich, 1887–9). Also involved in staging Guipet were the innovative director and dramatist Fritz Stavenhagen and the composers Max von Schillings, Ludwig Thuille, and Karl Freiherr von Kaskel.

31. Müller, *Albert von Keller,* pp. 84–85; see also the caption under the photograph of Guipet on stage in Schrenck-Notzing, "Albert von Keller," p. 209.

32. They included *Marie Madeleine als Kassandra* (Madeleine Guipet as Cassandra, 1904) and two versions of *Madeleine Guipet in Trance* (1904). Reproductions of all of these works, plus a photograph of Guipet performing one of her trance dances, can be found in Müller, *Albert von Keller,* pp. 84–85.

33. Schrenck-Notzing, *Traumtänzerin,* pp. 6–7, 10, and 76.

34. Georg Fuchs, *Der Tanz* (Stuttgart: Strecken & Schröder, 1906), pp. 12 and 21–24 (*Flugblätter für künstlerische Kultur* 6); see also Fuchs, *Sturm und Drang,* pp. 240–44. For a discussion of Fuchs's role in Munich modernism, see Peter Jelavich, *Munich and Theatrical Modernism: Politics, Playwriting, and Performance, 1890–1914* (Cambridge: Harvard University Press, 1985), pp. 187–208. Fuchs's responses to Guipet's trance dances must also be seen as part of the "culture of movement" discussed in August Nitschke, "Der Kult der Bewegung: Turnen, Rhythmik und neue Tänze," *Jahrhundertwende: Der Aufbruch in die Moderne, 1880–1930,* ed. August Nitschke et al. (Hamburg: Rowohlt, 1990), pp. 258–85. Guipet also resembled Isadora Duncan, Loïe Fuller, Maud Allan, and the creators of modern dance in other ways: none of these women had formal dance training, and all chose the music of Chopin, Liszt, Schubert, and Strauss to accompany them; see Gabriele Brandstetter, "Psychologie des Ausdrucks und Ausdruckstanz: Aspekte der Wechselwirkung am Beispiel der 'Traumtänzerin' Madeleine," in *Ausdruckstanz: Eine mitteleuropäische Bewegung der ersten Hälfte des 20. Jahrhunderts,* ed. Gunhild Oberzaucher-Schüller (Wilhelmshaven: Florian Noetzel Verlag, 1986), p. 207.

35. Richter, *Gabriel Max*, p. 265; trans. and quoted from Adolf Kohut, "Gabriel Max," *Westermanns illustrierte deutsche Monatshefte* 54 (May 1883): 173–86.

36. Hans Boventer, *Rilkes Zyklus 'Aus dem Nachlass des Grafen C. W.' Versuch einer Eingliederung in Rilkes Werk* (Berlin: Erich Schmidt Verlag, 1969), pp. 7–9 and 19. Boventer also reports (p. 4) that Rilke participated in séances at the home of his friend Princess Marie von Thurn und Taxis in 1912. Another account of Rilke's involvement with the occult is Ralph Freedman, *Life of a Poet: Rainer Maria Rilke* (New York: Farrar, Straus & Giroux, 1996), pp. 349–50 and 462–69.

37. R. F. Foster, *W. B. Yeats: A Life*: vol. 1, *The Apprentice Mage, 1865–1914* (Oxford: Oxford University Press, 1997), pp. 465–69. Mark Polizzotti, *Revolution of the Mind: The Life of André Breton* (New York: Farrar, Straus & Giroux, 1995), p. 102 and passim. For the connections between the symbolist movement in literature and the occult, see Alain Mercier, *Les Sources Ésotériques et Occultes de la Poésie Symboliste, 1870–1914: 2, Le Symbolisme Européen* (Paris: A.-G. Nizet, 1974), pp. 47–67.

38. For a psychological review of mediumistic art that draws heavily on German sources, see Elmar R. Gruber, "Mediumistic and Psychopathological Pictorial Expression: An Introductory Comparative Survey," *Confina Psychiat.* 23 (1980): 82–87. For the French case, see Françoise Will-Levaillant, "L'analyse des dessins d'aliénés et de médiums en France avant le Surréalisme," *Revue de l'Art* 50 (1980): 24–39. For the period after 1945, see José Pierre, "Raphael Lonné et le retour des médiums," *L'Oeil* 216 (December 1972): 30–43.

39. Hanns von Gumppenberg, *Lebenserinnerungen aus dem Nachlass des Dichters* (Berlin: Eigenbrödler, 1929), pp. 142–43; see also Karl-Wilhelm Wintzingerode-Knorr, *Hanns v. Gumppenbergs Künstlerisches Werk: Ein Beitrag zur Geschichte der deutschen Literatur der Wende vom 19. zum 20. Jahrhundert*, Ph.D. dissertation, Ludwig-Maximilians-Universität, Munich, 1958; and Hildegard Châtellier, "Entre religion et philosophie: Les approches du spiritisme chez Hanns von Gumppenberg," *Mystique, mysticisme, et modernité en Allemagne autour de 1900*, ed. Moritz Baßler and Hildegard Châtellier (Strasbourg: Presses Universitaires de Strasbourg, 1998), pp. 115–32.

40. Jelavich, *Munich*, pp. 34–35.

41. Gumppenberg, *Lebenserinnerungen*, pp. 144–53; Hanns von Gumppenberg, *Das dritte Testament: Eine Offenbarung Gottes* (Munich: M. Poessl, 1891), pp. 3–6. Note that *Schutzgeist* is one of the more common German terms for these spirits, though Gumppenberg also uses the term *Genius*. Sometimes these terms are translated into English as "control spirit."

42. Gumppenberg, *Lebenserinnerungen*, pp. 144–53; Gumppenberg, *Dritte Testament*, p. 3.

43. Gumppenberg, *Lebenserinnerungen*, p. 171; Hanns von Gumppenberg, *Der Prophet Jesus Christus, die Neue Religion, und andere Erläuterungen zum Dritten Testament Gottes* (Munich: M. Poessl, 1891), p. 10. Works developing his antimaterialist worldview include *Kritik des Wirklich-Seienden* (Critique of being, 1892), *Der fünfte Prophet* (The fifth prophet, 1895), *Grundlagen der wissenschaftlichen Philosophie* (Foundations of scientific philosophy, 1903), and *Philosophie und Okkultismus* (Philosophy and occultism, 1921).

44. Jelavich, *Munich*, pp. 166 and 176–77.

45. Robin Lenman, *Artists and Society in Germany, 1850–1914* (Manchester, Eng.: Manchester University Press, 1997), pp. 10–15.

46. In 1898 she married the writer Viktor Blüthgen, who wrote for bourgeois journals such as *Die Gartenlaube* and *Deutsche Monatsschrift* and was a successful author of children's verses and stories. For biographical information, consult *Deutsches Literatur-Lexikon* 1 (1968), s.v., "Blüthgen, Clara" and "Blüthgen, Viktor," pp. 593–95; also *An Encyclopedia of German Women Writers, 1900–1933: Biographies and Bibliographies with Exemplary Readings* 2 (1997), s.v., "Clara Blüthgen"; and *Lexikon deutschsprachiger Schriftstellerinnen, 1800–1945* (1986), s.v., "Blüthgen, Clara," pp. 33–34.

47. *Encyclopedia of German Women Writers*, s.v., "Clara Blüthgen," p. 29. According to this source (p. 32), there are no scholarly studies of Clara Blüthgen, a prolific writer.

48. Hans Freimark mentions that the first book took only two weeks: Hans Freimark, *Mediumistische Kunst mit einem Beitrag über den künstlerischen Wert mediumistischer Malereien von Eugen Johannes Maecker* (*Beiträge zur Geschichte der neueren Mystik und Magie* 2) (Leipzig: Wilhelm Heims, 1914), p. 77. Parts of Eysell-Kilburger's mediumistic poetry are reprinted in Smith, *Deutsches Literatur-Lexikon*. The German titles were *Klänge aus dem Jenseits: Ein Mysterium* and *Trance-Dichtungen*.

49. *Encyclopedia of German Women Writers*, "Clara Blüthgen," p. 29.

50. Freimark, *Mediumistische Kunst*, p. 76.

51. Eberhard Buchner, *Von den übersinnlichen Dingen: Ein Führer durch das Reich der okkulten Forschung* (Leipzig: Felix Meiner, 1924), p. 233.

52. Richard Baerwald, *Okkultismus, Spiritismus, und unterbewußte Seelenzustände* (Leipzig: B. G. Teubner, 1920), p. 40; Hans Freimark, *Das erotische Element im Okkultismus* (Pfullingen in Württemberg: Johannes Baum, 1922), pp. 54–57. Aßmann's choice of decoration had its parallels across the Atlantic. T. J. Jackson Lears has noted the fascination held by some American antimodernists for the Orient, particularly Japan, which they thought of as a "toyland" of "fairy-folk" and "sweet children": T. J. Jackson Lears, *No Place of Grace: Antimodernism and the Transformation of American Culture, 1880–1920* (Chicago, IL: University of Chicago Press, 1981), p. 149. For other trance artists, see Freimark, *Das erotische Element*, pp. 49–53 and passim; "Mediumistische Kunst," *Zentralblatt für Okkultismus* 8 (December 1914–January 1915): 283–87 and 311–15; and Max Moecke, "Medianyme Malerei," *Der Okkultismus* (October 1925): 30–34.

53. Suggested by Dieter Bassermann in Boventer, *Rilkes Zyklus*, pp. 40–41 and 152.

54. The standard work on Kandinsky's years in Munich from 1896 to 1914, when he returned to Russia, is Peg Weiss, *Kandinsky in Munich: The Formative Jugendstil Years* (Princeton, NJ: Princeton University Press, 1979); see also West, *The Visual Arts*, chapter 3, and Jill Lloyd, *German Expressionism: Primitivism and Modernity* (New Haven, CT: Yale University Press, 1991).

55. For his reading, see Ringbom, "Art in 'The Epoch of the Great Spiritual,'" pp. 416–17, and *The Sounding Cosmos*, pp. 36–39, 131, and passim. For his relation to Steiner, see Golding, *Paths to the Absolute*, p. 87. Note that Kandinsky never actually joined the Theosophical Society.

56. Lindsay and Vergo, *Kandinsky*, p. 197.

57. Ringbom, *Sounding Cosmos*, pp. 109, 128–30, and 206.

58. Lindsay and Vergo, *Kandinsky*, p. 160.

59. Golding, *Paths to the Absolute*, p. 98; see also Mario Ackermann, "Eine Sprache, die besser wirkt als Esperanto: Überlegungen zum Einfluß des Spiritismus auf Kandinsky," *Mystique, mysticisme, et modernité*.

60. Elsie Johna Badelt, *Das Mal-Phänomen Heinrich Nüßlein* (Magdeburg: Selbst-

verlag, n.d.), pp. 3, 10–20, 26, and 37. One doctor reported seeing Nüßlein perform a mummification; see Rolf Reißmann, "Der Seelenmaler im Herzogsbett," *Berliner Illustrierte Nachtausgabe (Beiblätter)*, 18 September 1935, p. 2. An undated sample of Nüßlein's automatic writing exists in the Eberhard Sammlung, Stadtbibliothek, Munich.

61. Georg Anschütz, "Phantasma und Kunst," *Schünemanns Monatshefte* 11 (November 1928): 1262–72; see also Reißmann, "Der Seelenmaler," p. 2.

62. Badelt, *Mal-Phänomen*, pp. 22–23; Kunstverein München, *Führer durch die Ausstellung "Geheimnisse der Inspiration: Gemälde, Aquarelle, und Zeichnungen okkult beeinflußter Maler"* (Munich, 1932); G. Senker, "Heinrich Nüßlein, ein supranormales Phänomenon," reprinted in Badelt, *Mal-Phänomen*, p. 41 (originally in *Leipziger Neueste Nachrichten*).

63. Badelt, *Mal-Phänomen*, pp. 29 and 33. The importance of rays, waves, and vibrations to this view of art may also have had something to do with popular conceptions of early-twentieth-century physics, particularly the discovery that the atom was divisible and the turn to the study of radiation through empty space. Ringbom, *Sounding Cosmos* considers this possibility with regard to Kandinsky, but then dismisses it after careful study of Kandinsky's sources. The same line of reasoning applies to Nüßlein. Perhaps a more fruitful avenue of historical research would be to examine early-twentieth-century Theosophy and physics as two manifestations of a new understanding of the nature of matter.

64. See, for instance, the reproductions in Anschütz, "Phantasma," pp. 1263 and 1268–69.

65. Wolfgang Heller, "Schneiderfranken, Joseph Anton," *Biographisch-Bibliographisches Kirchenlexikon*, ed. Friedrich Wilhelm Bautz (Herzberg: Verlag Traugott Bautz, 1995), pp. 569–72. Some additional biographical information can be found in Alfred Kober-Staehelin (Bô Yin Râ's publisher), *Meine Stellung zu Bô Yin Râ* (Basel: Kober'sche Verlagsbuchhandlung, 1931), p. 4, and Bô Yin Râ, *Aus meiner Malerwerkstatt* (Basel: Kober'sche Verlagsbuchhandlung, 1932), p. 17. Some of Schneiderfranken's landscapes are reproduced in full color in Rudolf Schott, *Der Maler Bô Yin Râ* (Zürich: Kober'sche Verlagsbuchhandlung, 1960).

66. Felix Weingartner, *Bô Yin Râ* (Basel: Rhein Verlag, 1923).

67. Bô Yin Râ, *Aus meiner Malerwerkstatt*, pp. 40–41, 64, and 71–72.

68. Ibid., pp. 55, 83–91, and 102.

69. Franz Marc, "Zur Kritik der Vergangenheit," *Okkultismus und Avantgarde*, pp. 274–76; Veit Loers and Pia Witzmann, "Münchens okkultistisches Netzwerk," *Okkultismus und Avantgarde*, p. 240.

70. Kunstverein München, *Führer durch die Ausstellung*, pp. 11 and 14. The Kunstverein was a group formed to help artists without steady customers find a suitable market for their works: Makela, *Munich Secession*, p. 165.

71. Pia Witzmann, " 'Dem Kosmos gehört der Tanzende': Der Einfluß des Okkulten auf den Tanz," *Okkultismus und Avantgarde*, pp. 600–25.

CHAPTER SIX: Occult Sciences and Their Applied Doubles

1. This chapter adapts its title from a sociological study of the occult by Leahey and Leahey, but takes its own approach; see Thomas Hardy Leahey and Grace Evans Leahey,

Psychology's Occult Doubles: Psychology and the Problem of Pseudoscience (Chicago, IL: Nelson-Hall, 1983).

2. Anson Rabinbach, *The Human Motor: Energy, Fatigue, and the Origins of Modernity* (Berkeley: University of California Press, 1990), p. 86. Rabinbach here defines social modernists as those dedicated to "applying new scientific modes of perception to social questions and bringing to bear a spirit of utopian and 'scientific' neutrality that was opposed to the forces that rent nineteenth-century society along lines of class and ideology." See also *Modernist Impulses in the Human Sciences, 1870–1930*, ed. Dorothy Ross (Baltimore, MD: Johns Hopkins University Press, 1994).

3. There is a huge body of literature devoted to the emergence of German social modernity. Historians have treated topics as diverse as the development of social insurance in Imperial Germany and its expansion in Weimar; the resulting emergence of a distinct "social realm" between state and economy that radically altered individuals' everyday life; the rise to power of a social-scientific class of experts, or social engineers, dedicated to "curing" social problems; and the enforcement as well as experience of social discipline; see, for instance: George Steinmetz, *Regulating the Social: The Welfare State and Local Politics in Imperial Germany* (Princeton, NJ: Princeton University Press, 1993); Detlev Peukert, *Grenzen der Sozialdisziplinierung: Aufstieg und Krise der deutschen Jugendfürsorge, 1878–1929* (Cologne: Bund, 1986), and Young-Sun Hong, *Welfare, Modernity, and the Weimar State, 1919–1933* (Princeton, NJ: Princeton University Press, 1998).

4. Detlev Peukert, *Max Webers Diagnose der Moderne* (Göttingen: Vandenhoeck & Ruprecht, 1989), p. 55.

5. K. R. v. Roques, "Strahlen-Urquell und Ende des Lebens," *Die Woche* 34 (24 September 1932): 1181–82.

6. See also Gustav Pohl, *Erdstrahlen als Krankheitserreger, Forschungen auf Neuland* (Diessen vor München: J. C. Huber, 1932).

7. Robert Proctor, *The Nazi War on Cancer* (Princeton, NJ: Princeton University Press, 1999), p. 137. The link between the occult and social modernity has received little attention in other national contexts. An exception is Richard Noakes, " 'Telegraphy Is an Occult Art': Cromwell Fleetwood Varley and the Diffusion of Electricity to the Other World," *British Journal for the History of Science* 32 (1999): 421–59.

8. Oscar A. H. Schmitz, "Über den Wert der Astrologie," *Süddeutsche Monatshefte* 24, no. 9 (1927): 163. A follower of Carl Jung, Schmitz was the first to bring astrology to a wide middle-class readership; see Oscar A. H. Schmitz, *Der Geist der Astrologie* (Munich: Müller, 1922).

9. James McKeen Cattell, "The Psychological Laboratory at Leipsic," *Mind* 13, no. 49 (1888): 45.

10. Wilhelm Hübbe-Schleiden, "Psychometrische Experimente," *Sphinx* 5, no. 27 (1888): 156–59. For a spiritualist take on psychometry, see Georg von Langsdorff, *Kurze Anleitung zur Erlernung der Psychometrie oder Entwicklung des in uns noch unerforschten sechsten Sinnes* (Leipzig: O. Mutze, 1898; Munich: Carussell-Verlag, 1981).

11. For the history of the measuring mania in psychology, see Joel Michell, *Measurement in Psychology: Critical History of a Methodological Concept* (Cambridge: Cambridge University Press, 1999).

12. For more on Aub's talent, see Annie Francé-Harrar, *So War's um Neunzehnhundert: Mein Fin de Siècle* (Munich: Albert Langen-Georg Müller, 1962), p. 136. Another

famous graphologist was Raphael Schermann of Vienna; see Oskar Fischer, *Experimente mit Raphael Schermann: Ein Beitrag zu den Problemen der Graphologie, Telepathie, und des Hellsehens* (Berlin: Urban & Schwarzenberg, 1924).

13. *Ueber einen Fall von Einfühlungsvermögen in die Seele des Menschen (Ludwig Aub): Aufsätze, Meinungen, Erklärungen* (Munich: Charakterologisches Sekretariat, n.d.), pp. 7–8 and 37.

14. Johannes Dingfelder, *Ludwig Aub als Hellseher und Hellfühler: Eine wissenschaftliche Studie über das Wesen der Graphologie und Psychometrie* (Munich: Fr. Seybolds Verlagsbuchhandlung, c. 1914), pp. 16 and 37.

15. *Ueber einen Fall,* pp. 13 and 49.

16. "Ludwig Aub," *Frankfurter Zeitung* 802, 30 November 1926, and "Ludwig Aub," *Münchner Neueste Nachrichten* 331, 30 November 1926, ZA Personen Aub, Ludwig, SdArMü. Many psychologists at the time, including such prominent representatives as Emil Kraepelin, spoke of the human body as a machine.

17. Alfred Gradenwitz, "Investigating Unknown Forces: The Unique Psychic Laboratory of Fritz Grunewald, at Charlottenburg," *Scientific American* (July 1922): 30. Note the similarities between this experimental set up and those of the time-motion studies being carried out by the "scientists of work" mentioned in the chapter introduction; Rabinbach, *The Human Motor,* figs. 20–26.

18. Busse also founded the *Institut für wissenschaftliche Graphologie* (Institute for scientific graphology), in 1894, and from 1898 edited the *Graphologische Monatshefte* (Graphological monthly). For further biographical information, see *Deutsches Literatur Lexikon: Biographisch-bibliographisches Handbuch* 2 (1969), s.v., "Busse," p. 419. Klages had studied with the philosopher Theodor Lipps, a member of Schrenck-Notzing's Psychological Society. Ulfried Geuter, *The Professionalization of Psychiatry in Nazi Germany* (Cambridge: Cambridge University Press, 1992), p. 95. Another key figure in the development of scientific graphology was the prominent child psychologist W. T. Preyer; see his *Zur Psychologie des Schreibens: Mit besonderer Rücksicht auf individuelle Verschiedenheiten der Handschriften* (Hamburg & Leipzig: L. Voss, 1895).

19. Hans Busse, "Graphologie und Okkultismus: Die Entwicklung der Graphologie zur exakten Wissenschaft," *Wissenschaftliche Zeitschrift für 'Okkultismus'* 1, nos. 2–3 (1899): 72–79.

20. *1. Kongress des Deutschen Bundes der gerichtlichen Schriftanverständigen und Berufsgraphologen (Sitz Berlin) am 6. und 7. September 1924 in Hotel Deutsches Haus in Leipzig, Königsplatz,* pp. 4–16.

21. Walter Benjamin, "Review of the Mendelssohns' *Der Mensch in der Handschrift,*" in *Walter Benjamin: Selected Writings,* vol. 2 (1927–34), ed. Michael W. Jennings, Howard Eiland, and Gary Smith (Cambridge, MA: Belknap Press, 1999), p. 131; originally published in *Die literarische Welt* (August 1928).

22. Richard Couvé, *Die Psychotechnik im Dienste der deutschen Reichsbahn* (Berlin: VDI, 1925); G. A. Jaederholm, *Psychotechnik der Verkaufs* (Leipzig: G. A. Gloeckner, 1926); Hans-Georg Gade, *Zur Psychotechnik des Flugzeugführers* (Berlin, 1928); William Stern, *Neue Beiträge zur Theorie und Praxis der Intelligenzprüfung* (Leipzig: J. A. Barth, 1925); David Katz, *Zur Psychologie des Amputierten und seiner Prothese* (Leipzig: J. A. Barth, 1921); Otto Lipmann, *Das Arbeitszeitproblem* (Berlin: Insitut für angewandte Psychologie, 1924).

23. Geuter, *Professionalization of Psychiatry,* pp. 83–94; Rabinbach, *The Human*

Motor, pp. 202–5, 259–62, 278–79, and passim. For more on the history of German psychotechnics, about which very little has been written, see *Untersuchungen zur Geschichte der Psychologie und Psychotechnik,* ed. Horst Grundlach (Munich: Profil, 1996).

24. *Ueber einen Fall,* pp. 7–8 and 57; Walter Benjamin, *Die literarische Welt* (August 1928), quoted in *Selected Writings,* p. 131; Anja and Georg Mendelssohn, *Der Mensch in der Handschrift* (Leipzig: E. A. Seemann, 1928).

25. Ellic Howe, *Astrology and the Third Reich: A Historical Study of Astrological Beliefs in Western Europe since 1700 and in Hitler's Germany, 1933–45* (Wellingborough, Northants.: Aquarian Press, 1984), pp. 95–100. This is the only study of German astrology available, and its focus is astrology's fate under the Nazis; see, however, the interesting comments by Paul Forman in "Weimar Culture, Causality, and Quantum Theory, 1918–27: Adaptation by German Physicists and Mathematicians to a Hostile Intellectual Environment," *Historical Studies in the Physical Sciences* 3 (1971): 1–115.

26. Hans Driesch, "Einführung," in H. von Klöckler, *Astrologie als Erfahrungswissenschaft* (Leipzig: Emmanuel Reinicke, 1926); from the series *Metaphysik und Weltanschauung,* ed. Hans Driesch and Werner Schingnitz.

27. Klöckler, *Astrologie,* the foreword and 191–92; see also part 2, where he presents his data.

28. Heinz Artur Strauß, "Zur Beurteilung der Einwände," *Süddeutsche Monatshefte* 24, no. 9 (1927): 173–76; Werner Achelis, "Astrologie und Menschenkunde," *Süddeutsche Monatshefte* 24, no. 9 (1927): 180–82. Both explicitly refrained from making any deterministic claims for astrological factors.

29. P. Phil. Schmidt, S.J., "Zur astrologischen Bewegung," *Klerusblatt* 16, no. 34 (1935): 579.

30. Karl Brandler-Pracht, *Erfolgreiches, glückliches Leben durch Beachtung der Tattwischen, und Astralen Einflüsse: Ein Schlüssel zur praktischen Verwendung der mit dem menschlichen Leben engverbundenen kosmischen Schwingungen, wodurch jedermann zum Herrn seines Geschickes werden kann* (Berlin-Pankow: Linser-Verlag, 1920).

31. Karl Brandler-Pracht, *Die astrologische Deutung: Diagnose und Prognose,* ed. Maria Brandler-Pracht (Berlin: Falken-Verlag Erich Sicker, n.d.), pp. 9–11.

32. See the folder on Michael Georg Conrad and Paul Jury, Monacensia Literaturarchiv, Stadtbibliothek München.

33. "Briefkasten," *Zentralblatt für Okkultismus* 12, no. 6 (1918): 284–87.

34. C. A. Browne, "Observations upon the Use of the Divining Rod in Germany," *Science* 73 (23 January 1931): 86.

35. Fanny Moser, *Der Okkultismus: Täuschungen und Tatsachen,* vol. 2 (Munich: Ernst Reinhardt, 1935), p. 606.

36. Hans Gross, *Handbuch für Untersuchungsrichter als System der Kriminalistik* (1893).

37. The history of forensic science has yet to be written: see *The Encyclopedia of Police Science* (1989), s.v., "Forensic Science," pp. 232–33.

38. Egbert Müller, *Der Spiritismus und die Criminal-Polizei: Mit Anhang über das Spiritistische um den Wende'schen Mord* (Berlin: Karl Siegismund, 1890).

39. "Verbot der Beschäftigung von sog. Kriminaltelepathen. Rd Erl. d. Pr. MdJ. vom 3.4.1929," PDM 7104, StArMü.

40. Moser, *Der Okkultismus,* pp. 610–11; Carl Pelz, *Das Hellsehen: Ein Kriminalfall* (Munich: Ludendorffs Verlag, 1937), pp. 7–8. Albert Hellwig, *Okkultismus und Ver-*

brechen: Eine Einführung in die kriminalistischen Probleme des Okkultismus für Polizeibeamte, Richter, Staatsanwälte, Psychiater, und Sachverständige (Berlin: P. Langenscheidt, 1929), pp. 29–30.

41. Ubald Tartaruga, *Aus dem Reiche des Hellsehwunders: Neue retroskopische Versuche* (Pfullingen in Württemburg: Johannes Baum, 1925?), pp. 25–26.

42. Hermann, "Die Iserlohner Hellseher-Experimente," *Kriminalistische Monatshefte* 10 (October 1928): 224.

43. Hans Knör, "Kriminal Telepathie," *Aus dem Rechtsleben* (weekly supplement to *Münchener Zeitung*) (4 April 1927), PDM 7107, StArMü.

44. Hellwig, *Okkultismus und Verbrechen.* The entire book is a critique of the practice.

45. Otto Seeling, *Der Bernburger Hellseher-Prozeß* (Berlin-Pankow: Linser-Verlag, 1925), pp. 28–30.

46. Seeling, *Hellseher-Prozeß* gives the fullest account of the trial from a sympathetic perspective; see also the newspaper clippings relating to this case assembled in PDM 7107, StArMü, and the discussion in Hellwig, *Okkultismus und Verbrechen,* pp. 245–46.

47. Seeling, *Hellseher-Prozeß,* pp. 39, 41, 43–44, and 51.

48. Hellwig, *Okkultismus und Verbrechen,* pp. 88–89.

49. Charles Rosenberg, "Holism in Twentieth-Century Medicine," in *Greater than the Parts: Holism in Biomedicine, 1920–1950,* ed. Christopher Lawrence and George Weisz (New York: Oxford University Press, 1998), pp. 340–41.

50. Hubert Knoblauch, *Die Welt der Wünschelrutengänger und Pendler: Erkundungen einer verborgenen Wirklichkeit* (Frankfurt: Campus Verlag, 1991), pp. 74–77.

51. Carl von Klinckowstroem, *Bibliographie der Wünschelrute* (Munich: Kommissions Verlag v. Ottmar Schönhuth, 1911), pp. 103–4; Carl von Klinckowstroem and Rudolf von Maltzahn, *Handbuch der Wünschelrute: Geschichte, Wissenschaft, Anwendung* (Munich: R. Oldenbourg, 1931), p. 72–75.

52. Klinckowstroem, *Bibliographie,* p. 110.

53. Ibid., p. 114; "Sitzungsprotokoll," *Bericht über die Tagung des Verbandes zur Klärung der Wünschelrutenfrage in Halle a. S., 18–20. September 1913* (Stuttgart: Konrad Wittwer, 1914), p. 8.

54. Klinckowstroem, *Bibliographie,* pp. 109–10, 114–17, 119, 122–23, 127, 131–32.

55. "Sitzungsprotokoll," p. 8; see also "Des Landrats von Uslar Arbeiten mit der Wünschelrute in Südwestafrika," *Schriften des Verbands zur Klärung der Wünschelrutenfrage* 1 (Stuttgart: Konard Wittwer, 1912).

56. "Mitglieder-Verzeichnis des Verbandes der Wünschelrutenfrage," *Schriften des Verbands zur Klärung der Wünschelrutenfrage* 3 (Stuttgart: Konrad Wittwer, 1912), p. 60.

57. Ibid., pp. 53–60.

58. The club also published the *Zeitschrift für Wünschelrutenforschung,* in print as early as 1923. In 1934, the group merged with other dowsing clubs to form the *Reichsverband für das Wünschelrutenwesen,* which was still in existence as late as 1938: Rep. 42, Acc. 2147, Nr. 27303, Landesarchiv Berlin.

59. "Wünschelrute und Erdstrahlen," *Münchner Tagblatt* 349 (15 December 1933): 4.

60. See, for example, A. Rothacker and H. Degler, "Das magische Reis und seine Probleme," *Hippokrates* (8 April 1937): 331–38.

61. Francé-Harrar, *Mein Fin de Siècle,* p. 138.

62. Carl von Klinckowstroem, *Von den Tricks der Medien* (Munich: A. Huber, 1932).

63. "Sitzungsprotokoll," p. 11.

64. Klinckowstroem and Maltzahn, *Handbuch der Wünschelrute,* pp. 125–26, 128, and plate 11 (between pp. 108–9). Maltzahn claimed to have experienced partial paralysis as well as disturbance of his breathing and heart beat during two separate sojourns at a hotel on the Rhine. His symptoms would disappear for a few days if he moved rooms, but then would always return stronger than ever a few days later. He also mentioned the experiences of a family whose members fell sick whenever they moved houses, despite neither side of the extended family having had a history of cancer. Without assuming that all cancer had its cause in water and land formations, Maltzahn nevertheless insisted that the siting of houses *(Örtlichkeit der Häuser)* could lead to the sickening of the human body.

65. See the essays by Kees Gispen (on engineers) and Vincent Clark (on architects) in *German Professions, 1800–1950,* ed. Geoffrey Cocks and Konrad H. Jarausch (New York: Oxford University Press, 1990); see also Kees Gispen, *New Profession, Old Order: Engineers and German Society, 1815–1914* (Cambridge: Cambridge University Press, 1989).

66. Gunda Wegner, "Das Leben des Georg von Langsdorff: Turner, Revolutionär, und Wissenschaftler," *Zeitschrift des Breisgau-Geschichtsvereins "Schau-ins-Land"* 3 (1992): 90.

67. Mathilde Scholl in Cologne to Wilhelm Hübbe-Schleiden in Göttingen, 27 March 1909, in Norbert Klatt, *Theosophie und Anthroposophie: Neue Aspekte zu ihrer Geschichte aus dem Nachlaß von Wilhelm Hübbe-Schleiden, 1846–1916, mit einer Auswahl von 81 Briefen* (Göttingen: Klatt, 1993), pp. 180–81.

68. Paul Zillmann, "Briefe über Mystik an einen Freund," *Neue Metaphysische Rundschau* 1, nos. 3–4 (1897): 198–99.

69. Marie Tonndorf, "Diätetische Winke," *Theosophie* 19, no. 3 (1931): 145–46.

70. Carsten Timmerman, "Constitutional Medicine, Neoromanticism, and the Politics of Antimechanism in Interwar Germany," *Bulletin for the History of Medicine* 75 (2001): 717–39; see also Michael Hau, "The Holistic Gaze in German Medicine, 1890–1930," *Bulletin for the History of Medicine* 74 (2000): 495–524.

71. Detlev Peukert, *The Weimar Republic: The Crisis of Classical Modernity,* trans. Richard Deveson (New York: Hill & Wang, 1989), pp. 135 and 138–39.

72. For a thoughtful review of terminological issues, see Robert Jütte, "The Historiography of Nonconventional Medicine in Germany: A Concise Overview," *Medical History* 43, no. 1 (1999): 342–58. My discussion uses the terms *conventional* (or *orthodox*) and *alternative,* and draws on Jütte's definition of conventional medicine as "the medical system which enjoys the approval, co-operation, and protection of a country's legal system and other supporting social institutions (e.g., sick funds, government licensing bodies, research agencies)" (p. 343).

73. Claudia Huerkamp, "Medizinische Lebensreform im späten 19. Jahrhundert: Die Naturheilbewegung in Deutschland als Protest gegen die naturwissenschaftliche Universitätsmedizin," *Vierteljahrschrift für Sozial-und Wirtschaftsgeschichte* 73, no. 2 (1986): 158–82.

74. For an excellent examination of how this law played out in Bavaria, see Michael Stolberg, "Alternative Medicine, Irregular Healers, and the Medical Market

in Nineteenth-Century Bavaria," *Historical Aspects of Unconventional Medicine: Approaches, Concepts, Case Studies,* ed. Robert Jütte, Motzi Eklöf, and Marie C. Nelson (Sheffield, Yorks.: European Association for the History of Medicine and Health Publications, 2001), pp. 139–62.

75. Wolfgang R. Krabbe, *Gesellschaftsveränderung durch Lebensreform: Strukturmerkmale einer sozialreformerischen Bewegung in Deutschland der Industrialisierungsperiode* (Göttingen: Vandenhoeck & Ruprecht, 1974), pp. 13–15. For further information on Lebensreform and the natural healing movement, see *Handbuch der deutschen Reformbewegungen, 1880–1933,* ed. Diethart Kerbs and Jürgen Reulecke (Wuppertal: Hammer, 1998); Robert Jütte, *Geschichte der Alternativen Medizin: Von der Volksmedizin zu den unkonventionallen Therapien von heute* (Munich: C. H. Beck, 1996); Cornelia Regin, *Selbsthilfe und Gesundheitspolitik: Die Naturheilbewegung im Kaiserreich, 1889–1914* (Stuttgart: Franz Steiner, 1995); and Karl E. Rothschuh, *Naturheilbewegung Reformbewegung Alternativbewegung* (Stuttgart: Hippokrates, 1983) (see the cautionary comments about this source in Jütte, "The Historiography," pp. 353–54).

76. "Ein Lourdes-Prozeß," *Münchner Neueste Nachrichten,* 26 November 1908; see also David Blackbourn, *Marpingen: Apparitions of the Virgin Mary in a Nineteenth-Century German Village* (Oxford: Oxford University Press, 1993), pp. 146–63 and passim for further connections between popular religion and unorthodox healing methods.

77. Dingfelder, *Ludwig Aub als Hellseher,* p. 38.

78. Gustav Zeller, "Mediale Diagnostik," *Der Okkultismus* 1, no. 2 (1925): 24. Such applications recall the seeress of Prevorst, who used her mesmeric skills to diagnose patients at a distance. For other examples of medical mediumism, see Zeller, "Mediale Diagnostik," p. 25; *Zentralblatt für Okkultismus* 5, no. 2 (1911): 127; and " 'Wunderheilungen' in einem Schwarzwalddorf: Ein ungewöhnlicher Fall von Hellseher-Diagnose: Wissenschaftliche Gutachten," *Zeitschrift für Seelenleben, Beilage* 32, no. 1 (1928): 7–8.

79. G. W. Surya, Okkulte Medizin: 5, *Okkulte Diagnostik und Prognostik,* 2nd ed. (Berlin-Pankow: Linser-Verlag, 1923). Surya's ideas inspired the founders of the Leipzig reform sanitarium Lichtort in 1932. In its healing regime, the institute used occult techniques, including graphology, astrology, and the sidereal pendulum; see Emmy Schumann, "Denkschrift zur Gründung des 'Lichtort-Kurheimes' in Leipzig," Friedrich Kallenberg, *Der Siegeszug des siderischen Pendels, 1911–1934* (Diessen vor München: Jos. C. Huber, 1934), pp. 160–64.

80. Although Heimsoth accepted the diagnostic insights of astrological character analysis for medical practice, he nevertheless professed little use for astrology's supposed predictive powers: Karl-Günther Heimsoth, "Astrologie und medizinische Charakterologie," *14 Vorträge über Astrologie: Gehalten auf dem VIII. Astrologen-Kongress Nürnberg, 1929,* ed. Hubert Korsch (Düsseldorf: Otto Fritz, 1929), pp. 47–50. Heimsoth, a psychoanalyst, also became chair in 1931 of the *Akademische Gesellschaft für astrologische Forschung.* This group included several men with medical and scientific degrees, among whom were the chemist Joachim Winkelmann, the soon-to-be astronomer Erich Winkel, the lawyers Ueberhorst and Winterberg (the defense attorney in several court cases on criminal mediumism), and Drs. Fritz Quade and Friedrich Schwab: "Satzung der Akademischen Gesellschaft für astrologische Forschung" (9 July 1924), Rep. 42, Acc. 2147, Nr. 26675, Landesarchiv Berlin. Heimsoth seems to have had more than a passing acquaintance with the radical Right as well; see his flattering

participant's portrayal of the Freikorps in *Freikorps greift an: Militärpolitische Geschichte und Kritik der Angriffs-Unternehmen in Oberschlesien, 1921* (Berlin: Kampf Verlag, 1930). For his correspondence with Ernst Röhm on Röhm's homosexuality and what Heimsoth made of it, see *Der Fall Röhm* (Berlin: Selbstverlag Dr. Helmut Klotz, c. 1932).

81. B. Wehdanner, "Psychoanalytik, Magnetopath, und Pendelforscher," PDM 7109, StArMü. For further medical applications of characterology, see the case of Erich Radloff/Emil Korrand in PDM 7107, StArMü; the case of Josef Hillenmeier in PDM 7109, StArMü; and the list of doctors practicing such techniques mentioned in A. Frank Glahn, *Glahns Pendel-Bücherei:* 1, *Der Gebrauch* (Memmingen: Uranus, 1936), pp. 105–6.

82. Erwin Liek, "Zünstige und unzünstige Wunderheiler," *Süddeutsche Monatshefte* 30 (November 1932): 82–84.

83. Jütte, *Geschichte der Alternativen Medizin*, pp. 42–45. For further information on this journal, see Detlef Bothe, *Neue Deutsche Heilkunde, 1933–1945: Dargestellt anhand der Zeitschrift "Hippokrates" und der Entwicklung der volksheilkundlichen Laienbewegung* (Husum: Matthiesen Verlag, 1991).

84. Dr. med. Hartung, "Okkulte Medizin," *Der Okkultismus* 1 (September 1925): 30. In 1925, Liek published a much-discussed article on "the crisis of medicine" in *Münchner Medizinische Wochenschrift* (Munich medical weekly).

85. Hartung, "Okkulte Medizin," p. 31.

86. Ibid., p. 32.

87. Ibid., p. 32.

88. Herbert Fritsche, *Iatrosophia: Metabiologische Heilung und Selbstheilung* (Leipzig: Richard Hummel Verlag, 1937). For his connections to Meyrink, see Meyrinkiana, file 1, 1 (Fritsche, Herbert), Handschriftenabteilung, Bayerische Staatsbibliothek.

89. Bernd Wedemeyer, " 'Zum Licht': Die Freikörperkultur in der wilhelminischen Ära und der Weimarer Republik zwischen Völkischer Bewegung, Okkultismus, und Neuheidentum," *Archiv für Kulturgeschichte* 81, no. 1 (1999): 190–91.

90. For a book-length study of Weissenberg, see Ulrich Linse, *Geisterseher und Wunderwirker: Heilssuche im Industriezeitalter* (Frankfurt am Main: Fischer, 1996); see also Frithjof Rohr, *Weißenberg-Heilpraktik* (Berlin-Lichterfeld: Karl Andrikowski, 1934), pp. 6–8.

91. Robert Proctor, *Racial Hygiene: Medicine under the Nazis* (Cambridge: Harvard University Press, 1988), p. 228; Proctor, *Nazi War*, pp. 55–57; see also chapter 9.

92. It is difficult to determine, moreover, exactly how sympathetic some of the supposed prophets of Nazi medicine actually were to the Third Reich. See the comments about the so-called "father of Nazi medicine," Erwin Liek, in Michael Kater, "Die Medizin im nationalsozialistischen Deutschland und Erwin Liek," *Geschichte und Gesellschaft* 16 (1990): 440–63.

93. Alexander Müller, *Kosmische und irdische Strahlen als Erreger der Krankheiten* (Hamburg: Steffens, 1930), p. 78.

94. *Psychomagnetisches-suggestives Heilinstitut München* (Prospekt) (Munich, c. 1910).

95. *Zentrale für praktischen Okkultismus* (n.p., n.d.), pp. 31–36.

96. G. Reinhardt, "Psychologische Diagnosen," *Zentralblatt für Okkultismus* 1, no. 8 (1908): 337. G. Reinhardt, "Psychologische Diagnosen," *Zentralblatt für Okkultismus* 1, no. 10 (1908): 433.

97. David Hollinger, "The Knower and the Artificer," *Modernist Impulses*, p. 26.

CHAPTER SEVEN: The Crimes of Anna Rothe

This chapter is a revised version of "The Culture of Knowledge in the Metropolis of Science: Spiritualism and Liberalism in Fin-de-Siècle Berlin," which appeared in *Wissenschaft und Oeffentlichkeit in Berlin, 1870–1930*, ed. Constantin Goschler (Wiesbaden: Franz Steiner Verlag, 2000), pp. 127–54.

1. The various accounts of Rothe's arrest agree on all details except the date, which some give as December 1901, others as March 1902. I have chosen to use the spring date documented in "Anna Rothe, das Blumenmedium," *Berliner Tageblatt*, 12 March 1903, and other contemporary periodicals. For the alternate date, see Hugo Friedlaender, *Interessante Kriminal-Prozesse von kulturhistorischer Bedeutung: Darstellung merkwürdiger Strafrechtsfälle aus Gegenwart und Jüngstvergangenheit* (Berlin: Hermann Barsdorf, 1910), p. 211.

2. "Anna Rothe, das Blumenmedium," *Berliner Tageblatt*, 12 March 1903.

3. Hugo Friedlaender, *Interessante Kriminal-Prozesse*, p. 211. "Prison for a Spiritualist," *New York Times*, 29 March 1903, p. 5; E. T. H., "Trial of a German Medium," *New York Times*, 11 April 1903, p. 2.

4. I borrow the term *epistemological anarchism* from Paul Feyerabend, *Science in a Free Society* (London: Verso, 1985), pp. 125–28.

5. For a general discussion, see Steven Shapin, "Science and the Public," in *Companion to the History of Modern Science*, ed. R. C. Olby (London: Routledge, 1990), pp. 990–1007.

6. For German liberalism, see my discussion in chapter 4.

7. Erich Bohn, *Der Fall Rothe: Eine criminal-psychologische Untersuchung* (Breslau: S. Schottlaender, 1901), p. 54.

8. Bohn, *Der Fall Rothe*, p. 3. Paladino had been investigated in 1892 in Milan by an international panel of experts whose ranks included the Italian doctor Cesare Lombroso, the French physiologist Charles Richet, the Italian astronomer Giovanni Schiaparelli, and the German philosopher Carl du Prel. The majority of the panel had been willing to sign a document testifying to Paladino's powers as a physical medium. Other famous physical mediums of the day included Henry Slade and D. D. Home (from the United States) and Mrs. Guppy, William Eglinton, and Florence Cook (from Britain).

9. M. J., "Anna Rothe," *Spiritistische Rundschau* 9, no. 4 (1902): 74–76. Corroboratory biographical information can be found in Bohn, *Der Fall Rothe*, pp. 2–3, and "Das Blumenmedium Anna Rothe vor Gericht," *Berliner Tageblatt*, 23 March 1903.

10. Bohn, *Der Fall Rothe*, pp. 2 and 88–89.

11. Ibid., pp. 8–14. Note that Bohn reprints the published protocols of many different séances, both of those he attended and others that he did not.

12. Liberal theology was a late-nineteenth-century movement across Europe and the United States that stressed the importance of personal experience in the formation of religious belief. Insisting on a fundamental methodological parallel between religion and science, adherents of liberal theology considered religion to be a mode of inquiry that—like science—should be empirical, rational, and tentative. Although this aspect of spiritualism has been explored in the American and British contexts, it has been almost completely neglected in the German one. For the classic discussion of liberal theology, see Ian Barbour, *Issues in Science and Religion* (New York: Harper & Row, 1971), pp.

104–8 and 126. For some discussion of the connections between spiritualism and German democratic impulses, see Ulrich Linse, *Geisterseher und Wunderwirker: Heilssuche im Industriezeitalter* (Frankfurt: Fischer, 1996), pp. 55–87.

13. Kap. 35, N146, Stadtarchiv Leipzig.

14. Egbert Müller, *Der Spuk von Resau* (Berlin: Karl Siegismund, 1889); Egbert Müller, *Stellung des Strafrichters zum Spiritismus und der Prozeß Valeska Töpfer* (Berlin: I. F. Conrads Buchhandlung, 1892); Albert Moll, *Der Spiritismus* (Stuttgart: Franckh'sche Verlagshandlung, 1925), pp. 58–59. For a fraud case in Munich, see Dr. Geipel, "Zwei Processe gegen spiritistische Medien," *Münchener Medizinische Wochenschrift* (4 May 1898): 664–67.

15. Bohn, *Der Fall Rothe*, pp. 34–36. Bohn reprints the reports sent to him by these two men.

16. Ibid., pp. 3 and 33; Erich Bohn, *Der Welt Spiegel*, 16 March 1902. Note that Rahn edited *Die übersinnliche Welt*. For a review of these and other exposures, see also C. W. Sellin, "Frau Rothe und die Wissenschaft," *Psychische Studien* 28 (November 1901): 687–706.

17. Bohn, *Der Fall Rothe*, p. 17.

18. Ibid., p. 150. The Latin translates as "so that no harm comes to the public."

19. Bohn was the chair of the Gesellschaft für psychische Forschung in Breslau. In 1896, he and his group broke with the national umbrella group of German occultists, the Verband Deutscher Okkultisten. Whereas the Breslau group regarded occult phenomena as a problem to be investigated according to the methods of the exact sciences, the Verband was involved in the attempt to make these phenomena the basis of a new worldview: "Näheres über den Okkultisten Verband," *Metaphysische Rundschau*, 1, no. 2 (1896): 186–87.

20. Bohn, *Der Fall Rothe*, pp. 29–30 and 124; see also Erich Bohn, "Der Fall Rothe," *Nord und Süd* 96 (February 1901): 223–56.

21. Ferdinand Maack, *Wie Steht's mit dem Spiritismus* (Hamburg: Xenologischer Verlag, 1901), pp. 13 and 65–72. Note that Maack includes an excellent bibliography of material published on Rothe's case after the appearance of Bohn's *Der Fall Rothe*.

22. Rudolf Müller, "Über Okkultismus als Erfahrungswissenschaft und sein Verhältnis zur Psychologie," *Wissenschaftliche Zeitschrift für Okkultismus* 1, nos. 2–3 (1899): 120. The journal that published this article was edited by Maack.

23. Bohn, *Der Fall Rothe*, pp. 59–64.

24. Ibid., p. 153.

25. Frances Haßmann, "Echt oder Unecht," *Nord und Süd* 96 (February 1901): 222.

26. For instance, see Stefan Zweig, *The World of Yesterday*, trans. by Harry Zohn (Lincoln: University of Nebraska Press, 1964), pp. 112–18; originally published as *Die Welt von Gestern: Erinnerungen eines Europäers* (Stockholm: Bermann-Fischer, 1942).

27. Friedlaender, *Interessante Kriminal-Prozesse*, p. 208. For the derogatory connotations that this phrase carried circa 1900, see Otto Ladendorf, *Historisches Schlagwörterbuch* (Strassburg: Karl J. Trübner, 1906), p. 297.

28. For a useful listing of many German occult groups from this period, see Hans-Jürgen Glowka, *Deutsche Okkultgruppen, 1875–1937* (Munich: Arbeitsgemeinschaft für Religions-und Weltanschauungsfragen, 1981).

29. R. Henneberg, "Ueber Spiritismus und Geistesstörung," *Archiv für Psychiatrie und Nervenkrankheiten* 34, no. 3 (1901): 998–1039.

30. *Spiritistische Rundschau* 9, no. 5 (1902): 117, and idem 9, no. 6 (1902): 141.

31. *Neue Metaphysische Rundschau* 1, no. 1 (1897), statement of purpose opposite the table of contents.

32. Egbert Müller, *Der Spiritismus und die Criminal-Polizei* (Berlin: Karl Siegismund, 1890). As early as 1890, Müller suggested that the local police use mediums to help apprehend criminals and urged the state to spend public funds to study other possible applications of occultism. Note that Müller abruptly converted to Roman Catholicism in 1897 and henceforth renounced spiritualism as demonism; see Egbert Müller, *Der Babelismus, der Kaiser, und die orthodoxe Theologie* (Berlin: Stuhr, 1903).

33. Egbert Müller, *Der Spuk von Resau*, 3rd ed. (Berlin: Karl Siegismund, 1889), pp. 52–53. Müller's liberal leanings come out further in his edited volume *Bismarck Assessed by His Contemporaries*. The book, he explained, gathered together the opinions of leading public figures like Ludwig Büchner, Moritz von Egidy, Theodor Fontane, Rudyard Kipling, Herbert Spencer, Émile Zola, and Cesare Lombroso so as to provide "the public" with a "living court" in which Bismarck's significance would be judged; see *Bismarck im Urteil seiner Zeitgenossen: Hundert Gutachten von Freund und Feind*, ed. Egbert Müller (Berlin: Gegenwart, c. 1895), p. 7.

34. Rudolf Steiner, *Theosophy: An Introduction to the Supersensible Knowledge of the World and the Destination of Man* (New York: Anthroposophic Press, 1923), p. viii.

35. Albert Moll, *Ein Leben als Arzt der Seele: Erinnerungen* (Dresden: Carl Reissner, 1936), pp. 100–101. Eventually, both Moltkes became followers of Steiner; see John C. G. Röhl, *The Kaiser and His Court: Wilhelm II and the Government of Germany* (Cambridge: Cambridge University Press, 1987), p. 64. Also see *Light for the New Millenium: Rudolf Steiner's Association with Helmuth and Eliza von Moltke: Letters, Documents, and After-Death Communications*, ed. T. H. Meyer (London: Rudolf Steiner Press, 1997).

36. Diethard Sawicki, *Leben mit den Toten: Geisterglauben und die Entstehung des Spiritismus in Deutschland, 1770–1900* (Paderborn: Ferdinand Schöningh, 2002), p. 337.

37. The others were Axel von Varnbüler and Kuno Moltke: Isabel Hull, *The Entourage of Kaiser Wilhelm II, 1888–1918* (Cambridge: Cambridge University Press, 1982), pp. 68–73; Röhl, *The Kaiser*, p. 66.

38. Henneberg, "Ueber Spiritismus und Geistesstörung," pp. 998–1039.

39. These included the philosopher Max Dessoir and the psychiatrist Albert Moll, both of whom belonged to Berlin's first psychical research circle, the Gesellschaft für Experimentalpsychologie (f. 1888), and maintained a combative relationship with the occult movement throughout their lives; see Max Dessoir, *Buch der Erinnerung* (Stuttgart: Ferdinand Enke, 1947), pp. 116–37, and Moll, *Ein Leben*, pp. 128–43.

40. Otto Riemann, *Ein aufklärendes Wort über den Spiritismus* (Berlin: R. J. Müller, 1901).

41. "Prediger D. Riemann gegen den Spiritismus," *Spiritistische Rundschau* 8, no. 2 (1900): 58–60; Bohn, *Der Fall Rothe*, pp. 71–72.

42. "Berliner Festwoche: Pastoral-Konferenz," *Neue Preussische Zeitung* 273 (14 June 1900). For more on Stoecker, see Andrew Lees, "Deviant Sexuality and Other 'Sins': The Views of Protestant Conservatives in Imperial Germany," *German Studies Review* 23, no. 3 (2000), 453–76.

43. "Berliner Festwoche: Pastoral-Konferenz," *Neue Preussische Zeitung* 275 (15 June 1900). Spiritualism continued to be a main topic of discussion among the assembled clergymen on the third and final day of the conference as well. The assembly proposed

but, due to insufficient numbers, was not able to pass a resolution condemning spiritualism as an error.

44. Hugh McLeod, introduction to *European Religion in the Age of Great Cities, 1830–1930*, ed. Hugh McLeod (London: Routledge, 1995), pp. 10–14.

45. Verband Deutscher Okkultisten, *Bericht über die Verhandlungen auf dem Dritten Congress des "Verbandes Deutscher Okkultisten," am 31. Mai und 1. Juni (Pfingsten) in München* (Selbstverlag, c. 1898), pp. 3–13.

46. Frederick Gregory, *Nature Lost? Natural Science and the German Theological Traditions of the Nineteenth Century* (Cambridge: Harvard University Press, 1992), p. 62.

47. Lay occultists can also be seen as belonging to German cultural Protestantism. Cultural Protestantism was a fin-de-siècle social movement hostile to the church hierarchy, sympathetic to such liberal ideals as the moral education of the individual, and dedicated to blending Protestant beliefs and scientific ideas for the improvement of German social and political life. Most recently, historians have studied this important social phenomenon as it was manifested in cultural sciences like theology, pedagogy, and economics circa 1900. Lay occultists belonged to a more populist and less-studied segment of cultural Protestantism; see Gangolf Hübinger, *Kulturprotestantismus und Politik: Zum Verhältnis von Liberalismus und Protestantismus im wilhelminischen Deutschland* (Tübingen: J. C. B. Mohr, 1994) and *Kultur und Kulturwissenschaften um 1900: Krise der Moderne und Glaube an die Wissenschaft*, ed. Rüdiger vom Bruch, Friedrich Wilhelm Graf, and Gangolf Hübinger (Stuttgart: Franz Steiner, 1989).

48. Dr. Riemann, "Die Entlarvungen des 'Blumenmediums' Anna Rothe und anderer 'Medien' und ihre Bedeutung für die spiritistische Bewegung," *Reformation* 1, no. 1 (1902): 9.

49. O. Henne am Rhyn, "Tragödien und Komödien des Aberglaubens: das Blumenmedium," *Die Gartenlaube* 12 (1902): 210–11.

50. Friedlaender, *Interessante Kriminal-Prozesse*, 218–37. Corroboratory evidence on all aspects of the trial can be found in the day-by-day coverage given in *Berliner Tageblatt*, 21 March–2 April 1903.

51. Friedlaender, *Interessante Kriminal-Prozesse*, pp. 218–19 and 233–34.

52. Ibid., pp. 218–21.

53. My thanks to Ben Hett for this information about Rothe's defense lawyers. The names of the two defense attorneys were Willy Thiele and Schwindt.

54. Friedlaender, *Interessante Kriminal-Prozesse*, p. 224.

55. Ibid., pp. 222–24.

56. Ibid., pp. 219 and 231.

57. Ibid., pp. 235–36.

58. Ibid., pp. 237–42.

59. E. T. H., "Trial," p. 2; Friedlaender, *Interessante Kriminal-Prozesse*, pp. 241–42.

60. Ibid., p. 2. For the response of the occult community, which echoed many of the opinions discussed in this section, see in particular Victor Blüthgen, "Vom Rothe-Prozess," *Psychische Studien* 30 (April 1903): 257–64; Fritz Freimar, "Ein Nachtrag zum Fall Rothe," *Psychische Studien* 30 (December 1903): 731–44; and Carl Obertimpfler, "Rand-Glossen zum Rothe-Prozess," *Die übersinnliche Welt* (1903): 187–92 and 229–35. Note that Blüthgen was the husband of the trance poet Clara Eysell-Kilburger, discussed in chapter 5.

61. "Anna Rothe & Co.," *Die Zukunft* 43 (4 April 1903): 44–45.

62. Caliban, "Die Betrügerin," *Die Gegenwart* 63, no. 14 (1903): 209–10.

63. Dr. jur. Grüttefien, "Der Fall Rothe in neuer Beleuchtung," *Berliner Tageblatt*, 4 April 1903.

64. Fedor von Zobeltitz, *Chronik der Gesellschaft unter dem letzten Kaiserreich* 2 (Hamburg: Alster, 1922), p. 34.

65. Max Dessoir, "Der Fall Rothe," *Die Woche* 14 (4 April 1903): 596–97.

66. Ibid., p. 597.

67. "Anna Rothe & Co.," *Die Zukunft* 43 (4 April 1903): 46.

68. Caliban, "Die Betrügerin," pp. 209–10.

69. Erich Sello, "Der Prozeß Rothe," *Die Zukunft* 43 (18 April 1903): 93. This is also an extended critique of the legal details of the trial.

70. "Der Kampf gegen die Dummheit," *Berliner Tageblatt*, 1 April 1903.

71. This is the major theme in James Sheehan, *German Liberalism in the Nineteenth Century* (Chicago, IL: University of Chicago Press, 1978).

72. See the earlier quoted passage in Bohn's introduction.

73. Otto Henne am Rhyn, *Eine Reise durch das Reich des Aberglaubens* (Leipzig: Max Spohr, 1893).

74. For information on the press of Max Spohr, see *Lexikon deutschen Verlage: Eine Chronik der deutschen Verlagsfirmen, enthaltend die Geschichte der Zeitungs-, Zeitschriften und Buchverlage, der Kunst-und Musikverlage, sowie der Katalogantiquare* (Leipzig: Curt Müller, c. 1930), p. 191.

75. Andreas Daum makes a related point in his recent study of scientific popularization, where he devotes systematic attention to the many channels and settings by which science and bourgeois culture grew together in nineteenth-century Germany; see Andreas Daum, *Wissenschaftspopularisierung im 19. Jahrhundert: bürgerliche Kultur, naturwissenschaftliche Bildung und die deutsche Öffentlichkeit, 1848–1914* (Munich: Oldenbourg, 1998).

CHAPTER EIGHT: Between Church and State

1. B. Wehdanner, "Psychoanalytik, Magnetopath, und Pendelforscher," PDM 7109, StArMü. When dangled over the body of a sick person, the sidereal pendulum supposedly swings in an irregular pattern that informs the investigator about the cause and cure of the patient's sickness. For expert opinion solicited by the Munich police on this practice, see the police report of 21 January 1926, PDM 7109, StArMü.

2. "Pendelforschung ist Strahlenforschung," PDM 7109, StArMü.

3. Alois Mager, "Der Katholizismus und die okkulten Strömungen," *Der Katholizismus als Lösung großer Menschheitsfragen* (Innsbruck: Verlagsanstalt Tyrolia, 1925), p. 103.

4. Traugott Konstantin Oesterreich, *Der Okkultismus im modernen Weltbild*, 3rd ed. (Dresden: Im Sibyllen-Verlag, 1923), pp. 14–18.

5. Carl du Prel, *Das Rätsel des Menschen: Einleitung in das Studium der Geheimwissenschaften* (Leipzig: Philipp Reclam, 1892), pp. 4–5.

6. Keith Yandell, "Protestant Theology and Natural Science in the Twentieth Century," in *God and Nature: Historical Essays on the Encounter between Christianity and Science*, ed. D. C. Lindberg and R. L. Numbers (Berkeley: University of California Press, 1986), pp. 448–50.

7. Paul Tillich, *The Religious Situation* (New York: Meridian Books, 1956), pp. 166–71; originally published as *Die religiöse Lage der Gegenwart* (Berlin: Ullstein, 1926).

8. M. Krawielitzki, *Gottesbund (Loge) Tanatra, Bund der Kämpfer für Glauben und Wahrheit (Horpeniten), Der Engel Jehovas* (Bad Blankenburg: Harfe, n.d.), pp. 6 and 11, CA AC-S 273, ADW.

9. W. B., "Okkultismus," in Walther Buntzel, *Handbuch für das kirchliche Amt* (Leipzig: J. C. Hinrichs'sche Buchhandlung, 1928), p. 439. For a similar distinction originally made by a Protestant commentator in 1912, see Paul Scheurlen, *Die Sekten der Gegenwart und neuere Weltanschauungsgebilde* (Stuttgart: Verlag der Evangelischen Gesellschaft, 1930).

10. The main goal of the *Apologetische Centrale* was to gather and disseminate information about groups, including occult ones, whose worldviews conflicted with Protestantism. It also provided a forum for the discussion of contemporary social issues.

11. Letter from Gerhard Richter to Apologetische Centrale, 14 November 1929, CA AC 216, ADW.

12. Letter to Herr Dr. Neustätter, CA AC 214, ADW.

13. Pfarrer Kircher, "Meine Antwort auf den neuesten Angriff der 'Horpena,'" CA AC-S 171, ADW. For legal proceedings against this group and its so-called Bombastus Factory, which manufactured healing products according to Paracelsian recipes, see Albert von Schrenck-Notzing, *Der Prozess der Bombastus-Werke und sonstige Beiträge zur forensischen und psychologischen Beurteilung spiritistischer Medien*, in *Sonderabdruck aus der Kriminalanthropologie und Kriminalistik*, ed. Hans Gross (Leipzig: F. C. W. Vogel, 1910).

14. Dora Hasselblatt, "Falsche Propheten," pp. 1 and 4–10, CA AC-S 45, ADW.

15. "Aus einem Briefe einer Anhängerin der Bo Yen Ra-Bewegung [*sic*]," CA AC-S 45, ADW.

16. Letter from Johannes Berger on 16 October 1928, CA AC 214, ADW.

17. *Aberglaube—was steckt dahinter?* CA AC-S 1, ADW.

18. The file dates these c. 1931: CA AC-S 319, ADW.

19. *Die Bereitschaft* (August 1928), CA AC-S 25, ADW. For more on the Protestant stance toward astrology, see Gerhard Richter, "Astrologie," in pamphlet *Stoffsammlung für Schulungsarbeit* 10 (n.d.), pp. 1–3, CA AC-S 26, ADW.

20. *Allgemeine Zeitung* (Augsburg), 122 (2 May 1853).

21. For a description of the official Roman Catholic position on spiritualism, see *The New Catholic Encyclopedia* 8 (1967), s.v., "Spiritism," pp. 576–77.

22. Rudolf Mader, "Karl du Prel in Beachtung und Urteil von Nichtokkultisten," *Zentralblatt für Okkultismus* 8, no. 2 (1914): 97; Mader quoted from *Die Stadt Gottes* 2 (1899–1900).

23. For a recent statement, see *The New Catholic Encyclopedia* 3, s.v., "Clairvoyance, Spiritual," p. 912.

24. A useful study of Roman Catholic modernism is Lester R. Kurtz, *The Politics of Heresy: The Modernist Crisis in Roman Catholicism* (Berkeley: University of California Press, 1986).

25. Josef Dörfler, *Der Spiritismus (Geistererscheinungen)* (Graz: Katholisches Glaubensapostolat, n.d.), CA AC-S 334, ADW.

26. Julius Beßmer, "Der Okkultismus von heute," *Stimmen der Zeit: Katholische Monatschrift für das Geistesleben der Gegenwart* 102 (February 1922): 338, 345–46, and 352–53.

27. P. Phil. Schmidt S. J., "Zur astrologischen Bewegung," *Klerusblatt* 16, no. 34 (1935): 577–79.

28. Dörfler, *Der Spiritismus*, CA AC-S 334, ADW.

29. Mager, "Der Katholizismus und die okkulten Strömungen," pp. 97, 103, and 111.

30. Beßmer, "Der Okkultismus von heute," pp. 338, 345–46, and 352–53.

31. Gregor v. Holtum, "Apologetik und Okkultismus," *Korrespondenz-und Offertenblatt für die gesamte katholische Geistlichkeit Deutschlands* (1926), 9:167–70.

32. Anton Seitz, *Okkultismus, Wissenschaft, und Religion: 1, Die Welt des Okkultismus* (Munich: Franz A. Pfeiffer, 1926), pp. 9–10 and 12–13; Anton Seitz, "Zum sogenannten wissenschaftlichen Okkultismus," *Bayerischer Kurier* 63, 4 March 1927; 70, 11 March 1927; 74, 15 March 1927; 77, 18 March 1927, ZA Okkultismus, SdArMü.

33. *Deutsches Literatur-Lexikon* 4 (1958), s.v., "Verweyen, Johannes Maria," p. 3118; see also the discussion of Verweyen in chapter 9 of Gerda Walther, *Zum anderen Ufer: Vom Marxismus und Atheismus zum Christentum* (Remagen: Otto Reichl, 1960).

34. Josef Kral, an editor and writer, and Alois Wiesinger, a Cistercian abbot, were prominent in this effort. There was also an International Society of Catholic Parapsychologists; see *The Encyclopedia of Occultism and Parapsychology* 3rd ed. (1991), s.v., "Wiesinger, Alois," "Kral, Josef," and "Humpfner, Winfried Goswin" (an Augustinian with an interest in parapsychology); see also "Programm und Geleitwort," *Erkenntnis und Glaube Christliche Monatsschrift für Parapsychologie, Seelenkunde, und Schicksalsforschung* 1 (15 July 1951).

35. For article 54, see *Das Polizeistrafgesetzbuch für das Königreich Bayern nach dem Stande der Gesetzgebung ab 1. Januar 1900*, annotated by Julius Staudinger (Munich: C. H. Beck, 1900), pp. 44–45.

36. Stellv. Generalkommando I. Bayer. Armeekorps. Bekanntmachung, PDM 3543, StArMü.

37. Albert Hellwig, "Astrologen vor Gericht," *Süddeutsche Monatshefte* 24, no. 9 (1927): 208–10.

38. Karl du Prel, *Der Somnambulismus vor dem königlichen Landgerichte München 1*, Monacensia Bibliothek und Literaturarchiv (Stadtbibliothek, Munich, n.d.), pp. 1–7.

39. Karl du Prel, "Okkultismus und Anarchismus," *Nachgelassene Schriften* (Leipzig: Max Altmann, 1911), pp. 110–11; originally published as "Die Philosophie der Geschichte," *Zukunft* (4 November 1894).

40. For information on the national crackdown on occult activities during the war, see Albert Hellwig, *Weltkrieg und Aberglaube: Erlebtes und Erlauschtes* (Leipzig: Wilhelm Heims, 1916); however, on Oesterreich's cautions about relying on Hellwig's opinions see T. K. Oesterreich, *Psychologisches Gutachten in einem Hellseherprozess* (Stuttgart: Verlag W. Kohlhammer, 1930).

41. Franz Heigl, Überwachung (19 May 1917), PDM 576, StArMü.

42. Franz Heigl an die K. Polizeidirektion (26 May 1917), PDM 576, StArMü.

43. Stellv. Generalkommando I. bayer. Armeekorps, Der Kommandierende General, gez. von der Tann (31 May 1917), PDM 576, StArMü. This disappearance could be due to the state's success in wholly shutting down Haugg's group; alternately, Haugg's

conflicts with the state may have ceased with the return of basic rights of speech and assembly during the 1920s.

44. No. 79859 P 1. Stellv. Generalkommando I. b. A. K. (19 July 1918), PDM 3543, StArMü.

45. Hanna Vogt-Vilseck to kg. Generalkommando (17 October 1918), PDM 3543, StArMü. For further information on this group, see Hans Schlosser to the Polizeidirektion München (12 May 1922); Betreff: Stark Leonhard (16 February 1923); and police form (9.9.1937), all in PDM 3543, StArMü.

46. PDM 678, 682, and 683, StArMü.

47. Vormerkung, PDM 5608, StArMü.

48. Scientific occultism also featured in court cases, but under the heading of fraud. In a 1927 case, for example, the Munich writer and amateur astrologer Max Kemmerich had to defend himself against charges of plagiarism made by Karl Gruber, a professor of biology at the Technical University in Berlin and a collaborator of Schrenck-Notzing; see the letter of Albert von Schrenck-Notzing in Munich on 5 September 1927 and the typescripts of Max Kemmerich, both at the Monacensia Literaturarchiv, Stadtbibliothek, Munich.

49. Urteil Max Grimm (1922), PDM 7111, StArMü. Grimm also published his own account of this sting as A. M. Grimm, *Uranus-Bücher* (Munich: Verlag A. M. Grimm, 1921).

50. Gauklertricks, PDM 7106, StArMü.

51. Report from Johann Knockl (29 November 1926), PDM 7106, StArMü.

52. Report on Margarethe Schicl (23 July 1927), PDM 7105, StArMü.

53. Polizeidirektion München an das Amtsgericht München (13 August 1923), PDM 7114, StArMü.

54. Astrologische Gesellschaft München an die Regierung von Oberbayern, Kammer des Innern, München: PDM 7114, StArMü.

55. Report from H. V. Seeliger, PDM 7105, StArMü. Seeliger used the ironic term *Beschränkte* to describe those with limited intelligence. This was a popular term with Munich literati, who expressed their antipathy toward the city's leading psychical researchers by using the nicknames "the swindled" *(Geprellten)* and "the limited" *(Beschränkten)* to refer to the investigative circles around du Prel and Schrenck-Notzing, respectively; see Hanns von Gumppenberg, *Lebenserinnerungen aus dem Nachlass des Dichters* (Berlin: Eigenbrödler, 1929), p. 108; see also M. G. Conrad, *Gelüftete Masken: Allerlei Charakterköpfe* (Leipzig: Wilhlem Friedrich, 1890), pp. 215–22.

56. H. v. Seeliger (17 July 1921), PDM 7105, StArMü.

57. See material on Karl Höcker in PDM 7113, StArMü. In a similar case that same year, the self-styled psychologist and character researcher Alfons Simon was charged with Gaukelei for having taught palmistry in a public lecture: Betreff Simon Alfons (16 November 1922), PDM 7113, StArMü.

58. Rev. Reg. 2. Nr. 315/1924. Urteil. In der Strafsache gegen die Sekretärsfrau Rosa Amann in München, PDM 7111, StArMü. Anz. Verz. Ziff. XIV 294/26. Berufg. Reg. Nr. 539/26, PDM 7111, StArMü.

59. Betreff Henkes Karl (27 October 1924), PDM 7113, StArMü.

60. Prof. Dr. Specht, Gutachten (7.11.30), PDM 7103, StArMü.

61. Betreff Fick Anton (20.9.31), PDM7113, StArMü.

CHAPTER NINE: The Spectrum of Nazi Responses

1. H. R. Trevor-Roper, *The Last Days of Hitler*, 5th ed. (London: Macmillan, 1978), pp. lix and 251.

2. Trevor-Roper included a footnote to the effect that Goebbels had in fact despised astrology and that the occult had also been the property of the regime's opponents, but these details seem to have eluded all but the most careful readers: Trevor-Roper, *Last Days*, pp. 94–96 and 112–14.

3. Walter Laqueur, foreword to Wilhelm Wulff, *Zodiac and Swastika: How Astrology Guided Hitler's Germany* (New York: Coward, McCann & Geoghegan, 1973), p. 8; originally published as Wilhelm Wulff, *Tierkreis und Hakenkreuz: Als Astrologe an Himmlers Hof* (Gütersloh: Bertelsmann, 1968).

4. Note that chapter 1 discusses the historiography of the Nazis and the occult. Particularly important is Nicholas Goodrick-Clarke's *The Occult Roots of Nazism: Secret Aryan Cults and Their Influence on Nazi Ideology* (New York: New York University Press, 1985), which investigates these links exhaustively.

5. Michael H. Kater, *Doctors under Hitler* (Chapel Hill: University of North Carolina Press, 1989), p. 37.

6. Robert Proctor, *The Nazi War on Cancer* (Princeton, NJ: Princeton University Press, 1999), p. 11.

7. The dowser was Gustav Freiherr von Pohl, a Dachau physician: Proctor, *Nazi War*, p. 137.

8. Goodrick-Clarke, *Occult Roots*, chapter 15; Ian Kershaw, *Hitler, 1889–1936: Hubris* (New York: W. W. Norton, 1998), pp. 50–52.

9. Proctor, *Nazi War*, pp. 250 and 257.

10. Peter Padfield, *Hess: Flight for the Führer* (London: Weidenfeld & Nicolson, 1991), pp. 230–31.

11. Proctor, *Nazi War*, pp. 55–57. For a short character study that explores the two sides of Himmler's character (rational bureaucrat and private mystic), see Joachim Fest, *The Face of the Third Reich: Portraits of the Nazi Leadership* (New York: Pantheon, 1970), pp. 111–24.

12. Felix Kersten, *The Kersten Memoirs, 1940–1945*, introduced by H. R. Trevor-Roper (New York: Macmillan, 1957), pp. 38, 148, and 152. The memoirs were originally published in German (1956).

13. Goodrick-Clarke, *Occult Roots*, pp. 177, 179, 180–83, 186–88, and 190.

14. The main point of Wulff's memoir seems to have been to right the wrongs committed against him by H.-R. Trevor-Roper. Wulff insisted that he had never been a Nazi, had never fulfilled any key function for top functionaries like Himmler, and had been an unwilling worker for the Nazi regime: Wulff, *Zodiac and Swastika*, p. 8.

15. Padfield, *Hess*, pp. 230–32.

16. "Grass eating" was presumably meant as a scathing reference to Hess's vegetarianism: Joseph Goebbels, *Die Tagebücher von Joseph Goebbels, 1, 1940–1941*, ed. Elke Fröhlich (Munich: K. G. Saur, 1998), pp. 310–12 and 315.

17. Witt in Munich to Tiessler in the Propagandaministerium Berlin on 16 May 1941, NS 18 file 497, BA Berlin.

18. Foreword to *Handbuch zur "Völkischen Bewegung," 1871–1918*, ed. Uwe Pusch-

ner, Walter Schmitz, and Justus H. Ulbricht (Munich: K. G. Saur, 1996), p. x; Uwe Puschner, *Die völkische Bewegung im wilhelminischen Kaiserreich: Sprache—Rasse—Religion* (Darmstadt: Wissenschaftliche Buchgesellschaft, 2001), pp. 9–10. Note also that although he was steeped in this milieu and took much from it, Hitler himself came to see the völkisch movement as a rival to Nazism and was especially critical of what he considered the excessive mystical religiosity of völkisch activists. This antipathy toward mysticism also informed his hostility to the occult.

19. For Freemasonry and the Third Reich, see Johannes Rogalla von Bieberstein, *Die These von der Verschwörung, 1776–1945: Philosophen, Freimaurer, Juden, Liberale, und Sozialisten als Verschwörer gegen die Sozialordnung* (Bern: Herbert Lang, 1976); and Ralf Melzer, *Konflikt und Anpassung: Freimaurerei in der Weimarer Republik und im "Dritten Reich,"* ed. A. Pelinka and H. Reinalter (Vienna: Braunmüller, 1999).

20. *The Encyclopedia of the Third Reich*, 2nd ed. (1991), s.v., "Freemasonry," pp. 294–95.

21. Alfred Rosenberg, " 'Deutsche' Freimaurerei," *Völkische Beobachter*, 20 March and 17 April 1921, reprinted in Alfred Rosenberg, *Kampf um die Macht: Aufsätze von 1921–1932*, ed. Thilo von Trotha, 4th ed. (Munich: Franz Eher, 1938), pp. 26 and 30.

22. Alfred Rosenberg, *The Myth of the Twentieth Century: An Evaluation of the Spiritual-Intellectual Confrontations of Our Age* (Newport Beach, CA: Noontide, 1982), pp. 124–25.

23. Günther Hartung, "Völkische Ideologie," in *Handbuch zur "Völkischen Bewegung,"* pp. 39–40.

24. Mathilde Ludendorff, *Ein Blick in die Dunkelkammer der Geisterseher: Moderne Medium-"Forschung": Kritische Betrachtungen zu Dr. von Schrenck-Notzing's "Materialisationsphaenomene"* (Munich: Ludendorffs Verlag, 1937), pp. 9–10 and 20–21. Note that this was earlier published under Ludendorff's first married name, as Mathilde von Kemnitz, *Moderne Mediumforschung: Kritische Betrachtungen zu Dr. von Schrenck-Notzings "Materialisationsphaenomene"* (Munich: J. F. Lehmanns Verlag, 1914).

25. Hartung, "Völkische Ideologie," pp. 39–40.

26. These essays were later collected and published as Mathilde Ludendorff, *Der Trug der Astrologie* (Munich: Ludendorffs Volkswarte Verlag, 1932), pp. 6 and 18.

27. Following Kraepelin, she called this a form of "induced insanity": Hermann Rewaldt, "Abwehrkampf gegen den Okkultismus," in *Mathilde Ludendorff: Ihr Werk und Wirken*, ed. General Erich Ludendorff (Munich: Ludendorffs Verlag, 1937), pp. 173, 179, and 184.

28. Rewaldt, *Mathilde Ludendorff*, pp. 176–77.

29. The Ludendorffs also founded the Deutsche Gotteserkenntnis (Community of believers), which was dedicated to the worship of ancient Germanic divinities and was adopted as the official religion of the Nazi state in 1939; see Ulrich Nanko, *Die Deutsche Glaubensbewegung: Eine historische und soziologische Untersuchung* (Marburg: Diagonal, 1993).

30. Knochen, a colonel in the SS, eventually became the head of the security police in occupied France from 1940 to 1944.

31. Melzer, *Konflikt und Anpassung*, pp. 181–83.

32. *The Encyclopedia of the Third Reich* 2 (1991), s.v., "Reich Security Main Office," p. 784.

33. "Sekten-Logen," R 58 file 1074, BA Berlin: "Schlagwortverzeichnis" (SD-Leipzig), RG-15.007M file 560, USHMM. Note that further archival sources probably exist in the recently published holdings of the SD. An index for this collection is planned for 2003, and this may be an excellent place to explore further the Nazi response to occultism; see *Regimekritik, Widerstand, und Verfolgung in Deutschland und besetzten Gebieten: Meldungen aus dem Geheimen Staatspolizeiamt, dem SD-Hauptamt, der SS, und dem Reichssicherheitshauptamt, 1933–1945,* ed. H. Boberach (Munich: K. G. Saur, 1999–2001).

34. "Das Sektenwesen" (SD-Hauptamt), RG-15.007M file 492, USHMM.

35. Ibid.

36. Ibid.

37. Detlef Garbe, *Zwischen Widerstand und Martyrium: Die Zeugen Jehovas im "Dritten Reich"* (Munich: Oldenbourg, 1993).

38. "Jahresbericht 1937 für das Referat II 1134—Sektenwesen" (SD-Hauptamt) and "Das Sektenwesen" (SD-Hauptamt), RG-15.007M file 492, USHMM.

39. Ibid.

40. "Das Sektenwesen" (SD-Hauptamt), RG-15.007M file 492, USHMM.

41. "Okkultistisches Schriftum" (SD-Hauptamt), RG-15.007M file 560, USHMM.

42. "Auflösung freimaurerlogenähnlicher Organisationen," *Ministerial-Blatt des Reichs-und Preußischen Ministeriums des Innern, Ausgabe A* 2 (98), Nr. 32 (11 August 1937), 1337–39. Some Theosophical groups had already been banned in 1936.

43. A few months later, Heydrich softened this initial order sufficiently to allow certain occult texts like Wilhelm Gundel's historical *Sternglaube, Sternreligion, und Sternorakel* off the black list: "Der Chef der Sicherheitspolizei in Berlin" (4 June 1941), R 58 file 1029, BA Berlin.

44. "Niederschrift über die Besprechung bei SS-Oberführer Nebe" (27 May 1940, Berlin) (RSHA), RG-15.007M file 109, USHMM.

45. This title comes from James Webb's path-breaking study of the occult movement in modern Europe, published as *The Occult Underground* (La Salle, IL: Open Court, 1974) and *The Occult Establishment* (La Salle, IL: Open Court, 1976). Webb and I use the phrase very differently, however. Whereas Webb postulates an occult "underground" that flourished in Germany in the years before 1933 and then emerged as an occult "establishment" following Hitler's rise to power, I argue that the occult movement was highly public and visible before 1933 and then was driven further and further underground after 1933.

46. Wolfgang von Weisl, "Querschnitt durch ein okkultes Zeitalter," *Querschnitt* (Berlin) 12 (1933): 846–51.

47. "Einladung" (RSHA), RG-15.007M file 387, USHMM.

48. "Auf der Suche nach einem neuen Lebensinhalt" (RSHA), RG-15.007M file 387, USHMM.

49. Johannes Baum Verlag to Hanns-Maria Clobes, 10 August 1937, and E. M. Däbritz to Archiv für Reinkarnation, 15 October 1937 (RSHA), RG-15.007M file 387, USHMM.

50. Erwin Schurig to Hanns-Maria Clobes, 25 June 1937 (RSHA), RG-15.007M file 387, USHMM.

51. "Leipziger Esoterische Studiengesellschaft Programm 1936" (SD-Leipzig), RG-15.007M file 560, USHMM.

52. The RSHA seems to have shared Issberner-Haldane's interest in the witch trials of the Middle Ages: it assembled several files with material from many different archives on just this topic; see, for instance, RG-15.007M files 484–485 and 656, USHMM.

53. "Vorbericht zu Ernst Issberner-Haldane Arisches Weistum" (SD-Hauptamt), RG-15.007M file 560, USHMM.

54. "Mazdaznan," *Judenkenner* 26 (14 August 1935), RG-15.007M file 411, USHMM.

55. "Sekten-Logen," R 58 file 1074, BA Berlin.

56. Telegram, 25 May 1937, to Gestapo in Berlin, R 58 file 887, BA Berlin.

57. Some sense of how this proceeded could be reconstructed by using the periodical lists published yearly in the *Bibliographie der deutschen Zeitschriften Literatur.*

58. From SS Frankfurt/Oder to Geheime Staatspolizeiamt, Berlin, 31 January 1935, R 58 file 887, BA Berlin.

59. HA Sipo, Berlin, Gestapo, RG-15.007M file 10, USHMM.

60. Ibid.

61. "Jahresbericht 1937 für das Referat 2 1134—Sektenwesen" (SD-Hauptamt), RG-15.007M file 492, USHMM.

62. "Sicherheitsdienst des Reichsführers-SS Linz" (9 September 1940) (SD-Linz), RG-15.007M file 431, USHMM.

63. Reichsministerium für Volksaufklärung und Propaganda in Berlin, 3 August 1939, R 58 file 887, BA Berlin.

64. Karl Schmeïng, "Justiz und Aberglaube," *Monatsschrift für Kriminalbiologie und Strafrechtsreform* 29 (1938): 382–88.

65. SD Abschnitt Bielefeld (8 March 1940), RG-15.007M file 618, USHMM.

66. Rolf Sylvéro in Leipzig to the Reichspropagandaleitung in Berlin, 21 August 1941; Gau-Propagandaamt Dresden to Reichsring Berlin, 21 August 1941; and W. A. Christiansen to the Reichspropagandaleitung, 28 August 1941, NS 18 file 497, BA Berlin.

67. For a personal account to be read with a very skeptical eye, see Erik Jan Hanussen, *Meine Lebenslinie* (Munich: Universitas Verlag, 1988), esp. pp. 139–44. Hanussen also shows up in the files of the Munich police department, which independently confirm some of these details; see PDM 7103, StArMü.

68. "Betreff: Fick Anton (20.9.31)," PDM 7113, StArMü; Hermann Steinschneider, *Der Leitmeritzer Hellseher-Prozeß Hanussen: Ausführliche Wiedergabe der sensationallen Gerichts-Verhandlung mit zahlreichen bisher unveröffentlichten Dokumenten* (Teplitz-Schönau: Selbstverlag, c. 1930).

69. *Hanussens B. W. Hellseher Zeitung* 31 (24 September 1932), Eberhard Sammlung, SdBMü.

70. Bruno Frei, "Hellseher," *Weltbühne* 29 (1933): 161–65.

71. Bella Fromm, *Blood and Banquets: A Berlin Social Diary* (New York: Carol Publishing, 1990), pp. 78–79.

72. Mel Gordon, *Hitler's Jewish Clairvoyant: Erik Jan Hanussen* (Los Angeles: Feral House, 2001), pp. 217, 226, 239–43, and 255–56. This source should be used with caution. Although Gordon uncovers new sources, he often uses them uncritically.

73. "Gefahrenzone Aberglaube," *Das Schwarze Korps* (7 October 1937), p. 12.

74. Karl Kamps, *Johannes Maria Verweyen: Gottsucher, Mahner, und Bekenner* (Wiesbaden: Im Credo-Verlag, 1955), pp. 40 and 46. Although factually accurate, this source has a strong Roman Catholic bias that affects its view of Verweyen and his Catholicism. For this reason, the source should be used with caution.

75. Johannes M. Verweyen, *Der Neue Mensch und Seine Ziele: Menschheitsfragen der Gegenwart und Zukunft,* 2nd ed. (Stuttgart: Walter Hädecke, 1930), p. 159.

76. Verweyen, *Der Neue Mensch,* p. 213; Kamps, *Johannes Maria Verweyen,* p. 66.

77. Kamps, *Johannes Maria Verweyen,* pp. 62 and 82.

78. Ibid., p. 6.

79. Pamphlet *Siemens-Studien-Gesellschaft* (SD-Hauptamt), RG-15.007M file 560, USHMM.

80. "Betr. Vortrag des Siemens-Studiengesellschaft" (13 October 1934), "Abschrift" (23 October 1934), and "Betr. Siemens Studiengesellschaft" (6 November 1934) (all from SD-Hauptamt), RG-15.007M file 560, USHMM.

81. "Abschrift Betr. Prof. Dr. Joh. E. Verweyen" and "Betrifft Siemens Studien Gesellschaft" (26 November 1934) (both from SD-Hauptamt), RG-15.007M file 560, USHMM.

82. Untitled report, pp. 21–22 and 63–64, 62 Di 1 20/1, BA Berlin.

83. Letter from E. K. Neumann in Leipzig to Dr. Bernhard Hörmann in Munich, 9 December 1940, NS 18 file 497, BA Berlin.

84. Rolf Sylvéro in Leipzig to the Reichspropagandaleitung in Berlin, 21 August 1941, and Gauhauptstellenleiter in Munich, 24 September 1941, NS18 file 497, BA Berlin.

85. Gauhauptstellenleiter in Munich, 24 September 1941, Denzel in Munich to the Reichspropagandaleitung in Berlin, 24 September 1941, Bernhard Hörmann in Munich to the Deutsche Arbeitsfront in Berlin, 5 June 1939, and NSDAP Reichsleitung in Berlin to Bernhard Hörmann in Munich, 16 January 1942, NS 18 file 497, BA Berlin.

86. One such lecturer was Franz-Wudia Falkenau: letter from DAF NSG Kraft durch Freude in Berlin to DAF NSG Kraft durch Freude in Munich, 16 October 1941, NS 18 file 497, BA Berlin.

87. Hans Weinert, *Hellsehen und Wahrsagen: Ein uralter Traum der Menschheit* (Leipzig: Helingsche Verlagsanstalt, 1943).

88. "Gefahrenzone Aberglaube," *Das Schwarze Korps* (30 September 1937), p. 12; "Die Spiritualisten und die Wissenschaft," *Die Gartenlaube* 2 (1861): 23–25.

89. "Gefahrenzone Aberglaube," *Das Schwarze Korps* (23 September 1937), p. 6.

90. Ibid., p. 12.

91. Ibid., p. 16.

92. For a dramatic indication of this drop off, compare the entries for terms like *Okkultismus* and *Theosophie* before and after 1937 in the *Bibliographie der deutschen Zeitschriftenliteratur.* The last (debunking) articles on occultism appeared in *Weltliteratur* 16 (August–September 1941); see especially Mandywel, "Höhere Welten," pp. 202–4, and Bernhard Hörmann, "Wünschelrute und Pendel bei Licht besehn," pp. 213–15.

93. Letter from M. Bormann in Munich to Dr. Goebbels on 30 June 1941, NS 18 file 211, BA Berlin: letter from Goebbels in Berlin to M. Bormann, 3 July 1941, NS 18 file 211, BA Berlin.

Conclusion: A Voice from the Beyond?

1. Willy K. Jaschke, *Maria: Eine Stimme aus dem Jenseits? Experimentelle Sitzungsergebnisse mit den Medien Luise Weber und Karl Schneider* (Bamberg: Kommissionsverlag W. E. Hepple'sche Buchhandlung, 1928), p. 13.

2. Ibid., p. 17.

3. Ibid., pp. 18–25.

4. Ibid., pp. 26–63; the train anecdote occurs on p. 46. Also, note that Karl Schneider was a real person: the younger brother of Willy and Rudi Schneider, two of Europe's best-known mediums in the 1910s and 1920s.

5. Ibid., pp. 90–94; the note from Maria is on p. 90.

6. David Blackbourn, *The Long Nineteenth Century: A History of Germany, 1780–1918* (New York: Oxford, 1997), pp. 304–5; see also Wolfgang Schivelbusch, *The Railway Journey* (Berkeley: University of California Press, 1986).

7. Dorothy Ross, "Modernism Reconsidered," in *Modernist Impulses in the Human Sciences, 1870–1930* (Baltimore, MD: Johns Hopkins University Press, 1994), pp. 1–2.

Selected Bibliography

ARCHIVAL SOURCES

Archiv, Diakonisches Werk, Evangelische Kirche in Deutschland, Berlin
(ADW)

Central-Ausschuss für die Innere Mission, Apologetische Centrale (CA AC)
214–16 Bildungs und Schülungsarbeit, Bd. 1–3, 1927–34
Central-Ausschuss für die Innere Mission, Apologetische Centrale-Sammlung (CA AC-S)
1–3 Aberglaube, 1928–36
25–29 Astrologie, 1927–36
45 Bô Yin Râ, 1924–31
159 Gesellschaft für psychische Forschung, 1931
171 Horpeniten (Bund der Kämpfer für Glaube und Wahrheit)
272–73 Okkultismus, 1925–37
318–19 Sekten, 1920–36
334 Spiritismus, 1922–33

Bayerische Staatsbibliothek, Munich (BSB)

Handschriftenabteilung
Nachlaß Gustav Meyrink (Meyrinkiana) 1, 1; xvia

Bundesarchiv Berlin (BA Berlin)

Bestand NS 18 Reichspropagandaleitung
211 Bekämpfung von Okkultismus (Erörterungen der Parteikanzler und Antwort
    Goebbels im Zusammenhang mit dem "Fall Hess"), June–July 1943
497 Okkultismus, 1941–43
Bestand R58 Reichssicherheitshauptamt
887 Überprüfung und Beanstandung von Veröffentlichungen in Zeitschriften. Reli-
    giöse und weltanschauliche Zeitschriften, 1935–42
1029 Maßnahmen gegen unpolitische Organisationen, 1934–1942
1074 Verzeichnis von Runderlassen über Sekten und Logen, 1934–43
Bestand 62 Di 1 Dienstellen Rosenberg
20/1 Theosophie-Anthroposophie

Evangelisches Zentralarchiv Berlin (EZB)

Bestand 1.A2 Deutscher Evangelischer Kirchenausschuß
465/1 Sonstige Religionsgemeinschaften, Freikirchen, Sekten, 1929–31
Bestand 1.C3 Allgemeine Tätigkeit der Kirchenkanzlei
298 Freidenker, Sekten, Gottlosenbewegung, 1935–42
Bestand 7. Generalia (Evangelisches Oberkirchenrat)
3946 Die spiritistische und scientistische Bewegung, 1901–34

Geheimes Staatsarchiv Preussischer Kulturbesitz (GSPK)

Bestand I Rep. 89 (2.2.1) Geheimes Zivilkabinett, jüngere Period, 1797–1918
15340 Scientismus und Spiritismus, 1902

Landesarchiv Berlin

Rep. 42, Acc. 2147 Amtsgericht Charlottenburg, 1879–1970
26390 Deutsche Okkultistische Gesellschaft, 1919–55
26675 Akademische Gesellschaft für Astrologische Forschung, 1925–55
27016 Verein für Pendelforschung, 1931–42
27303 Reichsverband für Wünschelrutenwesen, 1921–56
27591 Astrologische Gesellschaft, 1924–56
27703 Verein Magische Kunst, 1921–56

Niedersächsische Staats-und Universitätsbibliothek Göttingen

Nachlaß Wilhelm Hübbe-Schleiden (Cod WH-S)
416:1–2 Weltpolitik: neue Weltkultur, Weltreligion, Weltrasse, 1914
800:1 Satzung der Theosophischen Gesellschaft Leipzig, u.s.w.
800:2 Satzungen einzelner deutscher Ortsverbände und englischer Theosophischer
   Gesellschaften, u.s.w.
801 Rundschreiben verschiedener theosophischer und anthroposophischer Gesellschaften und Zweige, 1893–31
802:2 Zeitraum, 1914–22 (enth. Programm für die Theosophischen Ferienkurse im
   Sommer 1914 auf "Weisser Hirsch" bei Dresden), u.s.w.
807 Namen-und Adressenlisten von Personen, die zur Mitarbeit für die Sphinx gewon-
   nen werden sollten
812 Briefe und Materialien zur Theosophischen Societät Germania
812:1,16 Gebhard, Franz Gustav, 1884–87
812:2,1 Sammelmappe zur Geschichte der Theosophischen Societät Germania
815 Sammelmappe zur Internationalen Theosophischen Verbrüderung
821 Sammelmappe zum Orden des Sterns im Osten, 1912–16
826 Sammelmappe zum 1. Internationalen Okkultisten Kongreß, 1914
921 Sammelmappe zum Themenkreis "Theosophen und Kriegsgeschehen"
1012:1 Notizbuch, 1883–84

Staatsarchiv Munich (StArMü)

Polizeidirektion München (PDM)
576 Verein Freibund (Spiritismus)
674 Neu-Theosophische Vereinigung, 1887–1914
678 Theosophische Gesellschaft, 1894–1917
682 Theosophische Gesellschaft, 1904–17
683 Theosophische Loge, 1904–17
3543 Die Sucher, 1918–24, 1937
5433 Zentralstelle für Lebenserneuerung, 1929, 1936
5439 Zarathustrischer Bund, 1924, 1935
5608 Neuland, 1923–36
5610 Okkultistische Gesellschaft e.V., 1925–30
7103 Schwindel auf übersinnlichen Gebiet, 1930–40
7104 Hypnose, 1929–40
7105 Glücks-, Wahrsage-, Scherzbriefe, 1921–41
7106 Gauklertricks, 1924–37
7107 Hellseherei, 1924–47
7109 Pendel- und Wünschelrutengebrauch, 1924–40
7110 Spukerscheinungen, 1925–35
7111 Wahrsagerei und Kartenlegerei, 1935–41
7113 Handliniendeutung, 1922–35
7114 Astrologische Vereinigungen, 1923–37

Stadtarchiv Munich (SdArMü)

Zeitungsauschnitte
Aberglaube
Astrologie
Okkultismus
Personen Aub, Ludwig
Personen Schrenck-Notzing, Albert

Stadtbibliothek Munich

Sammlung Heinrich Eberhard (R C 4° 15 133)
Monacensia Literaturarchiv
Sammlung Hanns von Gumppenberg (L 2037)
Sammlung Karl du Prel
Sammlung Albert von Schrenck-Notzing

Stanford University Libraries (Department of Special Collections)

Janos Frecot Collection
Collection contains rare and ephemeral published sources noted in the footnotes

United States Holocaust Memorial Museum, Washington D. C.

RG-15.007M Records of the Reichssicherheitshauptamt
10 Monthly and daily reports of Gestapo activities, HA Sipo Berlin, Gestapo, 1939
109 Protocol for the conference with the SS chief how to use astrology to fight British imperialism in India, RSHA II B 3, 1940
346 Dr. Kittler correspondence concerning propaganda publishing houses. RSHA VII, Archive: Correspondence of Reichsschriftumskammer d.RMfVuP, UAbtl. für astrologische Wissenschaft, 1938–39
387 Personal correspondence among scholars concerned about the purity of race; correspondence regarding reincarnation and Theosophy, 1936–37
411 Photocopies concerning the organization of Anthroposophic societies, SD file on Organizations, Anthroposophy, 1933–34
431 The anthropologic society in the community Kirschlag Linz (section 2-B3); house search of the Anthroposophische Gesellschaft, 1940
484–5 Bibliography of mystical literature especially the witches trial; Rudolf Richter bibliography of literature on Hexenprozesse in Mitteldeutschland, 1936, 1941
492 Report about activities of sectarian religions; SDHA II 1134: SD V-man reports, extracts from Lageberichte und Jahresbericht 1937; correspondence with Gestapo, etc. regarding sectarian religious activities, 1935–44
560 Reports from various masonic lodges . . . Verbindungsstelle Leipzig reports on "related" occultist literature, especially Arisches Weistum, by Ernst Issberner-Haldane; advertisements for literature; Siemens Studien-Gesellschaft für Psychologische Wissenschaft, publications, 1938
618 Reports about the political adversaries activities on the German territory; SD Abschnitte reports of violations of public order, 1940
656 Excerpts from archival sources about the "witches trials" of the sixteenth and seventeenth century, 1936

PUBLISHED PRIMARY SOURCES

1. Kongreß des Deutschen Bundes der gerichtlichen Schriftanverständigen und Berufsgraphologen (Sitz Berlin) am 6. und 7. September 1924 in Hotel Deutsches Haus in Leipzig, Königsplatz. 1924.
Aeterna Bund. *Okkulte Probleme (Aeterna Bücher no. 1).* Munich: Aeterna, c. 1932.
Aksakow, Alexander. *Animismus und Spiritismus.* Leipzig: Oswald Mutze, 1890.
Andree, K. "Geisterklopfen und Tischrücken in den Hansestädten." *Allgemeine Zeitung (Beilage)* 94, 4 April 1853, pp. 1497–98.
"Anna Rothe & Co." *Die Zukunft* 43 (4 April 1903): 41–46.
"Anna Rothe, das Blumenmedium." *Berliner Tageblatt,* 12 March 1903.
Anschütz, Georg. "Phantasma und Kunst." *Schünemanns Monatshefte* 11 (November 1928): 1262–72.
Arnold, Hans. *Wie errichtet und leitet man spiritistischer Zirkel in der Familie: Ein Leitfaden für die selbständige Prüfung der mediumistischen Phänomenon.* Leipzig: M. Spohr, 1894.
"Auflösung freimaurerlogenähnlicher Organisationen." *Ministerialblatt des Reichs-und Preußischen Ministeriums des Innern, Ausgabe A* 2 (11 August 1937): 1337–39.

Badelt, Elsie Johna. *Das Mal-Phänomen Heinrich Nüßlein.* Magdeburg: Selbstverlag, n.d.

Baerwald, Richard. *Okkultismus, Spiritismus, und unterbewußte Seelenzustände.* Leipzig: B. G. Teubner, 1920.

Bastian, Adolf. "Spiritismus und Ethnologie." *Sphinx* 3 (1887): 87–90.

"Berliner Festwoche: Pastoral-Konferenz." *Neue Preussische Zeitung* 275, 14–15 June 1900.

Beßmer, Julius. "Der Okkultismus von heute." *Stimmen der Zeit* 102 (February 1922): 336–53.

Blüthgen, Victor. "Vom Rothe-Prozess." *Psychische Studien* 30 (April 1903): 257–64.

"Blumenmedium Anna Rothe vor Gericht, Das." *Berliner Tageblatt*, 23 March 1903.

Bô Yin Râ. *Aus meiner Malerwerkstatt.* Basel-Leipzig: Kober'sche Verlagsbuchhandlung, 1932.

Bohn, Erich. "Der Fall Rothe." *Nord und Süd* 96 (February 1901): 223–56.

———. *Der Fall Rothe: Eine criminal-psychologische Untersuchung.* Breslau: S. Schottländer, 1901.

Brandler-Pracht, Karl, and Maria Brandler-Pracht. *Die astrologische Deutung: Diagnose und Prognose.* Berlin: Falken-Verlag Erich Sicker, n.d.

Brandler-Pracht, Karl. *Erfolgreiches, glückliches Leben durch Beachtung der Tattwischen und Astralen Einflüsse: Ein Schlüssel zur praktischen Verwendung der mit dem menschlichen Leben engverbundenen kosmischen Schwingungen, wodurch jedermann zum Herrn seines Geschickes werden kann.* Berlin-Pankow: Linser, 1920.

Browne, C. A. "Observations upon the Use of the Divining Rod in Germany." *Science* 123 (23 January 1931): 84–86.

Brunn, Ludwig. "Der Prophet." *Sphinx* 7 (March 1889): 159–67.

Bry, Carl Christian. *Verkappte Religionen.* Gotha: Friedrich Andreas Perthes, 1924.

Buchner, Eberhard. *Sekten und Sektierer in Berlin.* Berlin: Hermann Seemann, n.d.

———. *Von den übersinnlichen Dingen: Ein Führer durch das Reich der okkulten Forschung.* Leipzig: Felix Meiner, 1924.

Büchner, Louis. *Force and Matter: Empirico-Philosophical Studies, Intelligently Rendered.* Ed. J. Frederick Collingwood. London: Trübner, 1864.

Buntzel, Walther, "Okkultismus." In *Handbuch für das kirchliche Amt,* ed. Walther Buntzel. Leipzig: J. C. Hinrichs'sche Buchhandlung, 1928.

Busse, Hans. "Graphologie und Okkultismus: Die Entwicklung der Graphologie zur exakten Wissenschaft." *Wissenschaftliche Zeitschrift für Okkultismus* 1, no. 1 (1899): 72–79.

Caliban. "Die Betrügerin." *Die Gegenwart* 14 (4 April 1903): 209–10.

Conrad, Michael Georg. *Gelüftete Masken: Allerlei Charakterköpfe.* Leipzig: Wilhelm Friedrich, 1890.

"Congress of Physiological Psychology at Paris, The." *Mind* 14 (October 1889): 614–16.

Crookes, William. "Address of the President before the British Association for the Advancement of Science, Bristol, 1898." *Science* 8 (4 November 1898): 610–12.

Deinhard, Ludwig. *Das Mysterium des Menschen im Lichte der psychischen Forschung: Eine Einführung in den Okkultismus: Mit einem Beitrag von Dr. Hübbe-Schleiden über das Problem der Wiederverkörperung.* Berlin: Reichl, c. 1910.

Dessoir, Max. *Buch der Erinnerung.* 2nd ed. Stuttgart: Ferdinand Enke, 1947.

———. "Der Fall Rothe." *Die Woche* 14 (4 April 1903): 595–97.

————. "Die Parapsychologie: Eine Entgegnung auf den Artikel 'Der Prophet.' " *Sphinx* 7 (1889): 341–35.

————. *Vom Jenseits der Seele: Die Geheimwissenschaften in kritischer Betrachtung.* Stuttgart: Ferdinand Enke, 1917.

Dessoir, Max, ed. *Der Okkultismus in Urkunden.* Berlin: Ullstein, 1925.

Dingfelder, Johannes. *Ludwig Aub als Hellseher und Hellfühler: Eine wissenschaftliche Studie über das Wesen der Graphologie und Psychometrie.* Munich: Fr. Seybolds Verlagsbuchhandlung, c. 1914.

du Prel, Carl. *Der Kampf ums Dasein am Himmel.* 3rd ed. Leipzig: E. Gunther, 1882.

————. *Nachgelassene Schriften.* Leipzig: Max Altmann, 1911.

————. *Die Philosophie der Mystik.* Leipzig: E. Gunther, 1885.

————. *The Philosophy of Mysticism,* trans. C. C. Massey. London: George Redway, 1889.

————. "Problem: Medium oder Taschenspieler? Der Stand der Streitfrage." *Sphinx* 1 (1886): 362–70.

————. *Das Rätsel des Menschen: Einleitung in das Studium der Geheimwissenschaften.* Leipzig: Philipp Reclam, 1892.

————. *Der Somnambulismus vor dem königlichen Landgerichte München* 1. Monacensia Bibliothek und Literaturarchiv. Stadtbibliothek, Munich.

————. *Der Spiritismus.* Leipzig: Philipp Reclam, 1893.

————. "Übersinnliche Gedankenübertragung: Komiteebericht der 'Psychologischen Gesellschaft' in München." *Sphinx* 5 (1888): 24–31.

Duboc, Julius. "Weibliche Philosophie." *Die Zukunft* 34 (2 March 1901): 366–73.

E. T. H. "Trial of a German Medium." *New York Times,* 11 April 1903, 2.

Engel, Leopold, ed. *Wahrheit-Sucher: Unparteiische Monatsschrift vereinter Wahrheit-sucher.* July 1896–June 1897.

Fischer, H. R. *100 Jahre 'Theosophische Gesellschaft': Ein geschichtlicher Überblick.* Calw/Württ.: Schatzkammerverlag Hans Fändrich, n.d.

Fischer, Oskar. *Experimente mit Raphael Schermann: Ein Beitrag zu den Problemen der Graphologie, Telepathie, und des Hellsehens.* Berlin: Urban & Schwarzenberg, 1924.

Flournoy, Théodore. *From India to the Planet Mars: A Case of Multiple Personality with Imaginary Languages.* Princeton, NJ: Princeton University Press, 1994.

Francé-Harrar, Annie. *So war's um Neunzehnhundert: Mein Fin de Siècle.* Munich-Vienna: Albert Langen-Georg Müller, 1962.

Frei, Bruno. "Hellseher." *Weltbühne* 29 (1933): 161–65.

Freimar, Fritz. "Ein Nachtrag zum Fall Rothe." *Psychische Studien* 30 (December 1903): 731–44.

Freimark, Hans. *Das erotische Element im Okkultismus.* Pfullingen in Württemberg: Johannes Baum, 1922.

————. *Mediumistische Kunst mit einem Beitrag über den künstlerischen Wert mediumistischer Malereien von Eugen Johannes Maecker. Beiträge zur Geschichte der neueren Mystik und Magie,* no. 2. Leipzig: Wilhelm Heims, 1914.

Freud, Sigmund. *The Interpretation of Dreams.* Ed. James Strachey. New York: Avon, 1965.

Friedlaender, Hugo. *Interessante Kriminal-Prozesse von kulturhistorischer Bedeutung: Darstellung merkwürdiger Strafrechtsfälle aus Gegenwart und Jüngstvergangenheit.* Berlin: Hermann Barsdorf, 1910.

Fritsche, Herbert. *Iatrosophia: metabiologische Heilung und Selbstheilung.* Leipzig: Richard Hummel, 1937.

Fromm, Bella. *Blood and Banquets: A Berlin Social Diary.* New York: Carol Publishing, 1990.

Fuchs, Georg. *Sturm und Drang in München um die Jahrhundertwende.* Munich: Georg D. W. Callwey, 1936.

———. "Der Tanz." *Flugblätter für künstlerische Kultur* 6 (1906): 3–43.

"Gefahrenzone Aberglaube." *Das Schwarze Korps* (September–October 1937).

Geipel, Dr. "Zwei Processe gegen spiritistische Medien." *Münchener Medizinische Wochenschrift* 39 (1898): 664–67.

Glahn, A. Frank. *Glahns Pendel-Bücherei.* Memmingen: Uranus, 1936.

Goebbels, Joseph. *Die Tagebücher von Joseph Goebbels, 1, 1940–1941.* Ed. Elke Fröhlich. Munich: K. G. Saur, 1998.

Gradenwitz, Alfred. "Investigating Unknown Forces: The Unique Psychic Laboratory of Fritz Grunewald, at Charlottenburg." *Scientific American* (July 1922): 30, 70.

Grimm, A. M. *Uranus Bücher.* Munich: A. M. Grimm, 1921.

Grimm, Elisabeth. *Geistige Inspiration durch Gottes Gnade gegeben am 20. Dezember 1926.* Forst: A. Stahn, 1926–27.

Groll, Jacques. "Aus der Kinderstube des modernen Spiritismus." *Spiritistische Rundschau* 10 (1902–3): 102–6.

Grüttefien. "Der Fall Rothe in neuer Beleuchtung." *Berliner Tageblatt* 173, 4 April 1903.

Gubalke, Max. *Bericht über die Verhandlungen auf dem Dritten Congress des "Verbandes Deutscher Okkultisten" am 31. Mai und 1. Juni (Pfingsten) 1898 in München.* Selbstverlag, c. 1898.

Gumppenberg, Hanns von. *Das dritte Testament: Eine Offenbarung Gottes: Seiner Zeit mitgeteilt von Hanns von Gumppenberg.* Munich: M. Poessl, 1891.

———. *Lebenserrinerungen aus dem Nachlass des Dichters.* Berlin: Eigenbrödler, 1929.

———. *Der Prophet Jesus Christus die Neue Religion und andere Erläuterungen zum Dritten Testamente Gottes.* Munich: M. Poessl, 1891.

Hanussen, Erik Jan. *Meine Lebenslinie.* Munich: Universitas, 1988.

Hartmann, Eduard von. "Die 'Grenzen der Philosophie': Eine Entgegnung auf Freiherrn Dr. von Goelers Aufsatz." *Sphinx* 5 (1888): 265–66.

———. *Der Spiritismus.* Leipzig: Wilhelm Friedrich, 1885.

Hartmann, Franz. "Autobiography of Franz Hartmann." *Occult Review* 7, no. 1 (1908): 7–35.

———. *Denkwürdige Erinnerungen aus dem Leben des Verfassers der "Lotusblüten": Mit besonderer Berücksichtigung der Geschichte der theosophischen Bewegung.* Calw (Württ.): Schatzkammerverlag Hans Fändrich, n.d.

Hartmann, William C. *Who's Who in Occultism, New Thought, Psychism, and Spiritualism.* New York: Occult Press, 1927.

Hartung, Erich. "Okkulte Medizin." *Der Okkultismus* 1, no. 1 (1925): 30–32.

Haßmann, Frances, "Echt oder Unecht." *Nord und Süd* (February 1901): 217–22.

Haupt Katalog, 1922. Berlin: Nirwana-Verlag für Lebensreform, 1922. Available at JFC.

"Der Hellseher Petzold vor Gericht." *Zentralblatt für Okkultismus* 5, no. 4 (1911): 248–50.

"Die Hellseherin bei der Mordaufklärung." *Kriminalistische Monatshefte* 8 (August 1928): 182–83.

Hellwig, Albert. "Gibt es nachweisbar echte Fälle von Kriminaltelepathie? Eine Betrachtung zum Insterburger Okkultistenprozeß." *Kriminalistische Monatshefte* 6 (June 1928): 121–23.

———. *Okkultismus und Verbrechen: Eine Einführung in die kriminalistischen Probleme des Okkultismus für Polizeibeamte, Richter, Staatsanwälte, Psychiater, und Sachverständige.* Berlin: P. Langenscheidt, 1929.

———. *Weltkrieg und Aberglaube: Erlebtes und Erlauschtes.* Leipzig: Wilhelm Heims, 1916.

Henne am Rhyn, Otto. *Eine Reise durch das Reich des Aberglaubens.* Leipzig: Max Spohr, 1893.

———. "Tragödien und Komödien des Aberglaubens: Das Blumenmedium." *Die Gartenlaube* 140, no. 12 (1902): 210–11.

Henneberg, R. "Ueber Spiritismus und Geistesstörung." *Archiv für Psychiatrie und Nervenkrankheiten* 34, no. 3 (1901): 998–1039.

Hermann. "Die Iserlohner Hellseher-Experimente." *Kriminalistische Monatshefte* 10 (October 1928): 221–24.

Holtum, Gregor. "Apologetik und Okkultismus." *Korrespondenz- und Offertenblatt für die gesamte katholische Geistlichkeit Deutschlands* 9 (1926): 167–70.

Honold, E. *Memoiren einer Spiritisten: Erlebte Wahrheiten gesammelt in 15jährigen okkultem Studium.* 4th–5th ed. Berlin: Prana, n.d.

Houdini, Harry. *A Magician among the Spirits.* New York: Harper & Brothers, 1924.

Hübbe-Schleiden, Wilhelm. "Aufruf und Vorwort." *Sphinx* 1 (1886): i–iv.

———. "Psychometrische Experimente." *Sphinx* 5 (1888): 156–59.

———. "Zöllners Zurechnungsfähigkeit und die Seybert-Kommission." *Sphinx* 4 (1887): 321–28.

James, William. *The Varieties of Religious Experience: A Study in Human Nature.* New York: Mentor Books, 1958.

———. *The Will to Believe and Other Essays in Popular Philosophy.* New York: Dover Publications, 1956.

Jaschke, Willy K. *Maria: Eine Stimme aus dem Jenseits? Experimentelle Sitzungsergebnisse mit den Medien Luise Weber und Karl Schneider.* Bamberg: Kommissionsverlag W. E. Hepple'sche Buchhandlung, 1928.

Jennings, Michael W., Howard Eiland, and Gary Smith, eds. *Walter Benjamin: Selected Writings.* Cambridge, MA: Belknap Press, 1999.

Jung, Carl Gustav. *Memories, Dreams, Reflections.* New York: Pantheon, 1961.

———. *Zur Psychologie und Pathologie sogenannter occulter Phänomene.* Leipzig: Oswald Mutze, 1902.

Kaesen, Wilhelm. "Spiritismus." *Theol. prakt. Quartalschrift* 1 (1923): 23–37.

Kallenberg, Friedrich. *P-Strahlen: das Neuland des siderischen Pendels.* Leipzig: Max Altmann, 1920.

———. *Der Siegeszug des siderischen Pendels, 1911–1934.* Diessen vor München: Jos. C. Huber, 1934.

Kandinsky, Wassily. *Kandinsky: Complete Writings on Art.* Ed. Kenneth C. Lindsay and Peter Vergo. New York: Da Capo, 1994.

Katalog zur Leihbibliothek. Berlin: Nirwana-Verlag für Lebensreform, 1925.

Kemnitz, Mathilde von. *Moderne Mediumforschung: Kritische Betrachtungen zu Dr. von Schrenck-Notzing's "Materialisationsphaenomene."* Munich: J. F. Lehmann, 1914.

Kern, Karl, ed. *Handbuch der Ariosophie.* Pforzheim: Verlag Herbert Reichstein, 1931–32.

Kersten, Felix. *The Kersten Memoirs, 1940–1945.* Trans. C. Fitzgibbon and J. Oliver. New York: Macmillan, 1957.

Keyserling, Hermann. *The Travel Diary of a Philosopher,* 2 vols. New York: Harcourt, Brace, 1925.

Kiesewetter, Karl. *Geschichte des Neueren Occultismus: Geheimwissenschaftliche Systeme von Agrippa von Nettesheym bis zu Carl du Prel.* Schwarzenburg: Ansata, 1977. Originally *Die Geheimwissenschaften: Die Entwicklungsgeschichte des Spiritismus von der Urzeit bis zur Gegenwart.* Leipzig: Wilhelm Friedrich, 1891–95.

Klinckowstroem, Carl von. *Bibliographie der Wünschelrute.* Munich: Kommissions Verlag v. Ottmar Schönhuth, 1911.

———. *Von den Tricks der Medien.* Munich: A. Huber, 1932.

Klinckowstroem, Carl von, and Rudolf Freiherr von Maltzahn. *Handbuch der Wünschelrute: Geschichte, Wissenschaft, Anwendung.* Munich: R. Oldenbourg, 1931.

Klöckler, Herbert von. *Astrologie als Erfahrungswissenschaft.* Leipzig: Emmanuel Reinicke, 1927.

"Klopfgeister und wandernde Tische." *Allgemeine Zeitung (Beilage)* 105, 15 April 1853, pp. 1674–75.

Kober-Staehelin, Alfred. *Meine Stellung zu Bô Yin Râ.* Leipzig: Kober'sche Verlagsbuchhandlung, 1931.

Korsch, Hubert, ed. *14 Vorträge über Astrologie: Gehalten auf dem 8. Astrologen-Kongress Nürnberg, 1929.* Düsseldorf: Otto Fritz, 1929.

Kratt, Gottfried. "Erinnerungen an Dr. Carl Freiherr du Prel." *Zentralblatt für Okkultismus* 5, no. 1 (1911): 31–36.

Kunstverein München. *Führer durch die Ausstellung Geheimnisse der Inspiration: Gemälde, Aquarelle, und Zeichnungen okkult beeinflußter Maler, mit 43 Abbildungen: Mitte August bis Mitte September 1932.* Available at BSB.

"Des Landrats von Uslar Arbeiten mit der Wünschelrute in Südwestafrika." *Schriften des Verbands zur Klärung der Wünschelrutenfrage,* vol. 1 (Stuttgart: Wittwer, 1912).

Langsdorff, Georg von. *Kurze Anleitung zur Erlernung der Psychometrie oder Entwicklung des in uns noch unerforschten sechsten Sinnes.* Munich: Carussell, 1981 (Leipzig: Oswald Mutze, 1898).

List, Guido von. *Urgrund: Eine Einführung in die Gedankenwelt des Wiener Forschers Guido von List.* Berlin-Lichterfelde: Guido von List Gesellschaft, 1935.

Lomer, Georg. *Neureligiöse Praxis.* Bad Schmiedeberg: F. E. Baumann, 1926.

Ludendorff, Erich, ed. *Mathilde Ludendorff: Ihr Werk und Wirken.* Munich: Ludendorffs Verlag, 1937.

Ludendorff, Mathilde. *Ein Blick in die Dunkelkammer der Geisterseher: Moderne Medium-"Forschung": Kritische Betrachtungen zu Dr. von Schrenck-Notzing's "Materialisationsphaenomene."* 2nd ed. Munich: Ludendorff, 1937. Retitled edition of Kemnitz (1914).

———. *Der Trug der Astrologie.* Munich: Ludendorffs Volkwarte-Verlag, 1932.

Maack, Ferdinand. *Wie Steht's mit dem Spiritismus?* Hamburg: Xenologischer Verlag, 1901.

Mackowsky, Hanns, August Pauly, and Wilhelm Weigand, eds. *Adolph Bayersdorfers Leben und Schriften aus seinem Nachlaß herausgegeben.* 2nd ed. Munich: F. Bruckman, 1908.

Mader, Rudolf. "Karl du Prel in Beachtung und Urteil von Nichtokkultisten." *Zentralblatt für Okkultismus* 8, no. 2 (1914): 94–97.

Mager, P. Alois, "Der Katholizismus und die okkulten Strömungen." In *Der Katholizismus als Lösung großer Menschheitsfragen,* pp. 97–116. Vienna-Munich: Verlagsanstalt Tyrolia, 1925.

Magische Unterweisungen des edlen und hochgelehrten Philosophie und Medici Philippi Theophrasti Bombasti von Hohenheim Paracelsus genannt. Leipzig: Im Wolkenwanderer Verlag, 1923.

Mann, Thomas, "Okkulte Erlebnisse." In *Gesammelte Werke,* vol. 10, pp. 135–71. Frankfurt: Fischer, 1974.

Marx, Karl, and Friedrich Engels. *Werke.* Berlin: Dietz, 1986.

"Mediumistische Kunst." *Zentralblatt für Okkultismus* 8, nos. 6–7 (1914–15): 283–87, 311–15.

Meyer, T. H., ed. *Light for the New Millennium: Rudolf Steiner's Association with Helmuth and Eliza von Moltke: Letters, Documents, and After-death Communications.* London: Rudolf Steiner, 1997.

"Mitglieder-Verzeichnis des Verbandes der Wünschelrutenfrage." *Schriften des Verbands zur Klärung der Wünschelrutenfrage* 3 (Stuttgart: Wittwer, 1912), pp. 53–60.

Moll, Albert. *Der Hypnotismus.* Berlin: Fischer, 1889.

———. *Ein Leben als Arzt der Seele: Erinnerungen.* Dresden: Carl Reissner, 1936.

———. *Der Spiritismus.* Stuttgart: Franckh'sche Verlagshandlung, 1925.

Moser, Fanny. *Der Okkultismus: Täuschungen und Tatsachen,* 2 vols. Munich: Ernst Reinhardt, 1935.

Müller, Alexander. *Kosmische und irdische Strahlen als Erreger der Krankheiten.* Hamburg: Steffens, 1930.

Müller, Egbert. *Der Spiritismus und die Criminal-Polizei: Mit Anhang über das Spiritistische um den Wende'schen Mord.* Berlin: Karl Siegismund, 1890.

———. *Der Spuk von Resau.* 3rd ed. Berlin: Karl Siegismund, 1889.

———. *Stellung des Strafrichters zum Spiritismus und der Proceß Valeska Töpfer.* Berlin: I. F. Conrads Buchhandlung (Paul Ackermann), 1892.

Müller, Rudolf. "Über Okkultismus als Erfahrungswissenschaft und sein Verhältnis zur Psychologie." *Wissenschaftliche Zeitschrift für Okkultismus* 1, nos. 2–3 (1899): 99–120.

"Näheres über den 'Okkultisten Verband.'" *Metaphysische Rundschau* 1, no. 2 (1896): 186–87.

Notzing, Albert von. "Telepathische Experimente des Sonderausschusses der Psychologischen Gesellschaft in München." *Sphinx* 4 (1887): 384–90.

Obertimpfler, Carl. "Rand-Glossen zum Rothe-Prozess." *Die übersinnliche Welt* (1903): 187–92 and 229–35.

Oesterreich, Traugott Konstantin. *Der Okkultismus im modernen Weltbild.* Dresden: Im Sibyllen-Verlag, 1923.

———. *Psychologisches Gutachten in einem Hellseherprozess.* Stuttgart: W. Kohlhammer, 1930.

Pelz, Carl. *Das Hellsehen: Ein Kriminalfall.* Munich: Ludendorff, 1937.

Pohl, Gustav. *Erdstrahlen als Krankheitserreger, Forschungen auf Neuland.* Diessen vor München: J. C. Huber, 1932.

"Prediger D. Riemann gegen des Spiritismus." *Spiritistische Rundschau* 8, no. 2 (1900): 58–60.

Preliminary Report of the Commission Appointed by the University of Pennsylvania to Investigate Modern Spiritualism in Accordance with the Request of the Late Henry Seybert. Philadelphia: J. B. Lippincott, 1920.

Price, Harry. *Rudi Schneider: A Scientific Examination of His Mediumship.* London: Methuen, 1930.

Prinzhorn, Hans. *Artistry of the Mentally Ill: A Contribution to the Psychology and Psychopathology of Configuration.* Trans. E. von Brockdorff. New York: Springer, 1972.

"Prison for a Spiritualist." *New York Times,* 29 March 1903, 5.

"Programm der psychologischen Gesellschaft in München." *Sphinx* 3 (1887): 32–36.

"Programm und Geleitwort." *Erkenntnnis und Glaube* 1 (15 July 1951): 1.

Psychomagnetisches suggestives Heilinstitut München. Pamphlet. Munich: c. 1910.

Reinhardt, G. "Psychologische Diagnosen." *Zentralblatt für Okkultismus* 1 (1908): 337 and 433.

Reißmann, Rolf. "Der Seelenmaler im Herzogsbett." *Berliner Illustrierte Nachtausgabe (Beiblätter),* 18 September 1935, p. 2.

"Report of the International Congress of Physiological Psychology." *Mind* 16, no. 61 (1891): 157–60.

Reventlow, Franziska zu. *Autobiographisches.* Munich: Albert Langen, 1980.

Riemann, Otto. "Die Entlarvungen des 'Blumenmediums' Anna Rothe und anderer 'Medien' und ihre Bedeutung für die spiritistische Bewegung." *Reformation* 1, no. 1 (1902): 7–10.

———. *Ein aufklärendes Wort über den Spiritismus.* Berlin: R. J. Müller, 1901.

Rohr, Frithjof. *Weißenberg-Heilpraktik.* Berlin-Lichterfeld: Karl Andrikowski, 1934.

Rosenberg, Alfred. *Kampf um die Macht: Aufsätze von 1921–1932,* Ed. Thilo von Trotha. 4th ed. Munich: Franz Eher, 1938.

———. *The Myth of the Twentieth Century: An Evaluation of the Spiritual-Intellectual Confrontations of Our Age.* Newport Beach, CA: Noontide, 1982.

Rothacker, A., and H. Degler. "Das magische Reis und seine Probleme." *Hippokrates* 14 (8 April 1937): 331–38.

Scheurlen, Paul. *Die Sekten der Gegenwart und neuere Weltanschauungsgebilde.* 4th ed. Stuttgart: Quell-Verlag d. Ev. Gesellschaft, 1930.

Schlund, P. Erhard. *Neugermanisches Heidentum im heutigen Deutschland.* Augsburg: Augsburg, 1978. Reprint of 2nd ed., Munich, 1924.

Schmeïng, Karl. "Justiz und Aberglaube." *Monatsschrift für Kriminalbiologie und Strafrechtsreform* 29 (1938): 382–88.

Schmidt. "Zur astrologischen Bewegung." *Klerusblatt* 16, no. 34 (1935): 577–79.

Schmitz, Oscar A. H. *Der Geist der Astrologie.* Munich: Müller, 1922.

Schopenhauer, Arthur. *Parerga and Paralipomena: Short Philosophical Essays,* vol. 1. Trans. E. F. J. Payne. Oxford, Eng.: Clarendon, 1974.

Schott, Rudolf. *Der Maler Bô Yin Râ.* Zürich: Kober'sche Verlagsbuchhandlung, 1960.

Schrenck-Notzing, Albert von. "Albert von Keller als Malerpsychologe und Metapsychiker." *Psychische Studien* 48 (April–May 1921): 193–215.

———. *Materialisationsphaenomene: Ein Beitrag zur Erforschung der mediumistischen Teleplastie.* Munich: E. Reinhardt, 1914.

———. *Der Prozess der Bombastus-Werke.* In *Sonderabdruck aus der Kriminalanthropologie und Kriminalistik,* ed. Hans Gross. Leipzig: F. C. W. Vogel, 1910.

———. *Die Traumtänzerin Magdeleine G.: Eine psychologische Studie über Hypnose und dramatische Kunst.* Stuttgart: Ferdinand Enke, 1904.

Schubert, Hermann. "The Fourth Dimension: Mathematical and Spiritualistic." *Monist* 3, no. 3 (1893): 402–49.

Sebottendorf, Rudolf von. *Bevor Hitler Kam.* Munich: Grassinger, 1933.

Seeling, Otto. *Der Bernburger Hellseher-Prozeß, mit Bild und Schriftprobe des Lehrers Drost nebst einem Vorwort von Rechtsanwalt Dr. Winterberg.* Berlin-Pankow: Linser, 1925.

Seiling, Max. *Mainländer, ein neuer Messias: Eine frohe Botschaft inmitten der herrschenden Geistesverwirrung.* Munich: Theodor Ackermann, 1888.

Seitz, Anton. *Okkultismus, Wissenschaft, und Religion,* 2 vols. Munich: Franz A. Pfeiffer, 1926–27.

Sellin, C. W. "Frau Rothe und die Wissenschaft." *Psychische Studien* 28 (November 1901): 687–706.

Sello, Erich. "Der Prozeß Rothe." *Die Zukunft* 43 (18 April 1903): 93–98.

Solden, Bert van. *Das astrologische Examen, 1, Die mündliche Prüfung.* Memmingen: Uranus, 1937.

"Spiritismus in Leipzig, Der." *Im Neuen Reich* (1878): 721–35.

"Spiritualisten und die Wissenschaft, Die: Tischdrehen. Tischklopfen. Tischschreiben." *Die Gartenlaube* 2 (1861): 23–25.

Steiner, Rudolf. *The Story of My Life.* London: Anthroposophical Publishing, 1928. Originally *Mein Lebensgang.* Dornach: Philosophisch-anthroposophischer Verlag, 1925.

———. *Theosophie: Einführung in übersinnliche Welterkenntnis und Menschenbestimmung.* Dornach: Rudolf Steiner, 1973.

———. *Theosophy: An Introduction to the Supersensible Knowledge of the World and the Destination of Man.* New York: Anthroposophic Press, 1923.

———. *Zur Geschichte und aus den Inhalten der ersten Abteilung der Esoterischen Schule, 1904–1914: Briefe, Rundbriefe, Dokumente, und Vorträge.* Dornach, Switzerland: Rudolf Steiner, 1984.

Steinschneider, Hermann. *Der Leitmeritzer Hellseher-Prozess Hanussen: Ausführliche Wiedergabe der sensationallen Gerichts-Verhandlung mit zahlreichen bisher unveröffentlichten Dokumenten.* Teplitz-Schönau: Selbstverlag, c. 1930.

Süddeutsche Monatshefte. Issue on astrology. June 1927.

Süddeutsche Monatshefte. Issue on fringe medicine. November 1932.

Surya, G. W. *Sammlung Okkulte Medizin.* Berlin-Pankow: Linser, 1921–25.

Tartaruga, Ubald. "Aus dem Reiche des Hellsehwunders: Neue retroskopische Versuche." *Die Okkulte Welt,* vol. 122, no. 3 (1925).

"Telepath als Detektiv, Der." *Zentralblatt für Okkultismus* 13, no. 11 (1920): 521–22.

"Therese (Claire) Reichart vor Gericht." *Münchner Neueste Nachrichten* 99, 10 April 1926, p. 7.

Tillich, Paul. *The Religious Situation.* Trans. H. Richard Niebuhr. New York: Meridian Books, 1956.

Tischner, Rudolf. *Geschichte der okkultistischen (metaphysischen) Forschung, von der Antike bis zur Gegenwart, 2, Von der Mitte des 19. Jahrhunderts bis zur Gegenwart.* Pfullingen in Württemberg: Johannes Baum, 1924.

Tonndorf, Marie. "Diätetische Winke." *Theosophie* 19, no. 3 (1931): 145–46.

Traub, Theodor, "Der Spiritismus." In *Kirchen und Sekten der Gegenwart,* ed. Ernst Kalb, 412–76. Stuttgart: Buchhandlung der Evang. Gesellschaft, 1905.

Ueber einen Fall von Einfühlungsvermögen in die Seele des Menschen (Ludwig Aub): Aufsätze, Meinungen, Erklärungen. Munich: Charakterologisches Sekretariat, n.d.

Verband Deutscher Okkultisten. *Bericht über die Verhandlungen auf dem Dritten Congress des "Verbandes Deutscher Okkultisten" am 31. Mai und 1. Juni (Pfingsten) 1898 in München.* Selbstverlag, c. 1898.

Verweyen, Johannes. *Der Neue Mensch und Seine Ziele: Menschheitsfragen der Gegenwart und Zukunft.* 2nd ed. Stuttgart: Walter Hädecke, 1930.

Wallace, Alfred Russel. "Wissenschaftliche und übersinnliche Anschauungen, ein Nachweis ihrer Übereinstimmung." *Sphinx* 1 (1886): 85–94.

Walther, Gerda, "A Plea for the Introduction of Edmund Husserl's Phenomenological Methods into Parapsychology." In *Proceedings of the First International Conference of Parapsychological Studies, 1953.* Clinton, MA: Colonial Press, 1955.

———. *Zum anderen Ufer: vom Marxismus und Atheismus zum Christentum.* Remagen: Otto Reichl, 1960.

Weingartner, Felix. *Bô Yin Râ.* Basel: Rhein, 1923.

Weisl, Wolfgang von. "Querschnitt durch ein okkultes Zeitalter." *Querschnitt* 12 (1933): 846–51.

Weltliteratur 16. Issue on occultism (August–September 1941).

Whistling, K. W. "Prof. Friedrich Zöllner." *Leipziger Illustrirte Zeitung* 2027 (6 May 1882): 374.

Woche, Die, 34. Issue on occultism (24 September 1932).

"'Wunderheilungen' in einem Schwarzwalddorf: Ein ungewöhnlicher Fall von Hellseher-Diagnose: Wissenschaftliche Gutachten." *Zeitschrift für Seelenleben (Beilage)* 32, no. 1 (1928): 7–8.

Wundt, Wilhelm. *Essays.* Leipzig: Wilhelm Engelmann, 1885.

"Wünschelrute und Erdstrahlen." *Münchner Tagblatt* 349, 15 December 1933, p. 4.

Zech, Elisabeth von. *Die Hellseherin Claire Reichert.* Munich: H. Frambold, n.d.

Zeller, Gustav. "Mediale Diagnostik." *Der Okkultismus* 1, no. 2 (1925): 23–26. Available at Stadtbibliothek München.

Zentrale für praktischen Okkultismus. n.p., n.d.

Zenz, Reinhold, ed. *Ist Hellsehen möglich? Der Insterburger "Hexen"-Prozeß gegen das kriminal-telepathische Medium Frau Günther-Geffers, mit 20 Abbildungen: Nach Prozeßberichten für die Königsberger Allgemeine Zeitung.* Königsberg: Königsberger Allgemeine Zeitung, 1928.

Zillmann, Paul. "Briefe über Mystik an einen Freund." *Neue Metaphysische Rundschau* 1, nos. 3–7 (1897–98): 196–201, 229–31, 328–32, 397–99.

———. "Die Wald-Loge und Akademie für okkulte Wissenschaft." *Neue Metaphysische Rundschau* 1, nos. 5–7 (1897–1898): 226–28.

Zobeltitz, Fedor von. *Chronik der Gesellschaft unter dem letzten Kaiserreich.* Hamburg: Alster, 1922.

Zöllner, Friedrich. "On Space of Four Dimensions." *Quarterly Journal of Science* 8 (April 1878): 227–37.

———. *Wissenschaftliche Abhandlungen.* 4 vols. Leipzig: L. Staackmann, 1878–81.

Zuckmayer, Carl. *A Part of Myself.* Trans. Richard and Clara Winston. New York: Harcourt Brace Jovanovich, 1966.

Zweig, Stefan. *The World of Yesterday.* Lincoln: University of Nebraska, 1943.

PUBLISHED SECONDARY SOURCES

Adorno, Theodor. "The Stars Down to Earth: The Los Angeles Times Astrology Column." *Telos* 19 (spring 1974): 13–90.

———. "Theses against Occultism." *Telos* 19 (spring 1974): 7–12.

Asendorf, Christoph. *Ströme und Strahlen: Das langsame Verschwinden der Materie um 1900.* Gießen: Anabas, 1989.

Ash, Mitchell G. *Gestalt Psychology in German Culture, 1890–1967.* Cambridge: Cambridge University Press, 1995.

Bade, Klaus J. *Friedrich Fabri und der Imperialismus in der Bismarckzeit. Revolution-Depression-Expansion.* Freiburg-im-Breisgau: Atlantis, 1975.

Bajohr, Frank, Werner Johe, and Uwe Lohalm, eds. *Zivilisation und Barberei: Die widersprüchlichen Potentiale der Moderne (Detlev Peukert zum Gedenken).* Hamburg: Christians, 1991.

Barrow, Logie. *Independent Spirits: Spiritualism and English Plebeians, 1850–1910.* London: Routledge & Kegan Paul, 1986.

Baßler, Moritz, and Hildegard Châtellier, eds. *Mystique, mysticisme, et modernité en Allemagne autour de 1900: Mystik, Mystizismus und Moderne in Deutschland um 1900.* Strasbourg: Presses Universitaires de Strasbourg, 1998.

Bauer, Eberhard. "Periods of Historical Development of Parapsychology in Germany: An Overview." *Research in Parapsychology 1991: Abstracts and Papers from the Thirty-Fourth Annual Convention of the Parapsychological Association* (1994): 123–27.

Ben-David, Joseph, and Randall Collins. "Social Factors in the Origins of a New Science: The Case of Psychology." *American Sociological Review* 31 (August 1966): 451–65.

Berman, Marshall, "Why Modernism Still Matters." In *Modernity and Identity,* ed. Scott Lash and Jonathan Friedman, 33–77. Oxford, Eng.: Blackwell, 1992.

Besser, Joachim. "Die Vorgeschichte des Nationalsozialismus in neuem Licht." *Die Pforte: Monatsschrift für Kultur* 21–22 (November 1950): 763–84.

Bibliographie der Zeitschriften des deutschen Sprachgebietes bis 1900. Stuttgart: Anton Hiersemann, 1977.

Blackbourn, David. *Marpingen: Apparitions of the Virgin Mary in a Nineteenth-century German Village.* Oxford: Oxford University Press, 1993.

———, and Geoff Eley. *The Peculiarities of German History: Bourgeois Society and Politics in Nineteenth-Century Germany.* Oxford: Oxford University Press, 1984.

Bock, Emil. *Rudolf Steiner: Studien zu seinem Lebensgang und Lebenswerk.* Stuttgart: Freies Geistesleben, 1961.

Boring, Edwin G. *A History of Experimental Psychology.* New York: Appleton-Century-Crofts, 1950.

Boventer, Hans. *Rilkes Zyklus "Aus dem Nachlass des Grafen C. W.": Versuch einer Eingliederung in Rilkes Werk.* Berlin: Erich Schmidt, 1969.

Braden, Charles S. *Spirits in Rebellion: The Rise and Development of New Thought.* Dallas, TX: Southern Methodist University Press, 1963.

Brandon, Ruth. *The Spiritualists: The Passion for the Occult in the Nineteenth and Twentieth Centuries.* New York: Alfred A. Knopf, 1983.

Brandstetter, Gabriele, "Psychologie des Ausdrucks und Ausdruckstanz: Aspekte der Wechselwirkung am Beispiel der 'Traumtänzerin' Madeleine." In *Ausdruckstanz: Eine mitteleuropäische Bewegung der ersten Hälfte des 20. Jahrhunderts,* ed. Gunhild Oberzaucher-Schüller, 199–211. Wilhelmshaven: Florian Noetzel, 1986.

Brinker-Gabler, Gisela, Karola Ludwig, and Angela Wöffen, eds. *Lexikon deutschsprachiger Schriftstellerinnen, 1800–1945.* Munich: Deutscher Taschenbuchverlag, 1986.

Brown, Michael F. *The Channeling Zone: American Spirituality in an Anxious Age.* Cambridge: Harvard University Press, 1997.

Bruch, Rüdiger vom, Friedrich Wilhelm Graf, and Gangolf Hübinger, eds. *Kultur und Kulturwissenschaften um 1900: Krise der Moderne und Glaube an die Wissenschaft.* Stuttgart: Franz Steiner, 1989.

Campbell, Bruce F. *Ancient Wisdom Revived: A History of the Theosophical Movement.* Berkeley: University of California Press, 1980.

Carlson, Maria. *"No Religion Higher Than Truth": A History of the Theosophical Movement in Russia, 1875–1922.* Princeton, NJ: Princeton University Press, 1993.

Celant, Germano. "Futurism and the Occult." *Art Forum* 19 (January 1981): 36–42.

"Clara Blüthgen." In *An Encyclopedia of German Women Writers, 1900–1933: Biographies and Bibliographies with Exemplary Readings,* ed. Brian Keith Smith. Lewiston, NY: Edwin Mellen, 1997.

Coon, Deborah. "Testing the Limits of Sense and Science: American Experimental Psychologists Combat Spiritualism, 1880–1920." *American Psychologist* 47 (February 1992): 143–51.

Cooter, Roger, and Stephen Pumphrey. "Separate Spheres and Public Spaces: Reflections on the History of Science Popularization and Science in Popular Culture." *History of Science* 32 (September 1994): 237–67.

Daim, Wilfried. *Der Mann, der Hitler die Ideen gab: Jörg Lanz von Liebenfels.* 3rd ed. Vienna: Ueberreuter, 1994.

Darnton, Robert. *Mesmerism and the End of the Enlightenment in France.* Cambridge: Harvard University Press, 1968.

Daum, Andreas. *Wissenschaftspopularisierung im 19. Jahrhundert: bürgerliche Kultur, naturwissenschaftliche Bildung und die deutsche Öffentlichkeit, 1848–1914.* Munich: R. Oldenbourg, 1998.

Decker, Hannah S. *Freud in Germany: Revolution and Reaction in Science, 1893–1907.* New York: International University Press, 1977.

Dixon, Joy. *Divine Feminine: Theosophy and Feminism in England.* Baltimore, MD: Johns Hopkins University Press, 2001.

During, Simon. *Modern Enchantments: The Cultural Power of Secular Magic.* Cambridge: Harvard University Press, 2002.

Eisner, Lotte. *Murnau.* Berkeley: University of California Press, 1964.

Eley, Geoff. *From Unification to Nazism: Reinterpreting the German Past.* Boston, MA: Unwin Hyman, 1986.

Eliade, Mircea. *Occultism, Witchcraft, and Cultural Fashions: Essays in Comparative Religion.* Chicago, IL: University of Chicago Press, 1976.

Ellenberger, Henri F. *The Discovery of the Unconscious: The History and Evolution of Dynamic Psychiatry.* New York: Basic Books, 1970.

Elsaesser, Thomas. *Weimar Cinema and After: Germany's Historical Imaginary.* London: Routledge, 2000.

Feyerabend, Paul. *Science in a Free Society.* London: Verso, 1985.

Forman, Paul. "Weimar Culture, Causality, and Quantum Theory, 1918–1927." *Historical Studies in the Physical Sciences* 3 (1971): 1–115.

Forster-Hahn, Françoise, ed. *Imagining Modern German Culture, 1889–1910.* Hanover, NH: University Press of New England, 1996.

Foster, R. F. *W. B. Yeats: A Life:* vol. 1, *The Apprentice Mage.* Oxford: Oxford University Press, 1997.

Freedman, Ralph. *Life of a Poet: Rainer Maria Rilke.* New York: Farrar, Straus & Giroux, 1996.

Galbreath, Robert. "The History of Modern Occultism: A Bibliographical Survey." *Journal of Popular Culture* 5, no. 3 (1971): 726–54.

———. "Spiritual Science in an Age of Materialism: Rudolf Steiner and Occultism," Ph.D. diss., University of Michigan, 1970.

Gauld, Alan. *A History of Hypnotism.* Cambridge: Cambridge University Press, 1992.

Gay, Peter. *Art and Act: On Causes in History: Manet, Gropius, Mondrian.* New York: Harper & Row, 1976.

Geuter, Ulfried, ed. *Daten zur Geschichte der deutschen Psychologie: Band I: Psychologische Institute, Fachgesellschaften, Fachzeitschriften und Serien, Biographien, Emigranten, 1879–1945.* Göttingen: Verlag für Psychologie, 1986.

Geuter, Ulfried. *The Professionalization of Psychiatry in Nazi Germany.* Cambridge: Cambridge University Press, 1992.

Glowka, Hans-Jürgen. *Deutsche Okkultgruppen, 1875–1937.* Munich: Arbeitsgemeinschaft für Religions-und Weltanschauungsfragen, 1981.

Godwin, Joscelyn. *The Theosophical Enlightenment.* Albany: State University of New York Press, 1994.

Golding, John. *Paths to the Absolute: Mondrian, Malevich, Kandinsky, Pollock, Newman, Rothko, and Still.* Princeton, NJ: Princeton University Press, 2000.

Goldstein, Jeffrey A. "On Racism and Anti-Semitism in Occultism and Nazism." *Yad Vashem Studies* 13 (1979): 53–72.

Goodrick-Clarke, Nicholas. *Black Sun: Aryan Cults, Esoteric Nazism, and the Politics of Identity.* New York: New York University Press, 2001.

———. *Hitler's Priestess: Savitri Devi, the Hindu-Aryan Myth, and Neo-Nazism.* New York: New York University Press, 1998.

———. "The Modern Occult Revival in Vienna, 1880–1910." *Durham University Journal* 80, no. 1 (1987): 63–68.

———. *The Occult Roots of Nazism: The Ariosophists of Austria and Germany, 1890–1935.* New York: New York University Press, 1985.

Gordon, Mel. *Hitler's Jewish Clairvoyant: Erik Jan Hanussen.* Los Angeles, CA: Feral House, 2001.

Götz von Olenhusen, Albrecht, ed. *Wege und Abwege: Beiträge zur europäischen Geistesgeschichte der Neuzeit: Festschrift für Ellic Howe zum 20. September 1990.* Freiburg: Hochschul, 1990.

Green, Martin. *Mountain of Truth: The Counterculture Begins: Ascona, 1900–1920.* Hanover, NH: University Press of New England, 1986.

Gregory, Frederick. *Nature Lost? Natural Science and the German Theological Traditions of the Nineteenth Century.* Cambridge: Harvard University Press, 1992.

————. *Scientific Materialism in Nineteenth-Century Germany*. Boston, MA: D. Reidel Publishing, 1977.

Hall, G. Stanley. *Founders of Modern Psychology*. New York: D. Appleton, 1912.

Harrington, Anne. *Reenchanted Science: Holism in German Culture from Wilhelm II to Hitler*. Princeton, NJ: Princeton University Press, 1996.

Hau, Michael. "The Holistic Gaze in German Medicine, 1890–1930." *Bulletin for the History of Medicine* 74 (2000): 495–524.

Hayman, Ronald. *A Life of Jung*. New York: W. W. Norton, 1999.

Hazelgrove, Jenny. *Spiritualism and British Society between the Wars*. Manchester, Eng.: Manchester University Press, 2000.

Hellge, Manfred. *Der Verleger Wilhelm Friedrich und das "Magazin für die Literatur des In-und Auslandes": Ein Beitrag zur Literatur-und Verlagsgeschichte des frühen Naturalismus in Deutschland*. Archiv für Geschichte des Buchwesens 16, nos. 4–5. Frankfurt-am-Main: Buchhändler-Vereinigung GmbH, 1976.

Henderson, Linda Dalrymple. *The Fourth Dimension and Non-Euclidean Geometry in Modern Art*. Princeton, NJ: Princeton University Press, 1983.

Herf, Jeffrey. *Reactionary Modernism: Technology, Culture, and Politics in Weimar and the Third Reich*. Cambridge: Cambridge University Press, 1984.

Herrmann, Dieter B. *Karl Friedrich Zöllner*. Leipzig: Teubner Gesellschaft, 1982.

Hieronimus, Ekkehard. *Lanz von Liebenfels: Eine Bibliographie*. Toppenstedt: Uwe Berg, 1991.

Howe, Ellic. *Astrology and the Third Reich: A Historical Study of Astrological Beliefs in Western Europe since 1700 and in Hitler's Germany, 1933–45*. Wellingborough, Northants.: Aquarian, 1984.

————, and Helmut Möller. "Theodor Reuss: Irregular Freemasonry in Germany, 1900–23." *Ars Quatuor Coronatorum* 91 (1978): 28–46.

Hübinger, Gangolf. *Kulturprotestantismus und Politik: Zum Verhältnis von Liberalismus und Protestantismus im wilhelminischen Deutschland*. Tübingen: J. C. B. Mohr, 1994.

————. "Liberalismus und Individualismus im deutschen Bürgertum." *Zeitschrift für Politik* 40, no. 1 (1993): 60–78.

————. "Der Verlag Eugen Diederichs in Jena: Wissenschaftskritik, Lebensreform, und völkische Bewegung." *Geschichte und Gesellschaft* 22 (1996): 31–45.

Huerkamp, Claudia. "Medizinische Lebensreform im späten 19. Jahrhundert: Die Naturheilbewegung in Deutschland als Protest gegen die naturwissenschaftliche Universitätsmedizin." *Vierteljahrschrift für Sozial- und Wirtschaftsgeschichte* 73, no. 2 (1986): 158–82.

Hughes, H. Stuart. *Consciousness and Society: The Reconstruction of European Social Thought*. New York: Vintage, 1958.

Hull, Isabel. *The Entourage of Kaiser Wilhelm II, 1888–1918*. Cambridge: Cambridge University Press, 1982.

Jardine, Nicholas, "*Naturphilosophie* and the Kingdoms of Nature." In *Cultures of Natural History*, ed. Nicholas Jardine, James A. Secord, and Emma C. Spary, 230–45. Cambridge: Cambridge University Press, 1996.

Jelavich, Peter. *Munich and Theatrical Modernism: Politics, Playwriting, and Performance, 1890–1914*. Cambridge: Harvard University Press, 1985.

Johnson, K. Paul. *The Masters Revealed: Madame Blavatsky and the Myth of the Great White Lodge*. New York: State University of New York Press, 1994.

Jones, Ernest. *The Life and Work of Sigmund Freud:* vol. 3, *The Last Phase, 1919–1939.* New York: Basic Books, 1957.

Jütte, Robert. *Geschichte der Alternativen Medizin: Von der Volksmedizin zu den unkonventionellen Therapien von heute.* Munich: C. H. Beck, 1996.

——. "The Historiography of Nonconventional Medicine in Germany: A Concise Overview." *Medical History* 43, no. 1 (1999): 342–58.

Jütte, Robert, Motzi Eklöf, and Marie C. Nelson, eds. *Historical Aspects of Unconventional Medicine: Approaches, Concepts, Case Studies.* Sheffield, Yorks.: European Association for the History of Medicine and Health Publications, 2001.

Kamps, Karl. *Johannes Maria Verweyen: Gottsucher, Mahner, und Bekenner.* Wiesbaden: Im Credo-Verlag, 1955.

Käss, Siegfried. *Der heimliche Kaiser der Kunst: Adolf Bayersdorfer, seine Freunde und seine Zeit.* Munich: tuduv Verlagsgesellschaft, 1987.

Kater, Michael. *Doctors under Hitler.* Chapel Hill: University of North Carolina Press, 1989.

Kerbs, Diethart, and Jürgen Reulecke, eds. *Handbuch der deutschen Reformbewegungen, 1880–1933.* Wuppertal: Peter Hammer, 1998.

Kerr, Howard, and Charles L. Crow, eds. *The Occult in America: New Historical Perspectives.* Urbana: University of Illinois Press, 1982.

Kershaw, Ian. *Hitler, 1889–1936: Hubris.* New York: W. W. Norton, 1998.

Klatt, Norbert. *Der Nachlaß von Wilhelm Hübbe-Schleiden in der Niedersächsischen Staats-und Universitätsbibliothek Göttingen: Verzeichnis der Materialien und Korrespondenten mit bio-bibliographischen Angaben.* Göttingen: Klatt, 1996.

——. *Theosophie und Anthroposophie: neue Aspekte zu ihrer Geschichte aus dem Nachlaß von Wilhelm Hübbe-Schleiden, 1846–1916 mit einer Auswahl von 81 Briefen.* Göttingen: Klatt, 1993.

Knoblauch, Hubert. *Die Welt der Wünschelrutengänger und Pendler: Erkundungen einer verborgenen Wirklichkeit.* Frankfurt: Campus, 1991.

Krabbe, Wolfgang R. *Gesellschaftsveränderung durch Lebensreform: Strukturmerkmale einer sozialreformerischen Bewegung in Deutschland der Industrialisierungsperiode.* Göttingen: Vandenhoeck & Ruprecht, 1974.

Kselman, Thomas A. *Death and the Afterlife in Modern France.* Princeton, NJ: Princeton University Press, 1993.

Kury, Astrid. *"Heiligenscheine eines elektrischen Jahrhundertendes sehen anders aus . . .": Okkultismus und die Kunst der Wiener Moderne.* Vienna: Passagen, 2000.

Langewiesche, Dieter. *Liberalism in Germany.* Princeton, NJ: Princeton University Press, 2000.

Latour, Bruno. *Science in Action: How To Follow Scientists and Engineers through Society.* Milton Keynes, Eng.: Open University, 1987.

Le Maléfan, Pascal. "Naissance du parapsychologique chez Max Dessoir, philosophe et médecin, 1867–1947." *Fr'en'esie* 10 (spring 1992): 237–48.

Leahey, Thomas Hardy, and Grace Evans Leahey. *Psychology's Occult Doubles: Psychology and the Problem of Pseudoscience.* Chicago, IL: Nelson-Hall, 1983.

Lears, T. J. Jackson. *No Place of Grace: Antimodernism and the Transformation of American Culture, 1880–1920.* Chicago, IL: University of Chicago Press, 1994.

Lenman, Robin. *Artists and Society in Germany, 1850–1914.* Manchester, Eng.: Manchester University Press, 1997.

Levinger, Matthew. *Enlightened Nationalism: The Transformation of Prussian Political Culture, 1806–1848.* New York: Oxford University Press, 2000.

Lexikon der deutschen Verlage: Eine Chronik der deutschen Verlagsfirmen, enthaltend die Geschichte der Zeitungs-, Zeitschriften und Buchverlage, der Kunst-und Musikverlage, sowie der Katalogantiquare. Leipzig: Curt Müller, c. 1930.

Linse, Ulrich, " 'Das Buch der Wunder und Geheimwissenschaften': Der spiritistische Verlag Oswald Mutze in Leipzig im Rahmen der spiritistischen Bewegung Sachsens." In *Das Bewegte Buch: Buchwesen und soziale, nationale und kulturelle Bewegungen um 1900,* ed. Mark Lehmstedt and Andreas Herzog, 219–44. Wiesbaden: Harrassowitz, 1999.

———. *Geisterseher und Wunderwirker: Heilssuche im Industriezeitalter.* Frankfurt-am-Main: Fischer, 1996.

Lukács, Georg. *The Destruction of Reason.* Trans. Peter Palmer. Atlantic Highlands, NJ: Humanities Press, 1981.

Makela, Maria. *The Munich Secession: Art and Artists in Turn-of-the-Century Munich.* Princeton, NJ: Princeton University Press, 1990.

McFarlane, James, "Berlin and the Rise of Modernism, 1886–1896." In *Modernism, 1890–1930,* ed. Malcolm Bradbury and James McFarlane, 105–19. New York: Penguin, 1976.

Martel, Gordon, ed. *Modern Germany Reconsidered, 1870–1945.* London: Routledge, 1992.

Mercier, Alain. *Les Sources Ésoteriques et Occultes de la Poésie Symboliste, 1870–1914.* Paris: Editions A.-G. Nizet, 1974.

Miers, Horst. *Lexikon des Geheimwissens.* Munich: Wilhelm Goldmann, 1993.

Moore, Laurence R. *In Search of White Crows: Spiritualism, Parapsychology, and American Culture.* New York: Oxford University Press, 1977.

Mosse, George L. *The Crisis of German Ideology: Intellectual Origins of the Third Reich.* New York: Universal Library, 1964.

———. "The Mystical Origins of National Socialism." *Journal of the History of Ideas* 22, no. 1 (1961): 81–96.

Müller, Oskar A. *Albert von Keller: 1884 Gais/Schweiz–1920 München.* Munich: Karl Thiemig, 1981.

Noakes, Richard J. " 'Telegraphy Is an Occult Art': Cromwell Fleetwood Varley and the Diffusion of Electricity to the Other World." *British Journal for the History of Science* 32 (1999): 421–59.

Noll, Richard. *The Jung Cult: Origins of a Charismatic Movement.* Princeton, NJ: Princeton University Press, 1994.

Okkultismus und Avantgarde: Von Munch bis Mondrian, 1900–1915. Schirn Kunsthalle, Frankfurt: Edition Tertium, 1995.

Oppenheim, Janet. *The Other World: Spiritualism and Psychical Research in England, 1850–1914.* Cambridge: Cambridge University Press, 1985.

Owen, Alex. *The Darkened Room: Women, Power, and Spiritualism in Late Victorian England.* Philadelphia: University of Pennsylvania Press, 1990.

———, "Occultism and the 'Modern Self' in Fin-de-Siècle Britain." In *Meanings of Modernity: Britain from the Late Victorian Era to World War II,* ed. Martin Daunton and Bernhard Rieger, 71–96. New York: Berg, 2001.

Padfield, Peter. *Hess: Flight for the Führer.* London: Weidenfeld & Nicolson, 1991.

Pascal, Roy. *From Naturalism to Expressionism: German Literature and Society, 1880–1918.* New York: Basic Books, 1973.

Peukert, Detlev. *Max Webers Diagnose der Moderne.* Göttingen: Vandenhoeck & Ruprecht, 1989.

———. *The Weimar Republic: The Crisis of Classical Modernity.* Trans. Richard Deveson. New York: Hill & Wang, 1989.

Polizzotti, Mark. *Revolution of the Mind: The Life of André Breton.* New York: Farrar, Straus & Giroux, 1995.

Proctor, Robert. *The Nazi War on Cancer.* Princeton, NJ: Princeton University Press, 1999.

———. *Racial Hygiene: Medicine under the Nazis.* Cambridge: Harvard University Press, 1988.

Pulzer, Peter G. *The Rise of Political Anti-Semitism in Germany and Austria.* New York: John Wiley & Sons, 1964.

Puschner, Uwe. *Die völkische Bewegung im wilhelminischen Kaiserreich: Sprache-Rasse-Religion.* Darmstadt: Wissenschaftliche Buchgesellschaft, 2001.

Puschner, Uwe, Walter Schmitz, and Justus H. Ulbricht, eds. *Handbuch zur "Völkischen Bewegung," 1871–1918.* Munich: K. G. Saur, 1996.

Rabinbach, Anson. "Eine andere Moderne?" *Central European History* 34 (2001): 579–85.

———. *The Human Motor: Energy, Fatigue, and the Origins of Modernity.* New York: Basic Books, 1990.

Repp, Kevin. *Reformers, Critics, and the Paths of German Modernity: Anti-Politics and the Search for Alternatives.* Cambridge: Harvard University Press, 2000.

Richter, Margaret Mary. "Gabriel Max: The Artist, the Darwinist and the Spiritualist," Ph.D. diss., New York University, 1998.

Ringbom, Sixten. "Art in 'The Epoch of the Great Spiritual': Occult Elements in the Early Theory of Abstract Painting." *Journal of the Warburg and Courtauld Institutes* 29 (1966): 386–418.

———. *The Sounding Cosmos: A Study in the Spiritualism of Kandinsky and the Genesis of Abstract Painting.* Abo, Finland: Abo Akademi, 1970.

Ringer, Fritz. *The Decline of the German Mandarins.* Hanover, NH: University Press of New England, 1990.

Rogoff, Irit, ed. *The Divided Heritage: Themes and Problems in German Modernism.* Cambridge: Cambridge University Press, 1991.

Röhl, John C. G. *The Kaiser and His Court: Wilhelm II and the Government of Germany.* Cambridge: Cambridge University Press, 1987.

———. *Young Wilhelm: The Kaiser's Early Life, 1859–1888.* Trans. Jeremy Gaines and Rebecca Wallach. Cambridge: Cambridge University Press, 1998.

Rohrkrämer, Thomas. *Eine andere Moderne? Zivilisationskritik, Natur, und Technik in Deutschland, 1880–1933.* Paderborn: Ferdinand Schöningh, 1999.

Rosenhagen, Hans. *Albert von Keller.* Bielefeld: Velhagen & Klasing, 1912.

Rosenthal, Bernice Glatzer, ed. *The Occult in Russian and Soviet Culture.* Ithaca, NY: Cornell University Press, 1997.

Ross, Dorothy, ed. *Modernist Impulses in the Human Sciences.* Baltimore, MD: Johns Hopkins University Press, 1994.

Sawicki, Diethard. *Leben mit den Toten: Geisterglauben und die Entstehung des Spiritismus in Deutschland, 1770–1900.* Paderborn: Ferdinand Schöningh, 2002.

Schmidt, Rudolf. *Deutsche Buchhändler, deutsche Buchdrucker.* Berlin: Frank Weber, 1902–8.

Schnurbein, Stefanie von. *Religion als Kulturkritik: Neugermanisches Heidentum im 20. Jahrhundert.* Heidelberg: Carl Winter Universitätsverlag, 1992.

Schorske, Carl. *Fin-de-Siècle Vienna: Politics and Culture.* New York: Vintage, 1961.

Schüler, Winfried. *Der Bayreuther Kreis von seiner Entstehung bis zum Ausgang der Wilhelminischen Ära: Wagnerkult und Kulturreform im Geiste völkischer Weltanschauung.* Münster: Aschendorff, 1971.

Shapin, Steven, "Science and the Public." In *Companion to the History of Modern Science,* ed. R. C. Olby, 990–1007. London: Routledge, 1990.

Sharp, Lynn L. "Spiritual Equality: Spiritism's Challenge to the Second Empire." *Proceedings of the Annual Meeting of the Western Society for French History* 18 (1991): 331–36.

———. "Women in Spiritism: Using the Beyond to Construct the Here and Now." *Proceedings of the Annual Meeting of the Western Society for French History* 21 (1994): 161–68.

Sheehan, James. *German Liberalism in the Nineteenth Century.* Chicago, IL: University of Chicago Press, 1978.

Shepard, Leslie, ed. *Encyclopedia of Occultism and Parapsychology.* 2nd and 3rd eds. Detroit: Gale Research. 1984–85 and 1991.

Smith, Woodruff D. *The Ideological Origins of Nazi Imperialism.* New York: Oxford University Press, 1986.

———. "The Ideology of German Colonialism, 1840–1906." *Journal of Modern History* 46 (December 1974): 641–62.

Spiegelberg, Herbert. *The Phenomenological Movement: A Historical Introduction,* 2 vols. The Hague: Martinus Nijhoff, 1960.

Spielvogel, Jackson, and David Redles. "Hitler's Racial Ideology: Content and Occult Sources." *Simon Wiesenthal Center Annual* 3 (1986): 227–46.

Spiritual in Art, The: Abstract Painting, 1890–1985. Los Angeles: Los Angeles County Museum of Art, 1986.

Stark, Gary D. *Entrepreneurs of Ideology: Neoconservative Publishers in Germany, 1890–1933.* Chapel Hill: University of North Carolina Press, 1981.

Staubermann, Klaus. "Tying the Knot: Skill, Judgement, and Authority in the 1870s Leipzig Spiritistic Experiments." *British Journal for the History of Science* 34 (2001): 67–79.

Stearns, Peter. "Stages of Consumerism: Recent Work on the Issues of Periodization." *Journal of Modern History* 69 (March 1997): 102–17.

Stern, Fritz. *The Politics of Cultural Despair: A Study in the Rise of the German Ideology.* Berkeley: University of California Press, 1961.

Sumser, Robert. "Rational Occultism in Fin de Siècle Germany: Rudolf Steiner's Modernism." *History of European Ideas* 18, no. 4 (1994): 497–511.

Szeemann, Harald, ed. *Monte Verità: Berg der Wahrheit: Lokale Anthropologie als Beitrag zur Wiederentdeckung einer neuzeitlichen sakralen Topographie.* Milan: Electa Editrice, 1978.

Thiel, Christian. "Zur Dynamik von Wissenschaft, Grenzwissenschaften, und Pseudo-wissenschaften in der Moderne." *Zeitschrift für Parapsychologie und Grenzgebiete der Psychologie* 30 (1988): 152–71.

Timmermann, Carsten. "Constitutional Medicine, Neoromanticism, and the Politics of Antimechanism in Interwar Germany." *Bulletin for the History of Medicine* 75 (2001): 717–39.

Tiryakian, Edward A. "Toward the Sociology of Esoteric Culture." *American Journal of Sociology* 78, no. 3 (1972): 491–512.

Tiryakian, Edward A., ed. *On the Margins of the Visible: Sociology, the Esoteric, and the Occult.* New York: John Wiley & Sons, 1974.

Treitel, Corinna, "The Culture of Knowledge in the Metropolis of Science: Spiritualism and Liberalism in Fin-de-Siècle Berlin." In *Wissenschaft und Öffentlichkeit in Berlin, 1870–1930,* ed. Constantin Goschler, 127–54. Stuttgart: Franz Steiner, 2000.

Trevor-Roper, H. R. *The Last Days of Hitler.* 5th ed. London: Macmillan, 1978.

Truzzi, Marcello. "Definition and Dimensions of the Occult: Towards a Sociological Perspective." *Journal of Popular Culture* 5, no. 3 (1971): 635–46.

Uhde-Bernays, Hermann. *Die Münchner Malerei im neunzehnten Jahrhundert, 2, 1850–1900.* Munich: F. Bruckmann, n.d.

Webb, James. *The Occult Establishment.* La Salle, IL: Open Court, 1976.

———. *The Occult Underground.* La Salle, IL: Open Court, 1974.

Wedemeyer, Bernd. "'Zum Licht': Die Freikörperkultur in der wilhelminischen Ära und der Weimarer Republik zwischen Völkischer Bewegung, Okkultismus, und Neuheidentum." *Archiv für Kulturgeschichte* 81, no. 1 (1999): 172–97.

Wegner, Gunda. "Das Leben des Georg von Langsdorff: Turner, Revolutionär, und Wissenschaftler." *Zeitschrift des Breisgau-Geschichtsvereins "Schau-ins-Land"* 111 (1992): 79–94.

Wehler, Hans-Ulrich. *Bismarck und der Imperialismus.* Cologne: Kiepenheuer & Witsch, 1969.

Wendelborn, Sören. "Die Entwicklung der Klinischen Psychologie im Berlin des ausgehenden 19. Jahrhunderts dargestellt am Beispiel Albert Moll, 1862–1939." *Psychologie und Geschichte* 6 (1994): 303–12.

Wessinger, Catherine, ed. *Women's Leadership in Marginal Religions: Explorations Outside the Mainstream.* Urbana: University of Illinois Press, 1993.

Winter, Alison. *Mesmerized: Powers of Mind in Victorian Britain.* Chicago, IL: University of Chicago Press, 1998.

Wintzingerode-Knorr, Karl-Wilhelm. "Hanns v. Gumppenbergs Künstlerisches Werk: Ein Beitrag zur Geschichte der deutschen Literatur der Wende vom 19. zum 20. Jahrhundert." Ph.D. diss., Ludwig-Maximilians-Universität München, 1958.

Woodward, William R., and Mitchell G. Ash, eds. *The Problematic Science: Psychology in Nineteenth-Century Thought.* New York: Prager, 1982.

Wulff, Wilhelm. *Zodiac and Swastika: How Astrology Guided Hitler's Germany.* New York: Coward, McCann & Geoghegan, 1973.

Zander, Helmut. *Geschichte der Seelenwanderung in Europa: Alternative religiöse Traditionen von der Antike bis heute.* Darmstadt: Wissenschaftliche Buchgesellschaft, 1999.

Names Index

Achelis, Werner (b. 1897), 141
Adorno, Theodor (1903–1969), 280n66
Agricola, Georgius (1494–1555), 150
Aigner, Eduard (b. 1871), 152–53
Aksakow, Alexander (1832–1903), 33, 39, 71, 108
Altmann, Max, 73
Amann, Rosa, 207
Andreas-Salomé, Lou (1861–1937), 49, 72
Arp, Hans (1886–1966), 109
Aßmann, Wilhelmine (pseud. Frieda Genthes), 122–24
Aub, Ludwig, 135–36, 139–40, 156
Aurelius, Marcus (121–180), 105

Balfour, Eleanor. *See* Sidgwick, Eleanor Balfour
Barrett, William F. (1844–1925), 150
Bastian, Adolf (1826–1905), 52
Bäumer, Gertrud (1873–1954), 51
Bayersdorfer, Adolf (1842–1901), 40, 62, 110, 283n27
Bellachini, Samuel (1827–1885), 4, 23
Benjamin, Walter (1892–1940), 139–40
Berger, Johannes, 196
Berman, Marshall, 50
Bernheim, Hippolyte (1840–1919), 33, 43, 47–48
Besant, Annie (1847–1933), 74, 125
Besser, Wilhelm, 39
Beßmer, Julius (1864–1924), 198–99
Beyer, Paul, 152
Binet, Alfred (1857–1911), 47–48
Bismarck, Otto von (1815–1898), 87, 90, 159
Blavatsky, H. P. (Helena Petrovna; 1831–1891), 53, 66, 74, 85, 95; fraud by, 83, 96
Bleibtreu, Karl (1859–1928), 72
Bleuler, Eugen (1857–1939), 29, 49

Bloch, Iwan (1872–1922), 45, 291n6
Blüthgen, Klara (pseud. Clara Eysell-Kilburger; 1856–1934), 121–22, 124
Böcklin, Arnold (1827–1901), 110
Böhme, Jakob (1575–1624), 159
Bohn, Erich, 172–74, 176, 181, 189
Bölsche, Wilhelm (1861–1939), 299n4
Bolyai, János, 8
Bormann, Martin (1900–1945), 217, 240
Bô Yin Râ. *See* Schneiderfranken, Joseph Anton
Braid, James (1795?–1860), 32, 35
Brandler-Pracht, Karl (1864–1939), 78, 141–42
Brentano, Franz Clemens (1838–1917), 35, 98
Bresch, Richard, 298n78
Breton, André (1896–1966), 119
Breuer, Josef (1842–1925), 48
Breuing, Katharina, 230
Brockdorff, Cay von (1844–1921), 99, 176
Brockdorff, Sophie von (1848–1906), 99, 176
Browne, C. A. (1870–1947), 143
Brunn, Ludwig, 46
Büchner, Ludwig (1824–1899), 32, 34–35
Bülow, Bernhard von (1849–1929), 91
Bülow, Werner von (1870–1947), 107
Bülow-Bothkamp, Cai von, 150
Buntzel, Walther, 195
Busse, Hans (1871–1920), 138–39

Cagliostro, Alessandro di Conte (Giuseppe Balsamo; 1743–1795), 53
Canetti, Elias (1905–1994), 290n56
Cattell, James McKeen (1860–1944), 134–36
Charcot, Jean-Martin (1825–1893), 32–33, 43, 46–47
Christiansen, W. A., 231

Clobes, Hanns-Maria, 226–28
Conrad, I. F., 70
Conrad, Michael Georg (1846–1927), 72, 119, 142
Cook, Florence (1856–1904), 111, 313n8
Courbet, Gustave (1819–1877), 110
Crookes, William (1832–1919), 5, 7, 29, 47–48, 71
Cyriax, Bernhard (b. 1820), 39

Däbritz, Max, 195–96
Dacqué, Edgar (1878–1945), 61
Dalberg, Otto (Clara Eysell-Kilburger's spirit guide), 121–22, 124
Damaschke, Adolf (1865–1935), 51
Daqué, Edgar, 140
Darwin, Charles (1809–1882), 53
Davis, Andrew Jackson (1826–1910), 38–39, 53, 71
Deinhard, Ludwig (1847–1917), 40
Delbouef, Joseph, 47
Dessoir, Max (1867–1947), 33, 44, 46, 61, 63, 152, 200; and experimental psychology, 47–48; on Freud, 49; and Rothe case, 184, 187; and women occultists, 64–65
Diederich, Mrs., 145
Diederichs, Eugen (1867–1930), 74
Dingfelder, Johannes, 136, 156
Doesburg, Theo van (1883–1931), 109
Dörfler, Josef (b. 1883), 198–99
Dove, Arthur (1880–1946), 109
Doyle, Arthur Conan (1859–1930), 126, 129, 144
Driesch, Hans (1867–1941), 140
Drost, August Christian (b. 1873), 145, 148–49
Dühring, Eugen (1833–1921), 10
Duncan, Isadora (1877–1927), 102, 118
du Prel, Albertine, 65
du Prel, Carl (1839–1899), 33, 40–43, 46, 48, 62, 206; and Catholic Church, 197–99; defense of occultism by, 202, 204, 208; and Kandinsky, 108; and periodicals, 52, 71, 83; publications of, 53, 70, 72, 74; on religion and science, 193–94; and Schrenck-Notzing, 44–45; and transcendent psychology, 50–51

Eckstein, Friedrich (1861–1939), 99
Eddy, Mary Baker (1821–1910), 53
Eglinton, William (1858–1933), 301n22, 313n8

Eisner, Kurt (1867–1919), 83–84
Ellis, Havelock (1859–1939), 291n61
Emmerich, Anna Katherina (1774–1824), 111, 301n19
Engels, Friedrich (1820–1895), 20
Ennemoser, Joseph (1787–1854), 35
Ernst, Max (1891–1976), 109
Eulenburg, Philipp zu (1847–1921), 66, 176
Eysell-Kilburger, Clara. *See* Blüthgen, Klara

Fabri, Friedrich (1824–1891), 87
Falk, Egbert. *See* Fuhrmann, Georg
Falk, Georg, 229
Fechner, Gustav Theodor (1801–1887), 3–4, 8, 15, 32, 44; and psychology, 21–22, 45
Ferenczi, Sandor (1873–1933), 49
Fichte, J. G. (1762–1814), 35
Flournoy, Théodore (1854–1920), 33, 48
Fontane, Theodor (1819–1898), 72
Forel, Auguste (1848–1931), 47–48, 291n61
Fox, Kate (1836–1892), 37
Fox, Maggie (1833–1893), 37
Francé-Harrar, Annie (b. 1886), 66
Frank, Hans (1900–1946), 213
Franzius, Georg (1842–1914), 150, 152
Frederick William III of Prussia (1770–1840), 35
Frei, Bruno (b. 1897), 233
Freud, Sigmund (1856–1939), 33, 36, 48–49, 51, 72
Frick, Ernst, 102
Friedchen (Anna Rothe's spirit guide), 169
Friedeberg, Raphael, 102
Friedrich, Wilhelm (1851–1925), 11, 72–74
Fritsche, Herbert (1911–1960), 159
Fuchs, Georg (1868–1949), 118
Fuhrmann, Georg (pseud. Egbert Falk; 1876–1949), 68
Fullerton, George (1859–1925), 15

Galton, Francis (1822–1911), 47, 107, 144
Gauss, Carl Friedrich, 8
Geben (Hanns von Gumppenberg's spirit guide), 120, 124
Gebhard, Franz (1853–1940), 62
Gebhard, Gustav (1828–1900), 62
Gebhard, Mary (1832–1892), 64
Genthes, Frieda. *See* Aßmann, Wilhelmine

Georgievitz-Weitzer, Demeter (pseud. G. W.
 Surya; 1873–1949), 156, 159
Gerber-Wieghardt, Mrs., 145
Gmelin, Eberhard (1753–1809), 282n10
Goebbels, Joseph (1897–1945), 211, 213–14, 216–
 17, 233, 240
Goethe, Johann Wolfgang von (1749–1832), 38,
 53, 64, 99, 176
Göler von Ravensburg, 62
Gollmann, Mr. (exorcist), 230
Goodrick-Clarke, Nicholas, 25–26
Graf, Oskar Maria (1894–1967), 102
Grau, Albin, 109
Greif, Martin (1839–1911), 283n27
Grimm, A. M. (b. 1892), 73, 205
Groll, Jacques, 31
Gross, Hans (1847–1915), 144
Gruber, Karl (1881–1927), 320n48
Grunewald, Fritz (1885–1925), 136–37
Grünewald, Karl, 230
Grüttefien, Ernst (b. 1866), 186
Gubalke, Max (1841–1900), 67, 178
Guipet, Madeleine (b. 1874), 49, 65, 114, 116–18,
 121
Gumppenberg, Hanns von (1866–1928), 65, 72,
 119–21, 124
Günther-Geffers, Else (Marie), 145–47
Guppy, Mary Jane (b. 1860), 313n8

Haeckel, Ernst (1834–1919), 111
Hahn, Diederich (1859–1918), 62
Hahnemann, Samuel (1755–1843), 159
Halbe, Max (1865–1944), 136
Hall, G. Stanley (1844–1924), 48
Hanussen, Erik Jan. *See* Steinschneider,
 Hermann
Harden, Maximilian (1861–1927), 72, 186, 188,
 289n34
Harnack, Adolf (1851–1930), 51
Hartleben, Otto Erich (1864–1905), 99
Hartmann, Eduard von (1842–1906), 24, 32–33,
 36, 39, 52; and du Prel, 41; and psychology,
 21–23; on Zöllner, 11, 13–15
Hartmann, Franz (1838–1912), 62–64, 66–67,
 71–72, 105; Theosophy of, 94–97, 99
Hartung, Erich, 158–59
Hasselblatt, Dora (1893–1975), 196

Hauffe, Friederike (Seeress of Prevorst; 1801–
 1829), 32, 35, 111
Haugg, Adolbert (b. 1878), 60, 203–4
Hegel, G. W. F., 98
Heigl, Franz, 203
Heimsoth, Karl-Günther, 156–57
Held, Hans Ludwig (1885–1954), 27
Hellpach, Willy (1877–1955), 45
Hellwig, Albert (1880–1950), 147–48, 201
Helmholtz, Hermann von (1821–1894), 8–11,
 21–23
Henkes, Karl, 207–8
Henne am Rhyn, Otto (1828–1914), 181, 189
Henneberg, Richard (1868–1962), 176–77, 184
Herrmann, Wilhelm, 179
Hess, Rudolf (1894–1987), 159, 240; flight to
 Britain of, 213–14, 216–17, 224, 231
Hesse, Hermann (1877–1962), 102
Hessel, Mrs., 145
Heydrich, Reinhard (1904–1942), 224
Heyse, Paul (1830–1914), 72
Hieronimus, Ekkehard, 26
Hildebrecht, Paul, 145
Himmler, Heinrich (1900–1945), 159, 211, 213–
 16, 225, 240; death of, 210
Hirschfeld, Magnus (1868–1935), 73
Hitler, Adolf (1889–1945), 25, 74, 159, 211, 216,
 218, 233, 240; and Ariosophy, 26, 104; death
 of, 210; and dowsing, 133, 213
Höcker, Karl, 206–7
Hoffmann, E. T. A. (1776–1822), 35, 53
Hollinger, David, 161
Holtum, Gregor von, 199
Home, D. D. (1833–1886), 313n8
Honigmann, Georg, 157
Honold, E., 54–55, 70
Höpfner, Walter, 231
Hornstein, Ferdinand von, 41
Hornstein, Robert (1833–1890), 283n27
Houdini, Harry (1874–1926), 165–66
Hübbe-Schleiden, Wilhelm (1846–1916), 27,
 40, 62, 101, 105, 135, 154, 227; and Franz Hart-
 mann, 94, 96–97; in India, 66; and modern-
 ism, 88, 90, 93; and nationalism, 87–89; on
 race, 87–88, 90–91, 103–4; and reform
 movements, 86, 90, 92–93; and *Sphinx*, 16,
 52, 71, 83–85, 89; and Theosophy, 86–93

Hubo, Bernhard (1851–1934), 62
Hufeland, Friedrich (1774–1839), 282n10
Husserl, Edmund (1859–1938), 49–50

Ibsen, Henrik (1828–1906), 72
Issberner-Haldane, Ernst (b. 1886), 73–74, 228

Jack the Ripper, 144
James, William (1842–1910), 24, 51, 88; and
     experimental psychology, 32, 46–48; and
     Leonora Piper, 33, 47
Janet, Pierre (1859–1947), 47–48
Jaschke, Willy, 243, 247–48
Jentsch, Max, 169, 187
Jung, Carl Gustav (1875–1961), 29–30, 33, 36,
     49, 51, 55, 102
Jury, Paul, 142

Kafka, Franz (1883–1924), 102
Kandinsky, Wassily (1866–1944), 16–17, 23–24,
     108–9, 111, 131; on color, 125–26; information
     problem of, 125; and Theosophy, 124–28
Kant, Immanuel (1724–1804), 7, 32, 72, 98; ide-
     alism of, 8–9, 20; occultism, 9; "thing in
     itself" of, 9, 20; transcendental subject of, 42
Kara Iki, 145
Kardec, Allan (1803?–1869), 72
Keller, Albert von (1844–1920), 40, 62, 110–11,
     118, 120; and Guipet, 116–17; and psychical
     research, 112–14
Keller, Helen (1880–1968), 53
Kemmerich, Max (1876–1932), 58, 320n48
Kern, Karl, 102–3
Kerner, Justinus (1786–1862), 32, 35, 53
Kersten, Felix (1898–1960), 214–15
Keyserling, Hermann (1880–1946), 93, 96
Kiesewetter, Karl (1854–1895), 72–74, 189
King, Kathie (Florence Cook's spirit guide), 111
Kircher, Mr., 195–96
Klages, Ludwig (1872–1956), 51, 138, 140, 208
Klee, Paul (1879–1940), 109
Klein, Christian Felix, 8
Klimt, Gustav (1862–1918), 114
Klinckowstroem, Karl von (1884–1969), 153
Klink, Else (1907), 131
Klint, Hilma af (1862–1944), 109
Klöckler, Herbert von (1896–1950), 140–41

Kluge, C. A. F. (1782–1844), 282n10
Knochen, Helmuth (b. 1910), 220
Kolrop, Mr., 220–22
Koot Hoomi, 92
Korsch, Hubert (1883–1942), 65, 78
Kraepelin, Emil (1856–1926), 208, 219
Krafft-Ebing, Richard von (1840–1902), 292n61
Kral, Josef (1887–1965), 319n34
Kratt, Gottfried, 69
Krawielitzki, M., 195
Kremer, Nikolaus, 152
Krishnamurti, Jiddu (1895–1986), 235
Kritzinger, H. H. (b. 1887), 206
Kröner, Walter, 156, 226
Kuhlenbeck, Ludwig (1857–1920), 83
Kürschner, Joseph (1853–1902), 99

Lagarde, Paul de (1827–1891), 83–84
Lampert, Carl, 239
Lang, Marie (1858–1934), 99
Langbehn, Julius (1851–1907), 74
Langsdorff, Georg von (1822–1921), 37–38, 67,
     69, 154, 183, 228
Lanz von Liebenfels, Jörg (1874–1954), 25–26,
     73, 104, 106, 159
Laqueur, Walter, 211, 215
Lauweriks, J. L. M. (1864–1932), 93
Lawrence, D. H. (1885–1930), 102
Leadbeater, Charles (1847–1934), 125
Lechter, Melchior (1865–1937), 299n4
Leixner, Otto von (1847–1907), 62
Leo, Alan (1860–1917), 53
Lessing, Theodor (1872–1933), 61, 88, 140
Liébault, Auguste Ambroise (1823–1904), 48
Liek, Erwin (1878–1935), 157–58
Liliencron, Detlev (1844–1909), 72
Lipps, Theodor (1851–1914), 48–49, 53, 61, 111
List, Guido von (1848–1919), 25, 53, 73–74, 104,
     215, 217
Lobatschewski, Nikolai Ivanovitch, 8
Loertzen, Erich, 244–47
Lombroso, Cesare (1836–1909), 47–48
Ludendorff, Erich (1865–1937), 219
Ludendorff, Mathilde (1882–1966), 218–20,
     225
Lukács, Georg (1885–1971), 279n59
Luther, Martin (1483–1546), 105, 159, 169

Maack, Ferdinand (1861–1930), 172–74, 176, 181
Machner, August, 175
Mager, Alois (1883–1946), 199
Magnin, Emile, 114, 116
Mailänder, Alois (1844–1905), 105
Malevich, Kazimir (1878–1935), 109
Maltzahn, Rudolf von, 153
Mann, Thomas (1875–1955), 36, 72, 109
Manteuffel, Hans von (1859?–1939), 62
Marc, Franz, 131
Massey, C. C. (b. 1838), 7
Matzinger, Lina, 40–42, 113–15, 117
Max, Emma von, 65
Max, Gabriel von (1840–1915), 40, 62, 110–12,
    118, 120
Maxwell, Herbert, 143
Meier-Parm, Christian, 78
Mendelssohn, Anja, 136, 140
Mensi von Klarbach, Alfred (1854–1933), 62
Mesmer, Franz Anton (1734–1815), 32, 35, 53
Meyer, Georg, 138
Meyrink, Gustav (1868–1932), 69, 109, 128, 130, 159
Migge, Mr., 145
Möckel, Erich, 145
Moll, Albert (1862–1939), 44, 63, 65, 176, 291n61
Moltke, Eliza von (1859–1932), 65, 100, 176, 183
Moltke, Helmuth von (1848–1916), 100, 176, 219
Moltke, Kuno (1847–1923), 66
Mondrian, Piet (1872–1944), 109
Morgner, Wilhelm (1891–1917), 131
Moser, Fanny (1872–1953), 143–44
Mosse, George, 25
Müller, Alexander, 160
Müller, Egbert, 144, 171, 175, 181
Müller, Élise-Catherin (pseud. Hélène Smith;
    1861–1929), 285n48
Münsterberg, Hugo von (1863–1916), 47
Murnau, Friedrich Wilhelm, 109
Mutze, Oswald (d. 1920), 7, 39; press of, 71–74
Myers, Frederic W. H. (1843–1901), 47–48

Narr, Regina, 202
Natge, Hans (1851–1906), 62
Nees von Esenbeck, Christian Gottfried (1776–
    1858), 38–39
Neumann-Kolmar, Eduard (pseud. Rolf Syl-
    véro), 231–32, 237–38

Neustätter, Otto (b. 1870), 195
Nielsen, Ejner (d. 1965), 136–37
Nietzsche, Friedrich (1844–1900), 18, 36, 53, 72,
    99, 234
Noë, Heinrich (1835–1896), 283n27
Nüßlein, Heinrich (b. 1879), 126, 128, 226

Oesterreich, Traugott Konstantin (1880–1949),
    193
Olcott, Henry Steel (1832–1907), 85, 88
Osswald, Kurt, 152

Paladino, Eusapia (1854–1918), 67, 168
Paracelsus (1493–1541), 70, 159
Peebles, J. M. (1822–1922), 95
Petzold, Mr., 145
Peukert, Detlev, 133
Pfänder, Alexander (1870–1941), 49–50
Pinkert, Mr., 171
Piper, Leonora (1859–1950), 33, 47
Pistor, Ernst, 229
Pius X, Pope, 198
Poessl, M., 72
Pohl, Gustav von (b. 1873), 133
Pollock, Jackson (1912–1956), 109
Preiswerk, Hélène (Helly), 29, 72
Prevorst, Seeress of. *See* Hauffe, Friederike
Prince, Morton (1854–1929), 48
Prinzhorn, Hans (1886–1933), 108–10, 131
Proctor, Robert, 213
Puppe, Georg (1867–1925), 184

Quade, Fritz (1884–1944), 311n80

Radloff, Erich, 312n81
Rahn, Max, 175
Rambacher, Adam, 31, 153, 156
Rathenau, Walter (1867–1922), 51
Reichardt, Johannes (b. 1897), 70
Reichart, Claire, 60–61
Reichenbach, Karl von (1788–1869), 32, 35
Reichstein, Herbert (1892–1944), 73–74, 105
Reil, Johann Christian (1759–1813), 282n10
Reingruber, Oskar, 131
Reuss, Theodor (1855–1923), 102
Reventlow, Franziska zu (1871–1918), 102, 109
Richet, Charles (1850–1935), 47–48

Riedlin, Gustav (b. 1863), 76
Riemann, Georg Friedrich, 8
Riemann, Otto (b. 1850), 177–79, 181
Rilke, Rainer Maria (1875–1926), 49, 109; spirit
  guide of, 119–21, 124
Ringbom, Sixten, 125
Rosenberg, Alfred (1893–1946), 74, 218
Rothe, Anna (1850–1907), 165–93, 241; back-
  ground of, 168–74; and class, 173, 247; expert
  opinion on, 201; followers of, 57, 176–77,
  182–85; and liberalism, 166–68, 182, 185–89;
  and religion, 172–73, 181–82, 188, 194, 223;
  trial of, 168, 180–85
Roth-Karoly, Mr. and Mrs., 145
Rudolph, Hermann (1865–1946), 102–3
Ruskin, John (1819–1900), 53

Sagittarius, Rudolf, 77
Savary, Mr., 145
Scheibner, Wilhelm (1826–1908), 4, 15
Scheler, Max (1874–1928), 49
Schelling, Friedrich (1775–1854), 34–35, 38, 53
Schermann, Rafael (b. 1879), 67
Schicl, Margarethe, 205
Schießl, Maria (b. 1867), 60
Schleiden, Matthias Jakob (1804–1881), 244
Schmitz, Oscar A. H. (1873–1931), 133–34
Schneider, Karl, 244
Schneider, Rudi (1908–1957), 49, 61, 65, 67, 226
Schneider, Willi (1903–1971), 67
Schneiderfranken, Joseph Anton (pseud. Bô
  Yin Râ; 1876–1943), 128, 130–31, 196, 221
Schopenhauer, Arthur (1788–1860), 13, 21, 32,
  35–37, 53; and du Prel, 41–43
Schreber, Daniel Paul (1842–1911), 72
Schrenck-Notzing, Albert von (1862–1929),
  43–47, 61–62, 65, 118, 120, 136, 200; attacks
  on, 219; and du Prel, 41–44, 202; and experi-
  mental psychology, 46–49; and Guipet, 114,
  116–17; and parapsychology, 41, 50; and Psy-
  chologische Gesellschaft, 40–41
Schurig, Erwin, 227–28
Schwab, Friedrich (b. 1878), 311n80
Schwab, Georg (b. 1899), 78
Schweitzer, Karl (1889–1965), 196
Sebottendorf, Rudolf von (1875–1945), 66–67
Seeliger, Hugo von (1849–1924), 206
Seeress of Prevorst. *See* Hauffe, Friederike

Seidl, Gabriel von (1848–1913), 116
Seidler, Lisbeth, 219
Seiling, Max (1852–1928), 105
Seitz, Anton (1869–1951), 199–200
Sellin, Albrecht W. (1841–1933), 62
Sellin, C. W. (1833–1910), 62, 181
Sello, Erich (1852–1913), 188
Seybert, Henry (1802–1883), 15
Sidgwick, Eleanor Balfour (1845–1936), 47–48
Sidgwick, Henry (1838–1900), 47–48
Siegismund, Karl (b. 1861), 175
Siegle, Gabriele, 65
Siemens, Otto, 235
Silbert, Maria (d. 1936), 67, 226
Simmel, Georg (1858–1918), 49
Slade, Henry (d. 1905), 8–12, 14, 67, 313n8;
  experiments with, 3–7, 17, 20, 22–23, 32, 37,
  39, 45, 47, 72; as fraud, 10, 15, 21
Smith, Hélène. *See* Müller, Élise-Catherin
Smith, Woodruff, 87
Sombart, Werner (1863–1941), 51
Specht, Gustav (b. 1860), 207–8
Spohr, Ferdinand, 292n60
Spohr, Max (1850–1905), 189; press of, 73
Spreti, Adolf von (1841–1925), 62
Spreti, Caroline von (1842–1915), 65
Stein, Heinrich von, 99
Steiner, Rudolf (1861–1925), 92, 97–101, 103, 131,
  219; color theories of, 125; mental exercises
  of, 100, 125; and science, 175–76
Steinschneider, Hermann (pseud. Erik Jan
  Hanussen, 1889–1933), 60, 67, 145, 208; and
  Nazi regime, 231–34, 237–38
Stenger, Ludwig, 78, 205
Stinde, Julius (1841–1905), 62
Stoecker, Adolf (1835–1909), 178–79
Stoll, Joseph, 226
Strauß, Heinz Artur (b. 1896), 77, 141
Streicher, Julius (1885–1946), 159
Strindberg, August (1849–1912), 53, 159
Sulzer, Georg, 183
Surya, G. W. *See* Georgievitz-Weitzer, Demeter
Sylvéro, Rolf. *See* Neumann-Kolmar, Eduard
Szabó, István, 60

Tartaruga, Ubald (b. 1875), 147
Teutschmann, Mrs., 230
Tillich, Paul (1886–1965), 194

Tingley, Katherine (1847–1929), 262n26
Tischner, Rudolf (1879–1961), 148, 157
Tolstoi, Leo (1828–1910), 53, 83
Tönnies, Ferdinand (1855–1936), 49
Töpfer, Valeska, 171
Traub, Theodor (1860–1928), 57
Trevor-Roper, Hugh, 210–11
Troeltsch, Ernst (1865–1923), 51
Trübner, Wilhelm (1851–1917), 40, 62
Twain, Mark (1835–1910), 105

Ueberhorst, Mr., 311n80
Uechtritz-Steinkirch, Karl Oswald Konstantin
    von (1824–1902), 62
Ulrici, Hermann (1806–1884), 11–13, 15
Ungewitter, Richard (1868–1958), 106, 159
Urban, Franz (1845–1917), 62
Urban, Hermann (1836–1916), 62

Varnbüler, Axel von (b. 1851), 66
Vaughan, Thomas (1622–1666), 297n64
Verweyen, Johannes Maria (1883–1945), 61, 140,
    200, 226, 231–32, 234–38
Virchow, Rudolf (1821–1902), 178–79
Vivekananda Paramahamsa Ramakrishna,
    Swami (1863–1902), 53
Vlcek, Mr., 226
Vogt, Karl (1817–1895), 40
Vogt-Vilseck, Hanna (b. 1876), 64, 204
Vollrath, Hugo (b. 1877), 63–64
Voß, Georg (1854–1932), 62

Wagner, Richard (1813–1883), 53, 63n2, 105, 234
Wallace, Alfred Russel (1823–1913), 52
Walther, Gerda (b. 1897), 50, 200
Weber, Ernst von (1830–1902), 62
Weber, Karl Maria von, 63n2, 67
Weber, Luise, 244
Weber, Max (1864–1920), 18–19, 51
Weber, William Edward (1804–1891), 3–5, 15
Wegener, Paul, 109
Wegert, Martin Friedrich, 131
Wehdanner, Balthasar (b. 1879), 156–57, 192–
    93
Wehler, Hans-Ulrich, 87
Weinert, Hans (b. 1887), 238
Weingartner, Felix (1863–1942), 128

Weisl, Wolfgang von (1896?–1948), 225–26
Weissenberg, Joseph (1855–1941), 60, 159, 223,
    226, 229, 239
Weißl, Frieda, 226
Weisthor, Karl Maria. *See* Wiligut, Karl Maria
Werner, Frank, 243–46
Weyrauch, Robert (1874–1924), 152
Wiene, Robert (1881–1938), 109
Wiesinger, Alois (1885–1955), 319n34
Wildhagen, Mrs., 151
Wilhelm II (1859–1941), 66, 176, 289n34
Wiligut, Karl Maria (pseud. Karl Maria
    Weisthor; 1866–1946), 215–16
Windischmann, Karl (1775–1839), 35
Winkel, Erich (b. 1894), 311n80
Winterberg, Mr., 311n80
Wittig, Gregor Konstantin (1834–1908), 7, 32,
    38–39
Wohlbold, Hans (1877–1949), 100
Wolfart, Karl Christian (1778–1832), 282n10
Wolff, Eugen, 18
Wolter, Karl, 171
Wulff, Wilhelm (1891–1980), 211, 215–16, 231
Wundt, Wilhelm (1832–1920), 4, 8, 14, 45; letter
    to Ulrici of, 11–13, 15; and psychology, 21–22,
    32, 44, 134
Würfl, Adolf, 136

Yeats, W. B. (1865–1939), 119

Zander, Helmut, 26
Zierer, Josephine, 78
Zillmann, Paul (1872–1940), 52–55, 71, 73–74,
    106, 154, 175
Zirngible, Änna, 78
Zobeltitz, Fedor von (1857–1934), 187
Zola, Émile (1840–1902), 72
Zöllner, Karl Friedrich (1834–1882), 28, 181, 244;
    academic credentials of, 8; anti-Semitism of, 7,
    10, 19, 278n48; experiments with Slade of, 3–7,
    17, 20, 22–23, 32, 37, 39, 45, 47, 72; on fourth
    dimension, 7–9, 14, 20, 23; and German pub-
    lic, 56; Hartmann on, 11, 13–15; Jung on, 29–
    30; and Kandinsky, 17, 108; knot experiment
    of, 5–6, 20; mental illness of, 11; and modern-
    ism, 19, 24; pragmatic occultism of, 24
Zuckmayer, Carl (1896–1977), 60

Subject Index

advertisements, 70, 76, 78, 160–61, 244, 247; and advice columns, 142–43

Adyar (India), 85, 96

afterlife, 12–14, 38, 91, 94, 177, 245; archive on, 226–27; and Rothe case, 170–71, 182. *See also* reincarnation

Akademie der Bildenden Künste, 110

alchemy, 53, 70

anarchism, 202–3

animal magnetism, 30, 34–36, 38, 43, 181; university chairs of, 32, 35

animism, 13, 39

Animismus und Spiritismus (Aksakow), 33, 108

anthropology, 141

Anthroposophical Society, 92, 100

Anthroposophy, 64, 77, 79, 101, 194, 219; under Nazi regime, 221, 225, 228, 230

anti-Semitism: and Ariosophy, 25–26, 103–7, 215; of Zöllner, 7, 10, 19, 278n48

antivivisectionism, 62, 63n2, 86, 156

Apologetische Centrale, 195–97

Ariosophy: and anti-Semitism, 25–26, 103–7, 215; and Hitler, 26, 104; masters in, 105; and nationalism, 25–26, 104, 107; and Nazi ideology, 84; under Nazi regime, 221, 225, 228–29; occultism in, 104–6; and presses, 73–74; vs. Theosophy, 104–7; and völkisch movement, 102–7, 217, 229

art, 24, 28, 62, 108–31; abstract, 126–28; and automatic writing, 122, 126; and Catholic Church, 110–11; and film, 109; and gender, 120–24; and modernism, 107; and photography, 113–15; and Psychologische Gesellschaft, 40, 110–18; realism in, 112, 128, 130; and science, 111, 116; self-focused, 131; spirit guides in, 118–24; and subjective experience, 108–10, 118; and Theosophy, 99, 109, 111, 124–31; trance, 110, 118, 121–24, 175. *See also* dance; Kandinsky, Wassily [Names Index]

Aryans, 25, 74, 90, 228; and Theosophy, 102–7

astrology, 7; and Ariosophy, 106; and Christianity, 194, 197–98; clubs for, 58–59, 64, 206; and the East, 66; and Himmler, 211, 225; and modernism, 134; and Nazi ideology, 213–17; under Nazi regime, 221, 225, 227–30, 233, 239–40; and occult economy, 69, 76; in periodicals, 52–53, 71; practical, 140–42, 152–53, 156, 160; practitioners of, 64–65, 77–78, 232; and presses, 73; and professionalism, 64, 77; prosecution of, 201; and the public, 56, 58; and race, 219, 239; and science, 204–6; scientific vs. intuitive, 140–42

atheism, 37, 69, 120, 200

Auferweckung der Tochter Jairi (Keller), 112–14

Augsburger Allgemeine Zeitung, 31

automatic writing, 3, 47, 119, 122, 126, 170, 245

Bavaria, 84; article 54 of police code in, 201–3, 205, 207–8, 244

Berlin: fraud cases in, 171; occultism in, 44, 55, 57–60, 77, 168, 174–80, 190; periodicals in, 10, 31, 152, 186, 188; religion in, 179; Rothe case in, 166–69, 180–85; University of, 32, 35

Berliner Tageblatt, 31, 152, 186, 188

Berliner Volkszeitung, 10

Berlin Secession, 122

Bhagavad Gita, 214, 216

Die Bilderschrift der Ario-Germanen (List), 105

Biochemie, 214

Blue Rider group, 131

bookstores, occult, 56, 69–70, 175. *See also* Appendix C

Bremen, 30–32

Breslau, 38

Britain, 86; Hess's flight to, 213–14, 216–17, 224, 231

Buddhism, 66, 77, 85, 111, 200

capitalism, 19, 51, 234

Catholic Church, 120, 248; and modern art, 110–11; and modernism, 198, 200; Nazi opposition to, 214–15, 219, 239; vs. occultism, 39, 57, 168, 193, 197–200; vs. science, 94; and Verweyen, 234–35

characterology, 64, 77, 140, 156, 175, 207. *See also* graphology

Chemnitz, 57

Christianity, 193–200; afterlife in, 227; and artists, 111; and astrology, 194, 197–98; vs. liberalism, 188; and magnetism, 157, 192, 196; and modernism, 51, 196; and Nazi regime, 220; in occultism, 57, 67; and parapsychology, 226; and psychology, 41; and Rothe case, 170, 183, 223; sects of, 94, 178, 220–21; and spiritualism, 67, 177–78, 195, 197; and Theosophy, 83, 195–97, 235; and völkisch movement, 217. *See also* Catholic Church; Protestantism

Christian Science, 197, 221, 225

Christian-Social Worker's Party, 178

cities, 18, 58–59, 77. *See also individual cities*

civilization, 51, 93, 167–68, 174, 188–89

clairaudience, 126

clairvoyance, 34, 36, 89, 95, 184; and Ariosophy, 104–5; and artists, 111; and Freud, 49; and Nazi ideology, 213, 216; under Nazi regime, 215, 228, 237; policing of, 202; practitioners of, 61, 98–100, 232; and science, 135

class, 60–66, 78, 175–76; and liberalism, 84; lower, 60, 175; in Rothe case, 173, 247; at séances, 65, 244, 247; and Theosophy, 61, 86. *See also* elite; middle class

clothing reform, 68, 72, 86, 90. *See also* Lebensreform

clubs: members of occult, 62–63; and occult economy, 76, 79; political, 167; professionals in occult, 61–64

clubs, occult, 7, 39, 57–59, 70–71; Abila, 13, 171; Astrologische Gesellschaft München, 58, 64, 206; Bund der Kämpfer für Glaube und Wahrheit (Horpena), 229–30; Bund für Seelenkultur, 67; Deutsche graphologische Gesellschaft, 137–38; Deutsche Kulturgemeinschaft zur Pflege der Astrologie, 61; Deutscher Bund der gerichtlichen Schriftanverständigen und Berufsgraphologen, 139; Esoterische Studiengesellschaft, 228; Friedensstadt, 60; Gesellschaft für Experimentalpsychologie, 33, 41, 44, 61–62; Gesellschaft für psychische Forschung, 58; Gnosis, 229; Horpena (Bund der Kämpfer für Glaube und Wahrheit), 229–30; Internationaler Verein der Wünschelrutenforscher, 152; Internationale Theosophische Verbrüderung, 101; International Theosophical Society, 88, 99; Liberal-Katholische Kirche, 235; Neugeist, 227; Neuland, 77, 204; Oschm-Rahmah-Johjihjah Lodge, 67–68; Siemens Studiengesellschaft für psychologische Wissenschaft, 235; Society for Psychical Research, 33, 47–49; Die Sucher, 64, 204; Uranus Gesellschaft für astrologische Forschung, 58; Verband deutscher Okkultisten, 67, 178; Verband zur Klärung der Wünschelrutenfrage, 152; Verein Freibund, 60; Wald Loge, 54. *See also* Appendix A; Gottesbund Tanatra; Mazdaznan; Psychologische Gesellschaft; Theosophische Societät Germania

Commission für Medienschutz, 173

communism, 232–33, 240; aristocratic, 204; and sects, 221–22, 224

communitarianism, 67–68, 102

Concerning the Spiritual in Art (Kandinsky). See *Über das Geistige in der Kunst*

consciousness, 30, 41–42, 91, 100–101, 200. *See also* unconscious

consumerism, 28, 57, 71, 74–80, 134

cosmic vibrations, 53, 125–26, 128–29, 136, 160

cosmopolitanism, 217–18, 226

Critique of Pure Reason (Kant), 32

culture: consumer, 28, 57, 71, 74–80, 134; entrepreneurs of, 74–76; experimentation with, 85, 125, 174, 248; German, 7, 11, 17–18, 83–85, 87; of knowledge, 189–91; mass, 28, 57, 76–80, 116, 132, 134, 139, 142–43, 161; occultism as alternative, 16, 242; and reform, 27; renewal of, 83–86; and spiritualism, 12–13, 16, 38

Dachau, 214
Daheim, 150
dance: eurhythmic, 131; trance, 55, 114–17
Darwinism, 111; Social, 90, 93, 103
dental hygiene, 38
De re metallica (Agricola), 150
Deutsche Arbeiterpartei, 25, 104
divining rod. *See* dowsing
dowsing, 7, 59, 69, 77, 232; and Hitler, 133, 213; and modernism, 150–51, 153–54; practical applications of, 153–54; in presses, 150, 152; and professionalism, 152–54, 193; scientific, 143–44, 150–54
dreams, 42, 44, 48–49
Dreams of a Spirit Seer (Kant), 72
Das dritte Testament (Gumppenberg), 120
The Duino Elegies (Rilke), 119, 124

the East, 53, 66–67, 214, 216; and Japanese style, 123–24. *See also* Buddhism
economy, German, 18, 91, 161, 218; and applied psychology, 139–40; industrialization of, 85, 87, 155
economy, occult, 74–80; and Ariosophy, 105; and astrology, 69, 76; in Berlin, 175; and clubs, 76, 79; and education, 7, 69, 76–80, 152, 160; health-related, 69; and modernism, 78–80, 134; services in, 76–80, 201–9, 230–33, 247–48; and spirit guides, 124; and Theosophy, 101
education: anti-occult, 13, 188–89; occult, 69, 76–80, 204, 235
Elements of Psychophysics (Fechner), 8, 32, 44
elite, 65–66; conservative, 87; and control of science, 189–91; and popular occultism, 78, 176; Protestant, 176, 178–80; and Rothe case, 183, 187; scientific-academic, 174–80
empiricism, 8–9, 11–13, 23–24
the Enlightenment, 14, 202
environmental issues, 150, 153
Essay on Spirit Seeing (Schopenhauer), 32
eugenics, 73, 90, 107, 144
exorcism, 230
expressionism, 16–17

feminism, 86, 99, 102
fingerprinting, 144

Force and Matter (Büchner), 32, 34
forensic science, 139, 143–50, 153–54
fortune telling, 7, 105, 230. *See also* palmistry
fourth dimension, 3–7, 10–11; as private property, 22–23; Zöllner on, 7–9, 14, 20
fraud, 232, 241, 246; forensic mediums as, 143, 145–46; Rothe as, 165–66, 170–74, 180–85; Slade as, 10, 15, 21; spiritualism as, 3, 12, 15–16, 39, 180–85, 244; and the state, 193, 201–2, 205, 207–8
Freemasons, 215, 234, 236; and Nazi regime, 217–21, 224; and occultism, 218–20, 223; and sects, 222, 224
Freiburg, 38
Freie literarische Gesellschaft, 99
From India to the Planet Mars (Flournoy), 33

Die Gartenlaube, 10, 150, 181, 189, 239
Gaukelei, 201–2, 205, 207–8
Gefahrenzone Aberglaube, 232, 238–40
Die Gegenwart, 41, 62, 186
gender, 61, 86, 105; and art, 120–24. *See also* women
geometries, non-Euclidean, 8–9
Germanenorden, 104
German Workers' Party (Deutsche Arbeiterpartei), 25, 104
Germany: ancient, 215, 228; civilization of, 188; colonialism of, 86–91; culture of, 7, 11, 17–18, 83–85, 87; democracy in, 194; economic expansion of, 91; fragmentation of, 90; industrialization of, 85; literature of, 97, 99; modernization of, 27, 56; Nazi, 27–28, 210–42; political developments in, 17–18, 30, 167; race in history of, 228–29; socioeconomic change in, 17–18, 38; unification of, 8, 19, 42, 85; universities in, 7, 19–20, 32, 35, 50, 61, 63; urbanization in, 18; Weimar, 27–28, 60–61, 72, 194, 212, 219, 223, 241; Weimar vs. Nazi, 230, 232, 234, 240; Wilhelmine, 26–28, 72, 167, 223, 241; Wilhelmine vs. Nazi, 234; and World War I, 17–18, 194; and World War II, 8, 210–11
Gesellschaft für modernes Leben, 119
God, 31, 34, 46, 50–51
Gottesbund Tanatra, 57, 195, 221; banning of, 229–30

Göttingen, 49

graphology, 7, 59, 69, 77, 152–53, 208; forensic, 139; professionals' interest in, 193; as science, 206–7; scientific vs. intuitive, 135–40, 142–43

Great White Brotherhood, 85, 100, 105

Hamburg, 58–59

Handschrift und Charakter (Klages), 140

healing, 7, 78, 133; and art, 126; and diet, 154, 158; faith, 222; herbal, 214, 230; holistic, 155, 159, 214; and hypnotism, 43–44, 48, 158; intuitive, 158; magnetic, 114, 154, 156–57, 160, 192; by mail, 160–61; natural, 148, 154–61, 212–14; and Nazi ideology, 212–14, 216, 230; and Rothe case, 169, 183; vs. specialization of medicine, 155; and trance, 55. *See also* health; Lebensreform; medicine

health, 69, 155, 247; businesses related to, 59; Jungborn sanitarium, 59. *See also* Appendix C; healing; Lebensreform; medicine

Hexenverbrennung (Keller), 114–15, 117

Hippokrates, 157

Die Hoffnungslosen, 41

holism: ecological, 150, 153–54; medical, 155, 159, 214

homeopathy, 155, 158, 213–14

homosexuality, 45, 73, 195, 222

humanitarianism, 218, 223, 236

hydropathy, 155

hyperspace, 9

hypnotism, 21, 32, 35, 52; and creativity, 40, 116–18; criticisms of, 223, 237; exhibitions on, 77; and forensic mediums, 145–48; and hysteria, 33, 43; practitioners of, 60, 78, 232; prosecution of, 203–4; research on, 41, 47; and Rothe case, 181, 184; therapeutic, 43–44, 48, 158

Illustrierte Frauenzeitung, 121

Im Neuen Reich, 10

India, 66, 85–86, 96

individualism: and liberalism, 84–85, 167; vs. mass culture, 142–43, 161; and modernism, 18, 133–34, 143; and natural healing, 155–56, 158–61; vs. Nazi ideology, 211; and Nazi regime, 234, 236; and rights, 167; spiritual, 68, 96, 98; vs. universal brotherhood, 100–101

industrialization, 85, 87, 155

institutes, occult, 7, 69, 76–80, 152, 160; Archiv für Reinkarnation, 226–27; Astrologische Zentralstelle, 77; Institut für wissenschaftliche Astrologie und Graphologie, 77; Institut für Wünschelruten-und Pendelforschung, 152; Psychomagnetisches-suggestives Heilinstitut, 160; Zentrale für praktischen Okkultismus, 101, 160. *See also* Appendix C

International Congress of Experimental Psychology (1892), 47

International Congress of Physiological Psychology (1889), 33, 46–47

internationalism, 211, 218, 222, 228, 231, 238

Interpretation of Dreams (Freud), 33, 48–49

Italy, 67

Jehovah's Witnesses, 195, 221–23

Jesus (Bô Yin Râ), 128, 130–31

Jesus Christ, 157, 192–93, 196, 199

Jews, 19, 53, 215, 228, 239; and Nazi ideology, 217–20; as occultists, 233–34; and sects, 222, 224. *See also* anti-Semitism

Jugendstil movement, 122, 125

Der Kampf ums Dasein am Himmel (du Prel), 42

Klänge aus dem Jenseits: Ein Mysterium (Eysell-Kilburger), 121

Kraft durch Freude, 231

Kriminalistische Monatshefte, 147

Kulturkampf, 167

Lebensreform, 51, 102, 234, 247; and natural healing, 155–56; and Nazi ideology, 212–13; and presses, 68–69, 72–73, 75–76. *See also* healing; health; medicine

lecture halls and schools, occult: Eclaros, 77; Erfolg Hochschule, 235. *See also* Appendix C

Leipzig, 7, 32, 71, 78; antispiritualism in, 13, 171; under Nazi regime, 228; occult clubs in, 58–59; population growth in, 18; spiritualism in, 38–39. *See also* Zöllner, Karl Friedrich [Names Index]

liberalism: and alternative worldviews, 241; and Hübbe-Schleiden, 92; and individualism, 84–85, 167; vs. the masses, 189; and Nazi

liberalism (*cont.*)
regime, 218, 234; political, 51; and presses, 7, 10, 168; and progress, 84–85, 167, 174, 189; and Protestantism, 13, 19; and reform movements, 73; and religion, 84, 170, 179, 188; and Rothe case, 166–68, 182, 185–89; and science, 167, 178, 190; and spiritualism, 172–73, 177, 179; vs. the state, 188–89; and superstition, 185–91; and Theosophy, 84–85
liberal theology, 313n12
libraries, occult, 32, 39, 56, 69, 76, 206, 226, 228. *See also* Appendix C
Liebenberg Circle, 66
lifestyles: modern, 76; transcendent, 50–55. *See also* Lebensreform
List Society, 104–6
literature: fantasy, 97, 104; German, 97, 99; occult, 226, 228; and spirit guides, 119–22
Die Lotse, 49
Lourdes, 156

Magazin für Literatur, 99
magnetism, 38, 52, 54, 60, 143, 196; clubs for, 59; exhibitions on, 77; and healing, 114, 154, 156–57, 160; and Jesus Christ, 157, 192; and Nazi ideology, 213, 216; under Nazi regime, 229; and the public, 175, 179; research on, 47. *See also* mesmerism
Malte Laurids Brigge (Rilke), 119
Maria: Eine Stimme aus dem Jenseits? (Jaschke), 243–48
Marxism, 200, 224
materialism, scientific: ambivalence towards, 245; and anti-Semitism, 19; and artists, 111, 120; and dowsing, 153; and healing, 157–58; and modernism, 18, 20; vs. Naturphilosophie, 35–36; and Nazi-era occultism, 228; vs. occultism, 176, 202–3, 227; opposition to, 16–17, 40–42, 46, 53, 94–95; and psychology, 22, 40, 44; vs. religion, 134, 178, 200; and Schrenk-Notzing, 44–45; and soul, 31, 34, 37, 46; vs. spiritualism, 13, 16, 23; and Theosophy, 86, 89; vs. the transcendent, 20, 23, 31, 34; and Zöllner, 16, 20, 22
Mazdaznan, 221, 229
medicine: crisis of, 157–58; holistic, 155, 159, 214; natural, 240; vs. naturopathy, 212–13;

and Nazi genocide, 213; professionalism in, 154–55, 203. *See also* healing; health; Lebensreform
mediums: vs. Anthroposophy, 101; as artists, 114–17; as artists' models, 110–18; and Catholic Church, 198; and class, 60–61, 175; control of, 177, 180; defense of, 173, 176–77, 182–85; vs. dowsing, 153–54; experimentation with, 95, 136–38, 144–46; forensic, 143–50, 153; fraud by, 3, 12, 15–16, 39, 143, 145–46, 165–66, 170–74, 180–85, 244; good faith of, 148–49, 185; materialization of objects by, 168–69, 171, 174, 177; and natural healing, 156; numbers of, 57; and psychology, 40–42, 53, 178; and the public, 173–74; rejection of, 137–38; and self-development, 55; in Theosophy, 85; from United States, 67; women as, 64–65, 114–17, 121
Mein Kampf (Hitler), 74
mental illness: and art, 108–9; of Hess, 213–14; and materialism, 42; occultism as cause of, 33, 43, 177, 181, 219; research on, 46, 72; of Rothe, 186–87; treatment of, 45, 66, 88; of Wiligut, 215; of Zöllner, 11
mesmerism, 35, 59, 155, 214
middle class, 31, 36, 61–65, 173, 175–76, 235; women of, 64–65, 121. *See also* petty bourgeoisie
mind/body problem, 21–22, 30, 42, 52
Modenwelt, 121
modernism: aesthetic, 72, 107, 109, 131; ambivalence towards, 50–51, 243–48; and anxiety, 18–19; and Catholic Church, 110–11, 198, 200; and consciousness, 101; diseases of, 133, 213; and dowsing, 150–51, 153–54; German, 17–18; and Hübbe-Schleiden, 88, 90, 93; and individualism, 18, 133–34, 143; and knowledge, 185, 188; and liminality, 114; and moral degeneration, 18–19; Munich as center of, 110–18, 125; and Nazi regime, 234, 240; and occult economy, 78–80, 134; and occultism, 27, 37, 93, 144, 225–27; and police code, 202; popular, 72–73; and presses, 71, 76; and professionalism, 19–20, 63–64, 132, 161; psychological, 17–24, 30, 72, 234, 279n57; and reform, 50–54; and religion, 51, 120, 194, 196, 198; and Rothe case, 172, 185; and science,

243–48; social, 132–34, 137, 139; social vs.
 psychological, 161; and technology, 18, 50–51,
 244–46; and Theosophy, 97, 100, 102; and
 worldviews, 90, 241
modernities, alternative, 51, 69, 103
modernization, 27, 56; subjects vs. objects of,
 50–51
monism, 200, 225–27, 234
Monte Verità (Switzerland), 59, 102
Münchner Moderne, 110–18
Munich, 44, 50, 67, 72, 77, 219; astrology in, 58,
 64, 206; as center of modernism, 110–18, 125;
 modern art in, 110–18; occult clubs in, 41,
 58–60; occultists in, 57, 64–65, 78; prosecution of occultism in, 202; Psychologische
 Gesellschaft in, 40–41; Schwabing subculture of, 59, 65–66, 243; University of, 50
Munich Secession, 110, 125

Nancy School of psychiatry, 33, 43
nationalism, 67, 93, 204, 228; and Ariosophy,
 25–26, 104, 107; and Hübbe-Schleiden, 87–
 89; and natural healing, 159–60
naturalist movement, 18, 72, 119–20
nature, 51, 54, 108, 131
Naturheilkunde, 68, 90, 155, 212–13
naturopathy. *See* Naturheilkunde
Naturphilosophie, 20–21, 34, 38, 43, 48; vs.
 materialism, 35–36
Nazi regime, 210–42; affinities with occultism
 of, 24–26, 84, 159, 211–16, 240–41; antipathy
 to occultism of, 216–20, 231–41; and Ariosophy, 25, 84, 221, 225, 228–29; and Catholic
 Church, 214–15, 219, 239; and eugenics, 107;
 ideological precursors of, 84, 87, 104; ideology of, 74, 86, 212–20; vs. liberalism, 218,
 234; murders by, 60, 220, 231, 233; opposition
 to, 235, 239; predictions about, 232–33; and
 public opinion, 238–41; secrecy of, 232, 240;
 suppression of occultism by, 7, 28, 58, 84,
 209, 211–14, 217, 220–25, 231–42, 246, 248;
 and underground occultism, 225–31, 241;
 worldview of, 211, 218, 222–23, 227
[Neue] Metaphysische Rundschau, 33, 71, 73–74,
 106, 175; vs. *Sphinx*, 52–53
neurasthenia, 45, 66, 88. *See also* mental illness
neurology, 13, 21

New Thought, 221, 227
New York Times, 166, 185
nudism, 155, 159
numerology, 105

occultism: applied, 24, 132–61, 246–47;
 attempts to debunk, 237–38; claims to objectivity of, 134–43; conversions to, 68–69; for-
 profit, 201–9, 230–33, 247–48; geographical
 spread of, 57–59; hostility to establishment
 of, 203–4; as mass movement, 57–68;
 nazification of, 228–29, 231; numbers
 involved with, 57, 223; policing of, 28, 165–
 91, 193, 200–208; popular, 174–75, 181–82,
 190; practice of, 24, 27–28, 70; scientific vs.
 vulgar, 199, 203–8; social relevance of, 133;
 tools of, 75
"Od" force, 35
*On the Psychology and Pathology of So-Called
 Occult Phenomena* (Jung), 33, 72
Ostara, 106

pacifism, 83, 86, 111, 221, 234, 238
palmistry, 59, 69, 206–7
pantheism, 198–99
parapsychology, 33, 59, 69, 193, 226; and Catholic Church, 199–200; and experimental
 psychology, 48; under Nazi regime, 227; and
 phenomenology, 49–50; and Schrenck-
 Notzing, 41, 50
Parerga and Paralipomena (Schopenhauer), 36
pendulum, 59, 69, 77, 192
periodicals: astrology in, 52–53, 71; in Berlin,
 10, 31, 152, 175, 186, 188; columns in, 142–43,
 161; and dowsing, 152; and German public,
 56; mass, 146; under Nazi regime, 226, 229–
 30; and Rothe case, 165–66; specialized, 71;
 and spread of occultism, 247; trade, 152
periodicals, occult: *Astrale Warte*, 229; *Astrologische Rundschau*, 71; *Erkenntnis und
 Glaube*, 200; *Hanussens B. W. Hellseher
 Zeitung*, 232; *Johannes Botschaft*, 229; *Lotusblüthen*, 71–72, 96; *Metaphysische Rundschau*, 175; *Neue Lotusblüthen*, 106; *[Neue]
 Spiritualistische Blätter*, 39; *Spiritistische
 Rundschau*, 175; *Sprechsaal*, 39; *Stein der
 Weisen*, 106; *Die übersinnliche Welt*, 171, 175;

periodicals, occult (*cont.*)
  Wissenschaftliche Zeitschrift für "Okkultismus," 138; *Zeitschrift für Seelenleben,* 67; *Zentralblatt für Okkultismus,* 142, 161. *See also* Appendix D; *[Neue] Metaphysische Rundschau; Psychische Studien; Sphinx*
pessimism, 13, 79
petty bourgeoisie, 60–61, 78
Phalanx group, 125
Phantastische Landschaft (Nüßlein), 128–29
phenomenology, 49–50, 200
philosophy, 13, 34, 36, 61; Eastern, 53, 66–67; irrationalist, 25; and psychology, 21–22, 40, 48; and Steiner, 97–98, 101; and Theosophy, 86; and Verweyen, 234–35
Philosophy of Mysticism (du Prel), 33
Philosophy of the Unconscious (Hartmann), 13, 32, 36
photography, 113–15
phrenology, 53
physics, 24; transcendental, 7–17
physiognomy, 207–8
Physiological Psychology (Wundt), 8
Picture with a Circle (Kandinsky), 126–27
police code, Bavarian: article 54 of, 201–3, 205, 207–8, 244
politics: and antipolitics, 51; German, 17–18, 30, 167; and Hanussen, 232–33; and Hübbe-Schleiden, 86, 92; liberal, 51; and occultism, 66–68; and presses, 74
positivism, 25
Potsdam, 66
the press: liberal, 7, 10, 167–68, 218; mass, 150, 152, 161, 167; national, 56, 66, 180; Nazi, 218
presses, occult, 7, 247; Max Altmann, 73; and Ariosophy vs. Theosophy, 105–6; in Berlin, 175; Cloud Traveler, 70; dowsing in, 150, 152; Eugen Diederichs, 74; on forensic mediumism, 149–50; Wilhelm Friedrich, 11, 72–74; and Lebensreform, 68–69, 72–73, 75–76; Oswald Mutze, 71–74; Nirwana-Verlag für Lebensreform, 75–76; and occult economy, 76, 79; M. Poessl, 72; and reform movements, 72–73, 76; specialized, 70–71; Max Spohr, 73; suppression of, 224–25, 229; and texts, 68–76; and völkisch movement, 73–74. *See also* Appendix B

Principles of Psychology (James), 33
private property, 22–23
professionalism: in dowsing, 152–54, 193; and expert opinion, 201–9; and graphology, 139; medical, 154–55, 203; and modernism, 19–20, 63–64, 132, 161; in occult economy, 77; and occultism, 61–64, 134, 144, 177, 179, 192–93; and psychology, 139–40; and Rothe case, 168, 174, 180–81, 184–86, 201; in science, 11, 241; in universities, 19–20
progress, social, 13, 92; and liberalism, 84–85, 167, 174, 189; and science, 166–67
Protestantism, 174–80, 194–97, 234; cultural, 51, 316n47; erosion of, 178; and intellectual elites, 176, 178–80; liberal, 13, 19; and sects, 224
Prussia, 32, 35
psyche, human: in art, 113, 118; Jung on, 29; and modernism, 245–46; occult powers of, 24; as private property, 22–23; research on, 171; and Rothe case, 172, 181; and science, 30, 40–50, 173; and spiritualism, 11–12
psychical research: and artists, 111–14, 116, 125; on astrology, 58; in Berlin, 175; on dowsing, 152; and experimental psychology, 39, 47–48; on hallucinations, 47; and hypnotism, 41, 43–44, 47; on magnetism, 47; on mediums, 116–17, 144–47; on mental illness, 46, 72; and middle class, 61; and modernism, 245; and Nazi regime, 219, 239–40; and objectivity, 136–38; organizations for, 40, 59, 69, 77; periodicals on, 71; policing of, 202, 204; and psychometry, 135; and Rothe case, 169–74, 180, 184; and science, 136–38, 171; and sexuality, 45; and spiritualism, 176–77; on unconscious, 14, 48, 246–47; of Zöllner, 3–7, 32, 37, 39, 45, 47, 72
Psychical Research, Society for, 33, 47–49
Psychische Studien, 7, 32, 39, 41, 71–72, 150, 171
psychoanalysis, 71
Psychologische Gesellschaft, 40–41, 43–45, 48–49, 61–62, 120; and art, 40, 110–18; founding of, 33; split in, 41
psychology, 21–23, 29–55, 193; applied, 139–40; and art, 110, 118; and Catholic Church, 199–200; criminal, 168; and dowsing, 153; and experience, 109; experimental, 8, 21, 32, 46–

48, 110, 139, 199; experimental vs. physiological, 44–45; expression, 140; of female experience, 111; and Freud, 33, 36, 48–49, 51, 72; and healing, 157–58; International Congress of Experimental (1892), 47; International Congress of Physiological (1889), 33, 46–47; and Jung, 29–30, 33, 36, 49, 51, 55, 102; and modernism, 30, 161; new, 21, 41, 45–46; and philosophy, 21–22, 40, 48; physiological, 8, 21–22, 33, 44–47; popular, 52–53; and professionalism, 61, 139–40, 208; vs. prophecy, 207; and religion, 42, 195, 198; and Rothe case, 172; scientific, 8–9, 135; self-focused, 235–36; sensory, 21; and spiritualism, 12–14, 39, 167, 177–78; on subjectivity, 55, 142; transcendent, 41–43, 45, 50–51, 202; on unconscious, 13, 21–22

psychometry, 134–36

psychophysics, 8, 32, 44–45

psychotechnicians, 140

the public, 56–80, 248; and astrology, 56, 58; and charismatic occultists, 232, 234; vs. experts, 187–88; and magnetism, 175, 179; and mediums, 148–50, 173–74, 179; Nazi "enlightenment" of, 238–41; and Rothe case, 185–89; and science, 166–67, 190–91; and Zöllner, 56

quantum theory, 23

race: in Ariosophy, 25–26, 67, 103–7; and astrology, 219, 239; and eugenics, 107; and Freemasons, 218; in German history, 228–29; and Hübbe-Schleiden, 87–88, 90–91, 103–4; vs. individualism, 236; and Nazi regime, 215, 223, 228; in presses, 73–74; purity of, 67, 83; and religion, 106–7; and sects, 222; in Theosophy, 88, 102–7, 223

Rasse-und Siedlungshauptamt (SS; Race and settlement main office), 215

realism, 112, 128, 130–31

Reformation, 181

reform movements, 91, 159, 248; and artists, 111; in Catholic Church, 198; clothing, 68, 72, 86, 90; cultural, 27; democratic, 87; and Hübbe-Schleiden, 86, 90, 92–93; liberal, 73; and modernity, 50–54; and natural healing, 155;

and presses, 68, 72–73, 76; prison, 86; and self-development, 68; sexual, 63, 73; and Theosophy, 84–86. *See also* Lebensreform

Reichsbote, 66

Reichssicherheitshauptamt (RSHA; Reich security main office), 220–25, 238–39

reincarnation, 195–96, 214, 226–27

religion: ancient German, 104, 215, 217; and Ariosophy, 103, 106–7; Eastern, 66–67, 214, 216; ecstasy in, 198; and German state, 167; and Hübbe-Schleiden, 88–89; and liberalism, 84, 170, 179, 188; vs. materialism, 134, 178, 200; and modernism, 51, 120, 194, 196, 198; and Nazi ideology, 214, 220–21; and occultism, 168, 193–200, 226, 241, 248; and personal experience, 190; and psychology, 42, 195, 198; and race, 106–7; and Rothe case, 170, 172–73, 181–82, 188, 194, 223; and science, 11–13, 43, 51, 92–93, 134, 179–80, 190–91, 193–200, 208–9, 241; and spirit guides, 120; and spiritualism, 190, 203; and Theosophy, 86; and Verweyen, 234–35. *See also* Catholic Church; Protestantism

The Religious Situation (Tillich), 194

Rembrandt als Erzieher (Langbehn), 74

revolutions of 1848, 30, 37–38

romanticism, 25

Rosicrucianism, 53, 221

RSHA. *See* Reichssicherheitshauptamt

Russia, 14

Salpêtrière Hospital (France), 32, 43

Salvation Army, 195

schools. *See* lecture halls and schools, occult

Schorers Familienblatt, 150

Schwabing, 59, 65–66, 243

Das Schwarze Korps, 233–34, 238–41

science: and animal magnetism, 36; and artists, 111, 116, 125; and astrology, 140–42, 204–6; authority of, 10–11, 135, 180–85, 187–88; vs. Catholic Church, 94; and dowsing, 143–44, 150–54; elite control of, 174–80, 189–91; and expert opinion, 193, 202; forensic, 139, 143–50, 153–54; and graphology, 135–40, 142–43, 206–7; and Hübbe-Schleiden, 91–92; and human psyche, 30, 40–50, 173; vs. Kantian idealism, 8–9; and liberalism, 167, 178, 190;

science (*cont.*)

  and modernism, 243–48; vs. natural healing, 155; and Nazi regime, 239–40; and occultism, 28, 40, 168, 192–200, 203–8, 227, 234, 241; vs. personal experience, 95, 182–83; professionalism in, 11, 174–80, 241; and progress, 166–67; and Protestantism, 176, 178–80; and psychical research, 136–38, 171; and psychology, 8–9, 30, 43, 135; and the public, 166–67, 190–91; and religion, 11–13, 43, 51, 92–93, 134, 179–80, 190–91, 193–200, 208–9, 241; and Rothe case, 170, 172, 180–85, 187–88; of siting homes, 153; and social problems, 132–34; spiritual, 176; and spiritualism, 13–15, 23–24, 167, 177, 180–85, 203; vs. spiritual values, 50–51; and Theosophy, 86, 91–92, 97–98, 100–101, 176; and the transcendent, 34, 43; of work, 132; worldview of, 94, 175, 190, 193, 233, 245. *See also* materialism, scientific

Science, 143

Scientific American, 136

SD. *See* Sicherheitsdienst

séances, 38, 55; and artists, 113, 116, 120; and Catholic Church, 197; and class, 65, 244, 247; Nazi regime on, 239; and psychology, 21–22, 49; of Rothe, 57, 165, 169; of Slade, 3–7. *See also* mediums; spiritualism

sects, 220–25

The Seeress of Prevorst (Kerner), 32, 35

self-development, 52–53, 131, 133–34, 142; and occult economy, 80; and psychology, 235–36; spiritual, 68, 90; and spiritualism, 54–55; and Theosophy, 93–102, 107, 120; vs. universal brotherhood, 93–94, 97, 100–101

sexuality, 45, 63, 70, 73, 114. *See also* homosexuality

Seybert Commission, 15–16, 33, 39

Sicherheitsdienst (SD; security service), 220–25, 230, 239

Social Democrats, 66, 84

social-insurance system, 155, 157

socialism, 10, 16, 18, 69, 86, 90, 110; attacks on, 167, 219

Die Somnambule (Keller), 114

somnambulism, 34, 38, 40

Sonderweg, 281n68

soul, 40, 54, 128, 157, 176; Kandinsky on, 125–26; and materialism, 31, 34, 37, 46; nightlife of, 30–40, 44, 50; world, 35

soul sickness, 24

Sphinx, 16, 71, 135, 150; and cultural renewal, 83–84; founding of, 33; and Hübbe-Schleiden, 16, 52, 71, 83–85, 89; on materialism, 16, 46; vs. *[Neue] Metaphysische Rundschau*, 52–53; and Psychologische Gesellschaft, 40–41

spirit guides, 118–24, 169; of Rilke, 119–21, 124

Der Spiritismus (du Prel), 70, 74

Der Spiritismus (Hartmann), 13, 33, 39

Die Spiritisten (Gumppenberg), 120

Spiritistischer Apport eines Bracelets (Keller), 114

spirit rapping, 31

spirit travel, 131

spiritualism: American, 30, 37, 67, 94; vs. Anthroposophy, 101; and art, 118, 122; and Catholic Church, 198–99; and Christianity, 67, 177–78, 195, 197; criticism of, 10–15, 33, 171, 176–77, 180–85; and culture, 12–13, 16, 38; exhibitions on, 77; as fraud, 3, 12, 15–16, 39, 180–85, 241, 244; German, 7–8, 30, 38–40, 66, 175; and Jung, 29–30, 49; and liberalism, 172–73, 177, 179; vs. materialism, 13, 16, 23; under Nazi regime, 7, 219, 221, 227–28; organizations for, 59, 69; and psychology, 12–14, 39, 167, 177–78; and race, 223; religious status of, 194; and science, 13–15, 23–24, 167, 177, 180–85, 203; and self-development, 54–55; vs. Theosophy, 95; vulgar, 177, 179, 189. *See also* mediums; séances

spiritual journeys, 66–68

spirit writing. *See* automatic writing

SS (Schutzstaffel), 219–21; symbolism of, 215–16

Die Stadt Gottes, 197–98

the state: and individual rights, 167; vs. liberalism, 188–89; vs. occultism, 193, 200–208, 241, 248; and Rothe case, 182, 185–91; and scientific opinion, 193. *See also* Germany; Nazi regime

Studien aus dem Gebiete der Geheimwissenschaften (du Prel), 108

subjectivity: in art, 108–10, 118; female spir-

itual, 111; liminal, 113–14; and modernization, 50–51; vs. objectivity, 134–43; in occultism, 51–52, 54, 101, 134; and psychology, 55,
142; and the transcendent, 42
Süddeutsche Monatshefte, 133, 141, 157
surrealism, 119

table turning, 7, 30–32, 34, 197, 239
Talmud, 105
Tannenbergbund, 219
technology, 103, 167; dangers of, 245–46; and
modernism, 18, 50–51, 244; occultism's use
of, 56; railroad, 56, 244–46
telepathy, 42, 49, 52, 78, 105, 228, 237
Theosophical Society, international, 88, 99
Theosophische Societät Germania (TSG), 33,
39–40, 62, 64, 83, 89
Theosophy, 7, 25, 28, 83–107, 175; adaptability
of, 84–85, 107; vs. Ariosophy, 104–7; and art,
99, 109, 111, 124–31; and Catholic Church,
197–99; and Christianity, 83, 195–97, 235;
and class, 61, 86; and Eastern religion, 66,
216; exhibitions on, 77; of Hübbe-Schleiden,
86–93; and Kandinsky, 124–28; and liberalism, 84–85; Masters in, 85, 88, 92, 95, 100,
105; and materialism, 86, 89; and modernism, 97, 100, 102; and natural healing, 154,
159; under Nazi regime, 221, 224–28; in
[Neue] Metaphysische Rundschau, 53; occultism in, 104–5; organizations for, 59, 69; periodicals on, 71; personal experience in, 96;
policing of, 204; and presses, 68–69, 73; and
the public, 179; race in, 88, 102–7, 223;
religious status of, 194; and science, 86, 91–
92, 97–98, 100–101, 176; vs. scientific astrology, 141; self-focused, 93–102, 107, 120; "sixth
root race" in, 102–3; universal brotherhood
in, 85–93, 102, 107, 228; in United States, 67;
and Verweyen, 234–35; women in, 64, 85–86,
99
Thule Society, 104
trains, 56, 244–46
trance, 44, 101; and art, 110, 118, 121–24, 175; and
dance, 55, 114–17
Trance-Dichtungen (Eysell-Kilburger), 121
the transcendent: and artists, 111; and healing,
158; and lifestyles, 50–55; vs. materialism, 20,

23, 31, 34; and pantheism, 198; in psychology,
41–43, 45, 50–51, 202; and Schopenhauer's
"will," 36; and science, 34, 43; and the self,
134; and worldview, 52, 89–91
transcendental physics, 7–17
Transcendental Physics (Zöllner), 7, 17, 108

Über das Geistige in der Kunst (Kandinsky), 16–
17, 108, 125
Über Land und Meer, 41
unconscious, 23, 31, 55, 181; and art, 108–31;
Catholic view of, 200; creative, 117–18;
Hartmann on, 13, 24, 32, 36; as Kant's transcendental subject, 42; and liminality, 114; vs.
positivism, 25; and psychology, 13, 21–22;
research on, 14, 48, 246–47; and
Schopenhauer's "will," 36
United States, 30, 37, 67, 94
universities, German, 7, 32, 35, 50, 61, 63; elite
in, 174–80; professionalization of, 19–20
Universum, 41

Vaterlandspartei, 204
vegetarianism, 68, 76, 86, 90, 212, 234; and nat-
ural healing, 154–55
Verein Deutscher Studenten, 62, 63n6
Verein zur Bekämpfung der Vivisektion, 63n2
Vienna, 97–99
Völkischer Beobachter, 218
völkisch movement, 25–27, 67, 215, 223; and
Ariosophy, 102–7, 217, 229; and Freemasons,
218–20; and natural healing, 159–60; and
presses, 73–74
Volksgemeinschaft, 220–22, 224, 236
Vossische Zeitung, 31

Weltbühne, 233
Weltpolitik, 91–92
Wissenschaft, 40, 52
Wissenschaftliche Abhandlungen (Zöllner), 5–7
Die Woche, 133, 152, 187
women: as artists, 114–17, 120–24; creativity of,
121; and feminism, 86, 99, 102; middle-class,
64–65, 121; new, 124, 150–51; in occultism,
64–65, 78, 114–17, 121; psychology of, 111;
rights of, 73, 85–86, 90; and Theosophy, 64,
85–86, 99

worldviews: Catholic, 200; and lifestyle, 52;
  modernist, 90, 241; Nazi, 211, 218, 222–23,
  227; and occult economy, 78–80; scientific,
  94, 175, 190, 193, 233, 245; sectarian, 220–
  23; transcendent, 52, 89–91; völkisch,
  220
World War I, 17–18, 93, 107, 194, 215
World War II, 8, 210–11. *See also* Nazi regime
Wotanism, 104

x-rays, 23

yoga, 53

Zentralbibliothek der okkulte Weltliteratur,
  226, 228
Zionism, 53
Zivilisationskritik, 51
Zukunft, 150, 186, 188, 202